IDKD Springer Series

Series Editors

Juerg Hodler, Department of Radiology, University Hospital of Zürich, Zurich, Switzerland

Rahel A. Kubik-Huch, Department of Radiology, Kantonsspital Baden, Baden, Switzerland

Justus E. Roos, Department of Radiology, Luzerner Kantonsspital, Lucerne, Switzerland

The world-renowned International Diagnostic Course in Davos (IDKD) represents a unique learning experience for imaging specialists in training as well as for experienced radiologists and clinicians. IDKD reinforces his role of educator offering to the scientific community tools of both basic knowledge and clinical practice. Aim of this Series, based on the faculty of the Davos Course and now launched as open access publication, is to provide a periodically renewed update on the current state of the art and the latest developments in the field of organ-based imaging (chest, neuro, MSK, and abdominal).

Juerg Hodler • Rahel A. Kubik-Huch
Justus E. Roos
Editors

Diseases of the Brain, Head and Neck, Spine 2024-2027

Diagnostic Imaging

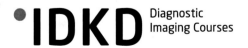 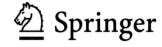

Editors
Juerg Hodler
University of Zurich
Zurich, Switzerland

Rahel A. Kubik-Huch
Department of Radiology
Kantonsspital Baden
Baden, Aargau, Switzerland

Justus E. Roos
Department of Radiology
Luzerner Kantonsspital
Lucerne, Switzerland

This book is an open access publication.

ISSN 2523-7829   ISSN 2523-7837   (electronic)
IDKD Springer Series
ISBN 978-3-031-50674-1   ISBN 978-3-031-50675-8   (eBook)
https://doi.org/10.1007/978-3-031-50675-8

Foundation for the Advancement of Education in Medical Radiology

This Springer imprint is published by the registered company Springer Nature Switzerland AG
The registered company address is: Gewerbestrasse 11, 6330 Cham, Switzerland

Paper in this product is recyclable

Contents

Part I

Brain/Skull Base/Head

Diseases of the Sella Turcica and Parasellar Region

W. Kucharczyk and L. A. Loevner

Abstract

Knowledge of the anatomy in the regions of the sella turcica, suprasellar cistern, and cavernous sinus paired with clinical history and presentation is important for accurate image interpretation. Focused diagnosis of lesions in these regions requires identifying the anatomic location in which a lesion arises, evaluation of specific imaging findings inherent to the lesion as well as in the surrounding structures, and correlation with clinical presentation (symptoms and signs).

It is important to determine whether a mass arises in the sella turcica versus the suprasellar cistern, and whether it involves both the sella turcica and suprasellar cistern.

Imaging features of a sellar mass that should be assessed include:

- Arising from or separate from the pituitary gland
- Cystic degeneration
- Size of the sella
- Infundibulum involved
- Stalk deviation
- Relationship to chiasm
- Edema optic pathways, hypothalamus
- Cavernous sinus—internal carotid artery
- Osseous remodeling, destruction

Keywords

Pituitary gland · Pituitary stalk · Sella turcica · Suprasellar cistern · Magnetic resonance imaging · CT imaging · Pituitary adenomas

W. Kucharczyk (✉)
Department of Radiology, University of Toronto, Toronto, ON, Canada
e-mail: w.kucharczyk@utoronto.ca

L. A. Loevner
Neuroradiology Division, Department of Radiology, University of Pennsylvania, Philadelphia, PA, USA

Learning Objectives
- Review anatomy of the sella turcica and parasellar regions.
- Illustrate distinguishing imaging findings of the most common lesions arising from the sellar and parasellar regions.
- Use imaging findings in conjunction with clinical signs and symptoms to develop a concise differential diagnosis and the "single best" diagnosis.

Key Points
- Knowledge of the anatomy of the pituitary gland, pituitary stalk, cavernous sinus, suprasellar cistern, optic chiasm, and arteries of the central skull base is essential for accurate diagnosis.

1.1 Introduction

A spectrum of pathology affects the pituitary gland/sella turcica and the surrounding regions. The most common abnormality is a pituitary adenoma, followed by Rathke cleft cyst and meningioma. Magnetic resonance imaging (MRI) is the imaging modality of choice in the evaluation of sellar and parasellar pathology. Patients are referred for MRI most often on the basis of clinical and laboratory findings; however, it is also common to discover lesions in these regions as incidental findings on imaging of the brain performed for other indications. Computed tomography (CT) may be used to supplement MRI findings such as to evaluate for intra-lesional calcifications or changes in adjacent bones (remodeling, destruction, or hyperostosis).

J. Hodler et al. (eds.), *Diseases of the Brain, Head and Neck, Spine 2024-2027*, IDKD Springer Series,
https://doi.org/10.1007/978-3-031-50675-8_1

1.2   Imaging Appearance of the Normal Pituitary Gland

The anterior lobe of the pituitary gland is isointense to brain on T1W and T2W imaging and demonstrates homogeneous enhancement following contrast administration (Fig. 1.1a, b). The posterior lobe of the pituitary gland is often hyperintense on T1-weighted imaging and positioned slightly behind the adenohypophysis, often within a cup-shaped depression of the dorsum sellae (Fig. 1.1a).

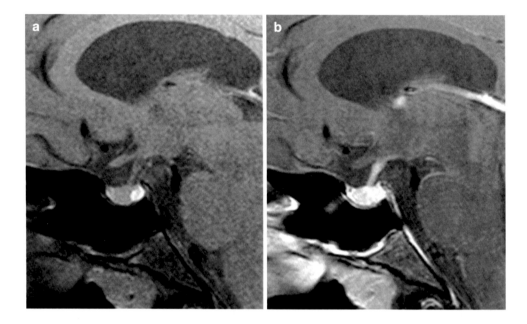

Fig. 1.1 Normal pituitary gland unenhanced T1-weighted MR (**a**). Contrast-enhanced T1-weighted MR (**b**)

1.3 Pituitary Adenomas

The imaging work-up of pituitary adenomas remains largely unchanged over the last decade with the exception of the ability to more routinely perform high resolution submillimeter thin imaging in select cases where adenomas are often not detected on conventional sequences/techniques (Cushing's disease). Unenhanced and enhanced T1-weighted images are obtained in the sagittal and coronal planes as well as a T2-weighted sequence in the coronal plane. Dynamic contrast-enhanced T1-weighted imaging is also often acquired to evaluate for microadenomas. If the conventional MR imaging is negative or equivocal, and the patient has unequivocal symptoms and signs (lab work, etc.), additional imaging utilizing sub-millimeter sequences may be indicated.

Pituitary microadenomas ($\leq$10 mm) are contained within the sella turcica and are often hypointense relative to the normal adenohypophysis on T1-weighted images. They are round in shape, and when over 5–6 mm in size often displaces the pituitary stalk away from the side of the lesion. Occasionally, pituitary adenomas may exhibit hyperintensity on T1-weighted images often reflecting internal hemorrhage. Such hemorrhage is more common in prolactinomas and may be spontaneous or following medicinal therapy such as bromocriptine. The signal intensity of microadenomas on T2W images varies, although if hyperintense relative to the normal gland, a microadenoma is likely. In the clinical and laboratory setting of excess growth hormone, a focal mass that is hypointense on T2-weighted images highly correlates with a diagnosis of a densely granulated GH-secreting adenoma. Following contrast administration, most pituitary adenomas show "differential enhancement" which means that they enhance but to a lesser degree than the normal surrounding avidly enhancing gland, so they appear relatively hypointense. Delayed contrast-enhanced imaging may inadvertently obscure microadenomas by virtue of their slower "wash-in" curve relative to normal pituitary. Dynamic contrast-enhancing imaging may be useful for some microadenomas, especially ACTH-secreting tumors.

Pituitary macroadenomas (defined as tumors greater than 10 mm in size) often extend beyond the confines of the sella, most often into the suprasellar cistern or the cavernous sinus. They may also grow inferiorly, invading the bone at the skull base and the sphenoid sinus. With trans-nasal endoscopic approaches being the mainstay in surgical management of sellar and parasellar pathology, the description of such extension is required in the preoperative imaging checklist.

Macroadenomas that grow superiorly into the suprasellar cistern are commonly bilobed "snowman" in shape, constrained at the waist by the diaphragma sella. Macroadenomas often are complex lesions with solid and cystic components resulting in heterogeneous signal on T1- and T2-weighted imaging. Cystic and/or necrotic components (caused by poor tumoral blood supply) exhibit variable signal, but often contain proteinaceous debris which may be hyperintense on T1-weighted images, and hypo- to hyperintense on T2-weighted imaging depending on the protein concentration. With macroadenomas, the neurohypophysis/stalk may be compressed, laterally displaced, or difficult to visualize. In some cases, compression of the infundibulum is disruptive such that the neurohypophyseal function is displaced upstream with a "new" bright spot more cephalad along the infundibulum.

Cavernous sinus involvement may be due to compressive growth and consequent medial and occasionally lateral dural reflection or may reflect true invasion of the sinus. Invasion is excluded if normal pituitary tissue is seen between the tumor and the sinus. On imaging, cavernous invasion is suggested when neoplasm is present lateral to the cavernous internal carotid artery (Knosp criteria grade 3A, 3B, and 4).

While prolactinomas and growth hormone (GH)-secreting adenomas are often located laterally in the sella turcica, ACTH-secreting adenomas in Cushing's disease are usually quite small in size, more difficult to detect, and are more often located in the midline. Because of the morbidity associated with this disease, ACTH-secreting lesions require the most detailed and exhaustive imaging with the intent to provide surgical management.

GH-secreting adenomas have the unique characteristic of exhibiting hypointensity on T2-weighted images in two-thirds of cases, usually the densely granulated subtype. Spontaneous infarction or necrosis of GH-secreting adenomas is not uncommon. Some cases of acromegaly detected late in the course of the disease exhibited an enlarged, partially empty sella turcica, lined with adenomatous tissue that proved difficult to analyze. Medical treatment based on octreotide analogs (somatostatin) decreases the size of the adenoma on average by 35% and brings the level of somatomedin C back to normal in 50% of cases.

Hemorrhage occurs in 20% of all pituitary adenomas, but it is usually occult. Pituitary apoplexy with severe headache, cranial nerve palsy, and significant hypopituitarism is generally caused by marked hemorrhage within a macroadenoma.

Surgery of the sella and parasellar region is usually undertaken via an endonasal transsphenoidal endoscopic approach for a number of reasons. Multiple instruments can be utilized including angled endoscopes. A nasoseptal flap can be harvested at the time of surgery to reconstruct the skull base and thus prevent CSF leaks. Furthermore, the exposure can be lateralized to resect parasellar lesions and can be extended posteriorly through the clivus to reach the prepontine cistern. Preoperative CT is routinely performed for intraoperative surgical navigation. CT also reveals bony anatomy including the location of sphenoidal sinus septae and their insertions, the presence of onodi cells, and the degree of aeration of the sphenoid sinus, all of which may influence the surgical approach, patient safety, and ultimately patient outcome.

1.4   Postoperative Sella Turcica

The surgical cavity immediately after endonasal transsphenoidal surgery is often filled with packing material. Surgicel is frequently used and is impregnated with blood and secretions. The presence of packing material, secretions, and adhesions usually keeps the surgical cavity from collapsing in the days and weeks following surgery. Blood, secretions, and packing material slowly involute over the following 2–3 months. Even after a few months, fragments of blood-impregnated surgicel can still be found in the surgical cavity. If the diaphragm is disrupted during surgery, fat or muscle implants are inserted by the surgeon to prevent the development of a cerebrospinal fluid fistula. Their resorption takes much longer. Implanted fat involutes slowly and may exhibit hyperintensity on the T1-weighted image up to 2–3 years after surgery. An MRI study performed 48 h after surgery checks for potential complications and may visualize what appears to be residual tumor, i.e., a mass of intensity identical to that of the adenoma before surgery that commonly occupies a peripheral portion of the adenoma. This early investigation is extremely helpful to interpret the follow-up MR examinations. Magnetic resonance imaging 2–3 months after surgery is essential to check for residual tumor. Subsequent surveillance MRIs, 1–2 years or more following surgical resection, may illustrate a progressively enlarging mass indicative of recurrent adenoma.

> **Key Points**
> - The most common lesions in the sella turcica are pituitary adenomas (microadenomas > macroadenomas), and many are visible on non-contrast MRI.

1.5   Rathke Cleft Cyst

Asymptomatic Rathke cleft cysts are a common incidental finding at autopsy and on MR imaging of the brain. These cysts are predominantly intrasellar in location. In an evaluation of 1000 autopsy specimens, 113 pituitary glands (11.3%) harbored incidental Rathke cleft cysts. Incidental Rathke cysts in a large autopsy series found 89% were localized at the center of the gland, with the remaining 11% predominantly lateral lesions. In that series, of all incidental pituitary lesions localized to the central part of the gland, 87% were Rathke cysts. Extrasellar Rathke cysts typically occur in the suprasellar cistern, usually midline and anterior to the stalk. Rathke cleft cysts are found in all age-groups. They share a common origin with some craniopharyngiomas in that they are thought to originate from remnants of squamous epithelium from the Rathke cleft. The cyst wall is composed of a single cell layer of columnar, cuboidal, or squamous epithelium on a basement membrane. The epithelium is often ciliated and may contain goblet cells. The cyst contents are typically mucoid, less commonly filled with serous fluid or desquamated cellular debris. Calcification in the cyst wall is rare.

Most Rathke cleft cysts are small and asymptomatic. Symptoms occur if the cyst enlarges sufficiently to compress the pituitary gland or optic chiasm and uncommonly, secondary to hemorrhage. The MR signal characteristics vary depending on the cysts contents (protein concentration of mucoid material), with approximately 60% hyperintense on unenhanced T1-weighted images (Fig. 1.2a), and 40% following the signal characteristics of CSF on T1-weighted and T2-weighted images. An "intra-cystic nodule" is diagnostic and is present in up to 75% of cases. These nodules are composed of mucinous material, protein, and cholesterol and are characteristically hypointense on T2-weighted imaging (Fig. 1.2b). The nodules may be hyperintense on T1-weighted imaging and do not enhance. Rathke cleft cysts do not enhance. Occasionally there may be thin marginal enhancement of the cyst wall. This feature can be used to advantage in difficult cases to separate these cysts from craniopharyngiomas.

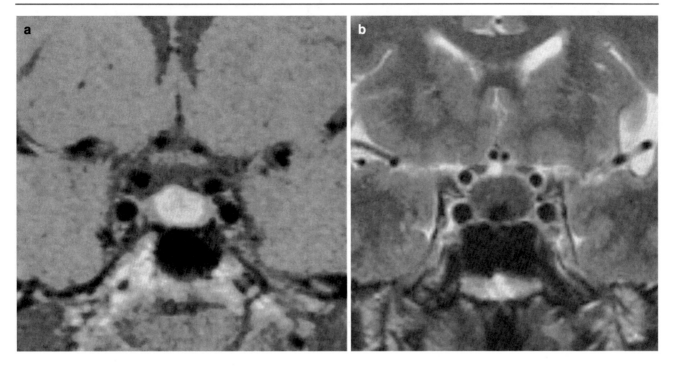

Fig. 1.2 Rathke cleft cyst. Coronal unenhanced T1-weighted MR (**a**). Coronal T2-weighted MR illustrating a hypointense central "intra-cystic nodule" (**b**)

1.6   Craniopharyngioma

Craniopharyngiomas are epithelial-derived neoplasms that occur in the region of the sella turcica and suprasellar cistern and less frequently in the third ventricle. Craniopharyngiomas account for approximately 3% of all intracranial tumors and show no gender predominance. Craniopharyngiomas are hormonally inactive lesions, although compression of the stalk may result in diabetes insipidus. They have a bimodal age distribution with more than half occurring in childhood or adolescence, with a peak incidence between 5 and 10 years of age. There is a second smaller peak in adults in the sixth decade of life. These tumors vary greatly in size and most often arise in the suprasellar cistern. Infrequently (5%), craniopharyngiomas are entirely intrasellar.

The most frequent craniopharyngioma is the classic *adamantinomatous* type, identified during the first two decades of life presenting with symptoms and signs of increased intracranial pressure including headache, nausea, vomiting, and papilledema. Visual disturbances due to compression of the optic apparatus are frequent but difficult to detect in young children. Others present with pituitary hypofunction because of compression of the pituitary gland, pituitary stalk, or hypothalamus. Rarely, *adamantinomatous* tumors are found outside the suprasellar cistern, including in the posterior fossa, pineal region, third ventricle, and nasal cavity (sphenoid sinus).

Adamantinomatous tumors are almost always cystic and usually have both solid and cystic components. Calcification is seen in the vast majority (~90%) of these tumors. These calcifications can often be identified on MRI as hypointense foci along the wall of the primary lesion; however, calcifications can be difficult to discern and in such cases CT will prove helpful. Extensive fibrosis and signs of inflammation are often found with these lesions, so that they adhere to adjacent structures including the vasculature at the base of the brain. Optic tract and hypothalamic edema on T2-weighted images is a common associated finding that is not usually seen with pituitary macroadenomas and meningiomas. Due to the inflammatory and fibrotic nature of craniopharyngiomas, recurrence is common, typically within the first 5 years after surgery.

On rare occasions, *adamantinomatous* craniopharyngiomas may be purely solid and completely calcified. These calcified types of tumors can be entirely overlooked on MRI unless close scrutiny is paid to subtle distortion of the normal suprasellar anatomy. Contrast administration shows a moderate degree of enhancement of the solid tumor.

Papillary craniopharyngiomas are typically found in adult patients. These tumors on MR imaging are solid and enhance, without calcification, and may be found within the third ventricle. Although surgery remains the definitive mode of therapy for all craniopharyngiomas, as papillary variants are encapsulated and are readily separable from nearby structures and adjacent brain, they are thought to recur much less frequently than the *adamantinomatous* type.

1.7   Meningioma

Approximately 10% of meningiomas occur in the parasellar region. These tumors arise from a variety of locations around the sella including the tuberculum sellae, planum sphenoidale, clinoid processes, medial sphenoid wing, and cavernous sinus. Meningiomas are usually slow growing and present because of compression on adjacent structures most commonly the pre-chiasmatic optic nerves and optic chiasm resulting in visual symptoms.

Meningiomas are most frequently isointense—and less commonly hypointense—to gray matter on unenhanced T1-weighted sequences. Approximately 50% remain isointense on the T2-weighted sequence, whereas 40% are hyperintense. Meningiomas enhance intensely and homogeneously, often with a trailing edge of thick dura "dural tail sign." Other diagnostic signs include visualization of a CSF cleft separating the tumor from the brain (and denoting its extraaxial location) and a clear separation of the tumor from the pituitary gland (thus indicating that the tumor is not of pituitary gland origin) (Fig. 1.3). A peripheral black rim occasionally noted at the edges of these meningiomas is thought to be related to surrounding veins. Hyperostosis and calcification are more apparent on CT scan. Vascular encasement is not uncommon, particularly with meningiomas in the cav-

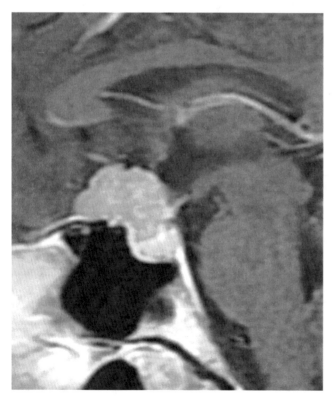

Fig. 1.3 Meningioma. Sagittal contrast-enhanced T1-weighted MR image shows the tumor centered on the planum sphenoidale and tuberculum sella and illustrates that it is separated from the pituitary gland

ernous sinus. The pattern of encasement is of diagnostic value. Meningiomas typically narrow the lumen of the encased artery (but do not occlude it). This is rare with other tumors most notably pituitary macroadenomas that grow laterally into the cavernous sinus.

1.8   Chiasmatic and Hypothalamic Gliomas

The distinction between chiasmatic and hypothalamic gliomas often depends on the predominant position of the lesion. In many cases, the origin of large gliomas cannot be definitively determined; therefore, hypothalamic and chiasmatic gliomas are discussed as a single entity. The vast majority (75%) of these tumors occur in the first decade of life, with equal prevalence in males and females. There is a definite association of optic nerve and chiasmatic gliomas with neurofibromatosis, more so for tumors that arise from the optic nerve rather than from the chiasm or hypothalamus.

Tumors of chiasmal origin are also more aggressive than those originating from the optic nerves and tend to invade the hypothalamus and floor of the third ventricle. Patients may experience monocular or binocular visual disturbances, hydrocephalus, or hypothalamic dysfunction. The appearance of the tumor depends on its position and direction of growth. It can be confined to the chiasm or the hypothalamus; however, because of its slow growth, the tumor usually attains a considerable size by the time of presentation, and the site of origin is frequently conjectural. Smaller nerve and chiasmal tumors are visually distinct from the hypothalamus, and their site of origin is more clear-cut. From the point of view of differential diagnosis, these smaller tumors can be difficult to distinguish from optic neuritis, which can also cause optic nerve enlargement. The clinical history is important in these cases (neuritis is painful, tumor is not) and, if necessary, interval follow-up of neuritis will demonstrate resolution of optic nerve swelling.

On T1-weighted images, these tumors are most often isointense while on T2-weighted images, they are moderately hyperintense. Calcification and hemorrhage are not features of these gliomas but cysts are seen, particularly in the larger hypothalamic tumors. Contrast enhancement occurs in about half of all cases. Because of the tumor's known propensity to invade the brain along the optic radiations, T2-weighted images of the entire brain are necessary. This pattern of tumor extension is readily evident as hyperintensity on the T2-weighted image; however, patients with neurofibromatosis (NF) present a problem in differential diagnosis. This relates to a high incidence of benign cerebral hamartomas and atypical glial cell rests in NF that can exactly mimic glioma. These both appear as areas of high signal intensity on T2-weighted images within the optic radiations. Lack of interval growth and possibly the absence of contrast enhancement are more supportive of a diagnosis of hamartoma while enhancement suggests glioma.

1.9   Metastases

Symptomatic metastases to the pituitary gland are found in 1–5% of cancer patients. These are primarily patients with advanced, disseminated malignancy, particularly breast and lung carcinoma. Intrasellar and juxtasellar metastases arise via hematogenous seeding to the pituitary gland and stalk, by extension of bone metastases and by CSF seeding. There are no distinctive MRI characteristics of metastases, although infundibular involvement is common, and bone destruction is a prominent feature of lesions that involve the skull base. Metastases involving the sella are not uncommonly misinterpreted as pituitary adenomas. In addition to evaluating the discriminating imaging features, metastases unlike adenomas are often associated with diabetes insipidus.

1.10   Infections

Infection in the suprasellar cistern and cavernous sinuses is usually part of a disseminated process or occurs by means of intracranial extension of an extracranial infection. The basal meninges in and around the suprasellar cistern are susceptible to tuberculous and other forms of granulomatous meningitis. The cistern may also be the site of parasitic cysts, in particular (racemose and subarachnoid) neurocysticercosis. In infections of the cavernous sinus, many of which are accompanied by thrombophlebitis, the imaging findings on CT and MRI consist of a convex lateral contour to the affected cavernous sinus with evidence of a filling defect after contrast administration. The intra-cavernous portion of the internal carotid artery may also be narrowed secondary to surrounding inflammatory change.

Infections of the pituitary gland itself are uncommon. Direct viral infection of the hypophysis has never been established, and bacterial infections are unusual. There has been speculation that cases of acquired diabetes insipidus may be the result of a select viral infection of the hypothalamic supra-optic and paraventricular nuclei. Tuberculosis and syphilis, previously encountered in this region because of the higher general prevalence of these diseases in the population, are now uncommon. Gram-positive cocci are the most frequently identified organisms in pituitary abscesses. Pituitary abscesses usually occur in the presence of other sellar masses such as adenomas, Rathke's cleft cysts, and craniopharyngiomas, indicating that these masses serve as predisposing factors to infection.

There are a few reports on CT of pituitary abscesses. These indicate that the lesion is similar in appearance to an adenoma. The correct preoperative diagnosis of abscess is difficult and rarely made. Non-contrast MRI demonstrates a sellar mass indistinguishable from an adenoma. Occasionally, pituitary abscesses are unrelated to primary pituitary lesions. In these cases, erosion of the bony sella from an aggressive sphenoid sinusitis may be the route of infection.

1.11   Noninfectious Inflammatory Lesions

Lymphocytic hypophysitis is an uncommon, noninfectious inflammatory disorder of the pituitary gland. It occurs almost exclusively in women and particularly during late pregnancy or in the post-partum period. The diagnosis should be considered in a peripartum patient with a pituitary mass, particularly when the degree of hypopituitarism is greater than that expected from the size of the mass. It is believed that, if untreated, the disease results in panhypopituitarism. Clinically, the patient complains of headache, visual loss, inability to lactate, or some combination thereof. Pituitary hormone levels are depressed. MRI shows diffuse enlargement of the anterior lobe without focal abnormality or change in internal characteristics of the gland. Thickening of the pituitary stalk may also be present.

Sarcoid afflicting the hypothalamic–pituitary axis usually manifests itself clinically as diabetes insipidus, or occasionally as a deficiency of one or more anterior lobe hormones. Low signal intensity on T2-weighted images is one finding that occurs in sarcoid with some frequency, but rarely in other diseases, with few exceptions (other granulomatous inflammatory diseases, lymphoma, some meningiomas). This low signal finding may aid in differential diagnosis. Also, the presence of multiple, scattered intra-parenchymal brain lesions should raise the possibility of the diagnosis, as should diffuse or multifocal lesions of the basal meninges. The latter are best defined on coronal contrast-enhanced T1-weighted images.

Tolosa-Hunt syndrome (THS) refers to a painful ophthalmoplegia caused by an inflammatory lesion of the cavernous sinus that is responsive to steroid therapy. Pathologically, the process is similar to orbital pseudotumor. Imaging in this disorder is often normal or may show subtle findings such as asymmetric enlargement of the cavernous sinus, enhancement of the prepontine cistern, or abnormal soft tissue density in the orbital apex. Hypointensity on T2-weighted images may be observed; since this observation is uncommon in all but a few other diseases (e.g., meningioma, lymphoma, and sarcoid), it may be helpful in the diagnosis. Clinical history allows further precision in differential diagnosis—meningioma does not respond to steroids while lymphoma and sarcoid have evidence of disease elsewhere in almost all cases.

1.12   Vascular Lesions

Saccular aneurysms in the sella turcica and parasellar area arise from either the cavernous or supra-clinoid segments of the internal carotid artery. It is extremely important to identify these lesions. Confusion with a solid tumor can lead to surgical catastrophes. Fortunately, their MRI appearance is distinctive. Aneurysms are well defined and lack internal signal on spin echo (SE) images, the so-called signal void created by rapidly flowing blood. This blood flow may cause artifacts on the image usually manifest as multiple ghosts in the phase-encoding direction, and in itself is a useful diagnostic sign.

Thrombus in the aneurysm lumen fundamentally alters these characteristics, the clot usually appearing multilamellated high signal on T1-weighted images, partially or completely filling the lumen. Hemosiderin from superficial siderosis may be visible in the adjacent brain manifest as low signal intensity on T2-weighted, gradient echo, or susceptibility-weighted images. MR or CT angiography is used to confirm the diagnosis, define the neck of the aneurysm, and establish the relationship of the aneurysm to the major vessels.

Carotid cavernous fistulas are abnormal communications between the carotid artery and the cavernous sinus. Most cases are due to trauma; less frequently they are "spontaneous." These spontaneous cases are due to a variety of abnormalities, including atherosclerotic degeneration of the arterial wall, congenital defects in the media, or rupture of an internal carotid aneurysm within the cavernous sinus. Dural arteriovenous malformations (AVMs) of the cavernous sinus are another form of abnormal arteriovenous (AV) communication in this region.

On MRI, the dilatation of the venous structures, in particular the ophthalmic vein and cavernous sinus, is usually clearly visible. The inter-cavernous venous channels dilate in both direct and indirect carotid cavernous fistulae and may also be seen on MR images. Furthermore, the internal character of the cavernous sinus is altered; definite flow channels become evident secondary to the arterial rates of flow within the sinus. The fistulous communication itself is most often occult on MRI. The pituitary gland has been noted to be prominent in cases of dural arteriovenous fistula without evidence of endocrine dysfunction. The exact mechanism of pituitary enlargement is not known, however venous congestion is a postulated cause.

Cavernous hemangiomas are acquired lesions and not true malformations and rarely may occur in the suprasellar cistern. They may have an atypical imaging appearance so some caution must be exercised in the differential diagnosis of parasellar masses. Even though cavernous hemangiomas in this location are rare, failure of the surgeon to appreciate their vascular nature can lead to unanticipated hemorrhage. Cavernous hemangiomas should be considered in the differential diagnosis of solid, suprasellar masses that do not have the classic features of more common lesions, in particular craniopharyngiomas or meningiomas. On MR imaging, T2-weighted images are helpful as hemangiomas are often markedly T2 hyperintense compared to meningiomas, and hemangiomas may have a peripheral dark rim.

Other vascular abnormalities of the sella include unilateral tortuous or bilateral "kissing" internal carotid arteries and medial trigeminal artery. While the former are relatively straightforward on imaging, the medial trigeminal artery is worth remembering. Much like with the intrasellar aneurysm, with the medial trigeminal artery, neurosurgical catastrophes can occur if the presence of an intrasellar artery is not identified. This artery will arise from the medial aspect of the cavernous carotid artery and will course directly posteriorly through the gland and through the dorsum sellae to reach the basilar artery. Approximately 40% of trigeminal arteries arise medially. In addition, patients with trigeminal arteries are at increased risk of associated intracranial aneurysm. Finally, congenital absence of the internal carotid artery and asymmetric pneumatization of the sphenoid and sella can pose confusing images.

> **Key Points**
> - Carotid artery aneurysms and anomalies can mimic intrasellar and parasellar mass lesions. Arterial lesions must be considered in the differential diagnosis of lesions in this area. MRA or CTA can be used to confidently confirm or exclude the presence of arterial lesions.

1.13   Additional Pathology in the Sellar and Parasellar Regions

Many other lesions may involve the sella turcica and parasellar region. These include mass lesions such as germinoma, epidermoid, dermoid, teratoma, schwannoma, chordoma, ecchordosis, choristoma, arachnoid cyst, hamartoma, IgG4-related disease, and Langerhans cell histiocytosis. Also, there are several important metabolic conditions that may cause pituitary dysfunction or MRI-observable abnormalities in and around the sella. These include diabetes insipidus, growth hormone deficiency, hemochromatosis, hypermagnesemia, and hypothyroidism. Space limitations preclude their further discussion in this synopsis.

1.14 Concluding Remarks

An understanding of the physiology of the pituitary gland and stalk, as well as the anatomy of the sella turcica and surrounding structures is important. There are 3 or 4 common pathologies that arise from each of these regions (sella turcica, suprasellar cistern, cavernous sinus). Knowledge of the anatomy, physiology, and familiarity with these pathologies results in high probability of correct imaging diagnosis.

> **Take-Home Messages**
> - The vast majority of lesions arising in the sella turcica are pituitary adenomas.
> - You do not want to miss aneurysms and arterial anomalies.
> - Anatomic relationships are key to arriving at a correct imaging diagnosis.
> - Knowledge of basic physiology and clinical presentation helps synch the diagnosis.

Further Reading

Araujo-Castro M, Acitores Cancela A, Vior C, Pascual-Corrales E, Rodrígue Berrocal V. Radiological Knosp, revised-Knosp, and Hardy–Wilson classifications for the prediction of surgical outcomes in the endoscopic endonasal surgery of pituitary adenomas: study of 228 cases. Front Oncol. 2022;11:807040.

Byun WM, Kim OL, Kim D. MR imaging findings of Rathke's cleft cysts: significance of intracystic nodules. AJNR Am J Neuroradiol. 2000;21(3):485–8.

Chapman PR, Singhal A, Gaddamanugu S, Prattipati V. Neuroimaging of the pituitary gland: practical anatomy and pathology. Radiol Clin N Am. 2020;58(6):1115–33.

Chatain GP, Patronas N, Smirniotopoulos JG, Piazza M, Benzo S, Ray-Chaudhury A, Sharma S, Lodish M, Nieman L, Stratakis CA, Chittiboina P. J Neurosurg. 2018;129(3):620–8.

Kucharczyk W, Peck WW, Kelly WM, Norman D, Newton TH. Rathke cleft cysts: CT, MR imaging and pathologic features. Radiology. 1987;165:491–5.

Langlois F, Varlamov EV, Fleseriu M. Hypophysitis, the growing spectrum of a rare pituitary disease. J Clin Endocrinol Metab. 2022;107(1):10–28.

Lundin P, Bergström K, Nyman R, Lundberg PO, Muhr C. Macroprolactinomas: serial MR imaging in long term bromocriptine therapy. AJNR Am J Neuroradiol. 1992;13:1279–91.

Manara R, Maffei P, Citton V, et al. Increased rate of intracranial saccular aneurysms in acromegaly: an MR angiography study and review of the literature. J Clin Endocrinol Metab. 2011;96(5):1292–757.

Nagahata M, Hosoya T, Kayama T, Yamaguchi K. Edema along the optic tract: a useful MR finding for the diagnosis of craniopharyngiomas. AJNR Am J Neuroradiol. 1998;19:1753–7.

Naylor MF, Scheithauer BW, Forbes GS, Tomlinson FH, Young WF. Rathke cleft cyst: CT, MR, and pathology of 23 cases. J Comput Assist Tomogr. 1995;19(6):853–9.

Oka H, Kawano N, Suwa T, Yada K, Kan S, Kameya T. Radiological study of symptomatic Rathke's cleft cysts. Neurosurgery. 1994;35(4):632–6.

Pinker K, Ba-Ssalamah A, Wolfsberger S, Mlynarik V, Knosp E, Trattnig S. The value of high-field MRI (3T) in the assessment of sellar lesions. Eur J Radiol. 2005;54(3):327–34.

Steiner E, Knosp E, Herold CJ, et al. Pituitary adenomas: findings of postoperative MR imaging. Radiology. 1992;185:521–7.

Teramoto A, Hirakawa K, Sanno N, Osamura Y. Incidental pituitary lesions in 1000 unselected autopsy specimens. Radiology. 1994;193:161–4.

Wolfsberger S, Ba-Ssalamah A, Pinker K, Mlynárik V, Czech T, Knosp E, Trattnig S. Application of three-tesla magnetic resonance imaging for diagnosis and surgery of sellar lesions. J Neurosurg. 2004;100(2):278–86.

Problem Solving Disorders of CSF

Tomas Dobrocky and Àlex Rovira

Abstract

Spontaneous Intracranial Hypotension (SIH)

Spontaneous intracranial hypotension (SIH) is a debilitating medical condition, which is perpetuated by the continuous loss of cerebrospinal fluid (CSF) at the level of the spine, and is the top differential diagnosis for patients presenting with orthostatic headache. Neuroimaging plays a crucial role in the diagnostic work-up and monitoring SIH, as it provides objective data in the face of various clinical symptoms and very often a normal opening pressure on lumbar puncture. Brain MRI frequently demonstrates typical signs of CSF depletion and includes homogenous dural enhancement, venous distention, subdural collections, and brain sagging. Three types of CSF leaks may be distinguished: (1) ventral dural leaks due to microspurs, (2) leaking spinal nerve root cysts, (3) or direct CSF venous fistula. The quest for the leak may be the fabled search for the needle in the haystack, scrutinizing the entire spine for a dural breach often the size of pin. The main role of spine imaging is the correct classification and precise localization of CSF leaks. Precise localization of the CSF leak site is crucial to successful treatment, which is generally a targeted percutaneous epidural patch or surgical closure when conservative measures fail to provide long-term relief.

Obstructive Hydrocephalus. Communicating Hydrocephalus. Normal Pressure Hydrocephalus

Modern imaging techniques play an essential role for understanding of the anatomy of the cerebrospinal fluid (CSF) spaces and ventricular system, as well as the hydrodynamics of CSF flow, and consequently in the assessment of the different types of hydrocephalus. Obstructive (non-communicating) hydrocephalus is a complex disorder resulting from an obstruction/blockage of the CSF circulation along one or more of the narrow apertures connecting the ventricles, being the most common type of hydrocephalus in children and young adults. On the other hand, communicating hydrocephalus is defined as a cerebrospinal fluid flow circulation abnormality outside the ventricular system that produces an increase in the ventricular size. Most cases are secondary to obstruction of CSF flow between the basal cisterns and brain convexity and include common conditions such as subarachnoid hemorrhage and meningitis (infectious and neoplastic). In a subset of communicating hydrocephalus, no CSF obstruction can be demonstrated as occurs in normal pressure hydrocephalus (NPH), a complex entity with poorly understood cerebrospinal fluid dynamics. Neuroradiology plays an essential role in the diagnosis of hydrocephalus, and in distinguishing this condition from other causes of ventriculomegaly.

Keywords

Spontaneous intracranial hypotension · SIH · CSF leak · CSF venous fistula · Epidural blood patch · Hydrocephalus · Normal pressure hydrocephalus · Cerebrospinal fluid disorders · Dementia · MRI · CT

T. Dobrocky (✉)
Department of Diagnostic and Interventional Neuroradiology, Bern, Switzerland
e-mail: tomas.dobrocky@insel.ch

À. Rovira
Section of Neuroradiology, Department of Radiology, Hospital Universitari Vall d'Hebron, Barcelona, Spain
e-mail: alex.rovira.idi@gencat.cat

© The Author(s) 2024
J. Hodler et al. (eds.), *Diseases of the Brain, Head and Neck, Spine 2024-2027*, IDKD Springer Series,
https://doi.org/10.1007/978-3-031-50675-8_2

2.1 Spontaneous Intracranial Hypotension (SIH)

Learning Objectives
- To get acquainted with clinical symptoms, underlying pathomechanism in spontaneous intracranial hypotension (SIH).
- To recognize typical brain imaging findings in SIH and be able to use the Bern SIH score.
- To recognize three spinal CSF leak types and be aware of different myelography techniques.
- To be familiar with treatment options in SIH patients.

Key Points
- Typical brain imaging findings of SIH include dural enhancement, distension of intracranial veins and sinuses, subdural collections, pituitary enlargement, and effacement of subarachnoid cisterns.
- The Bern SIH score is a 9-point, brain MRI-based score, allowing stratification of the likelihood of a spinal CSF leak.
- Low opening pressure on lumbar puncture is not a reliable marker of SIH.
- Non-enhanced MRI of the entire spine, with fat suppression, is important to screen for spinal longitudinal extradural CSF (SLEC) collection and guide further diagnostic steps.
- Spinal CSF leaks do not always occur at the level of prominent disc protrusions or a large nerve root cyst.
- Three types of CSF leaks can be distinguished; (1) ventral dural tears due to an osteogenic microspur, (2) leaking spinal nerve cyst, (3) CSF venous fistula.

According to the International Classification of Headache Disorders (ICHD-3), low opening pressure on lumbar puncture (<6 cm CSF) or classical imaging signs of intracranial hypotension (brain OR spine MRI) is required to fulfill the diagnostic criteria for SIH [1]. Despite the fact that "hypotension" is included in the term "SIH," a low opening pressure on lumbar puncture is only present in about one-third of patient [2, 3]. Consequently, neuroimaging plays a crucial part in the work-up of patients with clinical suspicion of SIH. It is important to distinguish SIH from other pathologies which may be associated with CSF depletion, like postdural puncture headache (PDPH), rhinorrhea, or CSF loss after surgical interventions, since diagnostic work-up, therapeutic approach, and outcome differ.

2.1.1 Clinical Presentation

The incidence of SIH is 5/100,000 and is almost equal to the incidence of aneurysmatic subarachnoid hemorrhage [4]. Women are twice as often affected than men. The classic clinical hallmark of SIH is orthostatic headache, with an increasing intensity in the upright position and decreases when recumbent. This is most likely due to stretching of pain sensitive fibers in the dura mater, which is more pronounced in the upright position. However, the orthostatic character phenotype may become less apparent in the subacute and chronic stage of the disease, and other non-orthostatic forms including thunderclap, non-positional, exertional, cough related, and "second-half-of-the-day" may occur [5]. Other clinical symptoms include neck pain, tinnitus, changes in hearing, vertigo, nausea, and diplopia. Some of these symptoms are believed to be due to brain sagging which causes stretching of cranial nerves. Other rare presentations of SIH include endocrine disorders due to pituitary enlargement, decreased level of consciousness or coma, which are most likely due to outflow restriction with consecutive thrombosis of the internal cerebral veins [6–8].

2.1.2 Etiology

In total, approximately 100–150 mL of CSF circulates in the intracranial and intraspinal compartments. The CSF encloses the brain parenchyma and spinal cord, providing protection, buoyancy, and a conduit for clearing of metabolic waste products. The CSF is sealed within the confines of the dura while a meticulous balance between production and resorption is maintained. Perturbations of production or resorption disturb this equilibrium and cause symptoms. According to the Monro-Kellie doctrine, the total volume within the confines of the skull is constant and is the sum of the volumes of blood, CSF, and brain parenchyma. Volume loss in one compartment is compensated by a reciprocal volume increase in one or both other compartments. In patients with SIH, the loss of CSF leads predominantly to increased blood volume, which may be appreciated as distension of veins and hyperemia on brain and spine imaging [9, 10].

It is important to note that even though the classical clinical presentation is headache, the underlying cause of the disease is exclusively to be found at the level of the spine. CSF leaks at the level of the skull base are typically not associated with SIH symptoms [11]. Three types of CSF leaks can be distinguished (Table 2.1) [12, 13]. Type I leaks are due to an osteogenic microscope (endplate osteophyte or calcified disc protrusion) penetrating the dura. Type II leaks are due to a leaking spinal nerve cyst. Type III leaks are the so-called CSF venous fistulas which represent a direct communication between the intrathecal space and the epidural/paraspinal vein [14, 15]. In type I and II leaks, a spinal lon-

gitudinal extradural CSF collection (SLEC) is invariably present, thus they may be considered as "wet leaks". On the other hand, type III leaks do not demonstrate a spinal longitudinal extradural CSF collection and thus may be considered "dry leaks".

Table 2.1 Etiology of SIH, brain MRI-based quantitative SIH score (Bern score), typical spine MRI findings

Etiology	Brain MRI imaging	Spine MRI imaging
Type 1: Osteogenic microspur (endplate osteophyte, calcified disc protrusion) Type 2: Leaking nerve root cyst Type 3: CSF venous fistula	Brain SIH score (Bern score) • Major criteria (2 points) 1. Venous distention 2. Pachymeningeal enhancement 3. Suprasellar cistern (≤4 mm) • Minor criteria (1 point) 4. Subdural fluid collection 5. Prepontine cistern (≤5 mm) 6. Mamillopontine distance (≤6.5 mm)	Screen for spinal longitudinal epidural CSF collection (SLEC) SLEC positive ("wet leaks") Type 1 or type 2 leaks SLEC negative ("dry leaks") Type 3 leaks
	Other findings: pituitary enlargement, (infratentorial) superficial siderosis, calvarial hyperostosis	Start with a T2w fat-suppressed MRI Spine MRI has no localizing value for CSF leaks

2.1.3 Diagnostic Work-Up

2.1.3.1 Brain MRI

The diagnostic work-up of SIH patients usually starts with a brain MRI. As proposed by Schievink, the most typical findings include subdural fluid collections, enhancement of the pachymeninges, engorgement of venous structures, pituitary hyperemia, and sagging of the brain (mnemonic: SEEPS) [16] (Fig. 2.1). Additional imaging signs which may be usually be found in long-standing (untreated) SIH include superficial siderosis, calvarial hyperostosis, or enlargement of paranasal sinuses [17, 18].

In 2018, a 9-point, brain MRI-based SIH score (bSIH) allowing stratification of the likelihood of finding a spinal CSF leak in patients with clinically suspected SIH was proposed (Table 2.1) [10]. The score comprises 3 major (2 points each) and 3 minor (1 point each) signs. The major signs are pachymeningeal enhancement, distention of venous sinuses, and effacement of the suprasellar cistern (≤4.0 mm). The minor signs are subdural fluid collection, effacement of the prepontine cistern (≤5.0 mm), and reduced mamillopontine

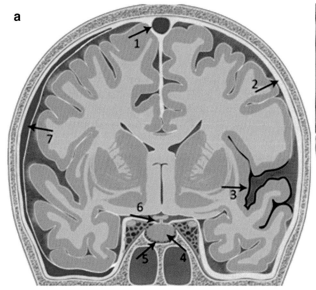
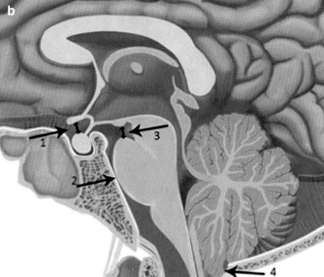
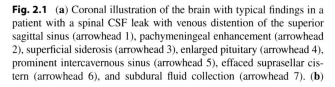

Fig. 2.1 (a) Coronal illustration of the brain with typical findings in a patient with a spinal CSF leak with venous distention of the superior sagittal sinus (arrowhead 1), pachymeningeal enhancement (arrowhead 2), superficial siderosis (arrowhead 3), enlarged pituitary (arrowhead 4), prominent intercavernous sinus (arrowhead 5), effaced suprasellar cistern (arrowhead 6), and subdural fluid collection (arrowhead 7). (b) Sagittal illustration of the posterior fossa with typical findings in patients with a CSF leak with effaced suprasellar cistern (arrowhead 1; pathologic ≤4 mm), effacement of the prepontine cistern (2; pathologic ≤5 mm), decreased mamillopontine distance (3; pathologic ≤6.5 mm), and low-lying cerebellar tonsils (arrowhead 4). (Reprinted from Dobrocky et al., JAMA 2019)

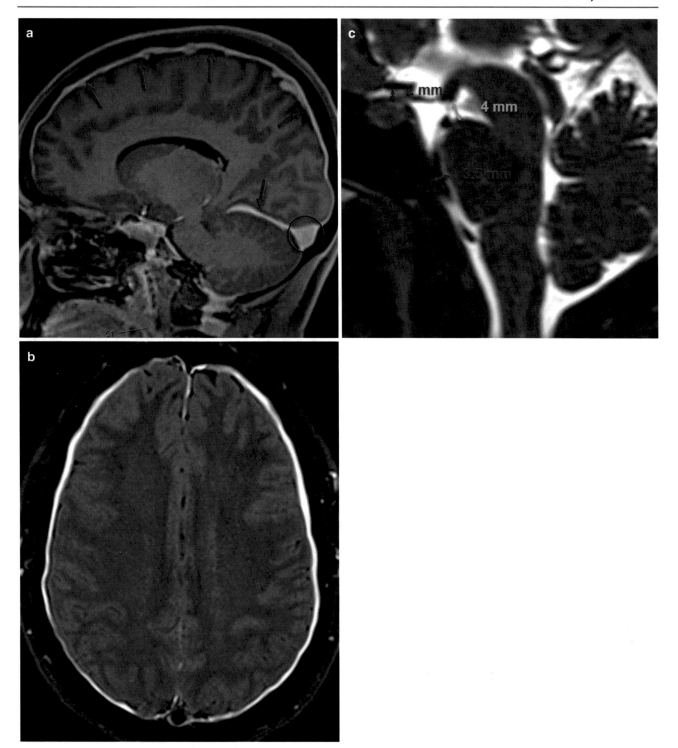

Fig. 2.2 (**a**) Gadolinium-enhanced brain MRI in the sagittal plane demonstrating homogenous and smooth pachymeningeal enhancement and distension of the transverse sinus. (**b**) Flair image in the transversal plane demonstrating bilateral subdural collections. (**c**) T2-weighted MRI in the sagittal plane demonstrating effaced CSF cisterns; suprasellar cistern 2 mm, (pathologic ≤4 mm), prepontine cistern 3.5 mm (pathologic ≤5 mm), mamillopontine distance 4 mm (pathologic ≤6.5 mm)

distance (≤6.5 mm) (Fig. 2.2). Based on the bSIH score ≤2, 3–4, and ≥5, the probability of the myelographic discovery of a CSF leak or CSF venous fistula is low, intermediate, and high, respectively [10, 19].

More recently, the score has been referred to as the Bern SIH score. It has been used as a quantitative tool for therapy monitoring after surgical closure of CSF leaks as well as after endovascular treatment of CSF venous fistulas [20, 21].

2.1.3.2 Spine Imaging

Identification and precise localization of a CSF leak are the main goals of spine imaging. This remains challenging since the quest for the leak may be the fabled search for the needle in the haystack, scrutinizing the entire spine for a dural breach often the size of pin. Various imaging modalities have been used for the spine work-up: unenhanced spine MRI, intrathecal gadolinium-enhanced spine MRI, conventional dynamic myelography, postmyelography CT, dynamic CT myelography, and digital subtraction myelography [22]. Even though a detailed discussion of these techniques is beyond the scope of this chapter, each modality has its unique strengths (spatial/temporal resolution) and shortcomings (intrathecal application of contrast, radiation exposure) which need to be considered.

A non-enhanced MRI of the entire spine should be the first diagnostic step in case of a positive brain MRI or in case of high clinical suspicion of SIH [23]. The spine study should include T2-weighted, fat-suppressed, high-resolution images (Fig. 2.3a) which help to identify any epidural collection of CSF and thus distinguish between "wet leaks" (SLEC +) and "dry leaks" (SLEC −), which guides further diagnostic steps.

In case of intractable SIH, not responding neither to conservative therapy nor to non-targeted epidural blood patch (EBP), the precise localization of a spinal CSF leak is crucial. As previously reported, non-enhanced MRI has no localizing value (accuracy less than 40%) [24]. The reasons for poor accuracy of leak localization on spine MRI are multiple. First, the epidural CSF collection usually spans several vertebral levels and does not allow to pinpoint the culprit lesion at a specific vertebral level [25]. Second, several suspicious culprit lesions are encountered in most patients, including multiple disc protrusions and nerve root cysts. However, in the overwhelming majority of patients, there is only a single site of CSF leakage.

For precise CSF leak localization, three dynamic myelography techniques are available: conventional dynamic myelography (CDM), digital subtraction myelography (DSM), and dynamic CT myelography (DCTM) [26–28]. The practice in different centers may vary according to local availability and expertise. In SLEC positive patients (type 1 and 2), a diagnostic technique with a high temporal resolution is mandatory. Patient positioning should be adapted according to the suspicious findings on spine MRI, prone for suspected ventral osteo-discogenic microspur (type 1 leak) or lateral decubitus for suspected rupture of a spinal nerve root cyst (type 2 leak) [27]. The spinal level where contrast starts to spill from the intrathecal into the epidural compartment when contrast has reached the level of the dural breach needs to be captured during the exam (Fig. 2.3c).

Imaging of CSFVF has evolved over the past few years, and different variations of the technique have been proposed. Lateral decubitus and sustained inspiration during myelography have been reported to increase the diagnostic yield [29, 30]. A CSFVF may be appreciated as an opacified tubular structure ("hyperdense paraspinal vein sign") extending from a nerve root cyst into an epidural or paravertebral vein [15, 31, 32].

2.1.4 Treatment

A three-tier therapeutic model with increasing level of invasiveness for treatment of SIH patients is generally applied, including conservative treatment (bed rest or caffeine), percutaneous treatment with epidural patching (targeted or non-targeted), and surgical or endovascular closure of the CSF leak or fistula.

Conservative measures reported in the literature include bed rest, oral hydration, and oral caffeine administration, however, are unlikely to provide long-term relief in most SIH patients.

When conservative measures fail, non-targeted or targeted image-guided epidural blood patches may be applied. Untargeted epidural blood patch (EBP) is a minimally invasive, readily available, effective symptomatic therapy providing short-term relief in a substantial number of SIH patients. However, according to a recent cohort study, the success rate of permanently sealing a spinal CSF leak is low (<30%), which in turn might explain the high rate of delayed symptom recurrence [33].

Response rates after one EBP reported in the literature range between 36 and 88%. The reason for striking difference in EBP efficacy is manifold. First, the technique varies substantially between studies and depends on the amount (low or high volume), type of injected substance (autologous blood or fibrin), number of injected levels, the way of delivery (targeted vs non-targeted), or the way of application (imaging guided vs blind). Second, several studies do not differentiate between SIH leak type, PDPH, and other possible etiologies of orthostatic headache. Third, the outcome measures are heterogeneous and mainly report short-term improvement in headache severity (<3 months). However, long-term follow-up and objective measures are usually neglected.

Ultimately, in cases of intractable SIH, microsurgical exploration and closure of the dural breach are the treatment of choice [34, 35]. In order to limit the extent of bone removal during surgery, pinpointing the site of dural dehiscence to one vertebral level on dynamic imaging is mandatory for the success of this approach. Recently, Brinjikji et al. proposed a

Fig. 2.3 (**a**) T2-weighted, fat-saturated sagittal image demonstrating a CSF collection in the dorsal epidural space - spinal longitudinal epidural CSF collection (SLEC). The posterior dura is clearly visible (red arrows). (**b**) Lateral decubitus myelography demonstrating a type 2 leak with an abnormally enlarged nerve root cyst (red circle) at the level T11 with spilling of intrathecal contrast into the adjacent epidural space (green arrows). (**c**) Conventional dynamic myelography in prone position showing the spill of intrathecal contrast (blue arrow) into the ventral epidural space (red arrow) at T12. (**d**) Postmyelography CT demonstrating a microspur (red arrow) originating at the dorsal endplate and penetrating the dura

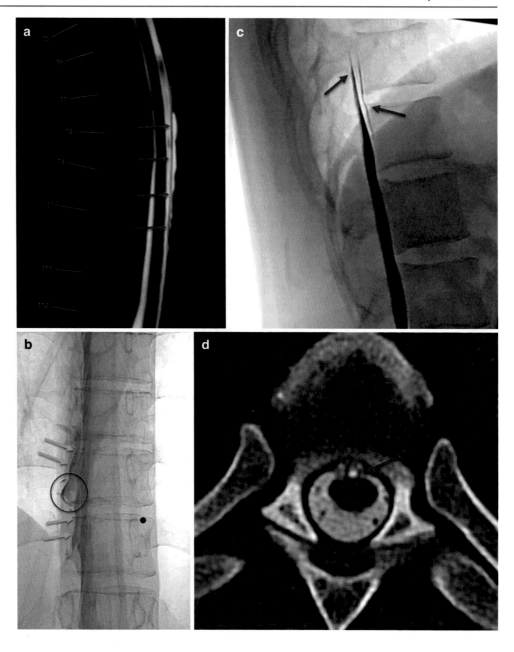

transvenous embolization of CSF venous fistulas with very promising results [36].

A recent systematic review on the efficacy of EBP or surgery in SIH patients including 139 studies reported an overall low level of the strength of evidence [37]. In total, 38% studies did not clearly meet the ICHD-3 criteria, CSF leak type was unclear in 78% studies, while nearly all (85%) reported patient symptoms using unvalidated measures. A prospective randomized clinical trial is necessary to clarify the effectiveness of epidural blood patching and surgery in SIH patients.

2.1.5   Concluding Remarks

Due to the growing awareness among headache specialist including, but not limited to, neurologists, neuroradiologists, and neurosurgeons, SIH is increasingly recognized. It typically presents with orthostatic headache and when left untreated may leave the patient psychologically burdened or in despair. Unlike insinuated by the term SIH, true hypotension is an unreliable marker of the disease, underlying on the importance of recognition of objective, however often subtle imaging signs. A meticulous and standardized diagnostic work-up of patients is mandatory in order detect imaging signs of the disease and provide effective therapy.

Take-Home Messages (3–5)
- The **Bern SIH** (bSIH) score is 9-point, brain MRI-based scale that stratifies the likelihood of finding a spinal CSF leak in patients with suspected SIH.
- **Three pathologies** at the level of the spine that may cause SIH: (1) osteogenic microspurs, (2) leaking nerve root cysts, (3) CSF venous fistulas.
- **Non-enhanced MRI** of the entire spine with **fat suppression** is important to screen for spinal longitudinal extradural CSF collection **(SLEC)** and guide further diagnostic steps.
- Spinal CSF leaks do not always occur at the level of prominent disc protrusions; **myelography** with intrathecal contrast and **high temporal resolution** is generally required for leak localization (as opposed to conventional spine MRI).
- **Individualized** treatment approach according to the **leak type** seems warranted (epidural blood patch, microsurgical closure of the leak, transvenous embolization in case of a CSF venous fistula).

2.2   Obstructive Hydrocephalus. Communicating Hydrocephalus. Normal Pressure Hydrocephalus

Learning Objectives
- To gain knowledge on the different types of hydrocephalus.
- To know the MRI protocol required in the diagnostic work-up of suspected hydrocephalus.
- To recognize the typical radiological features of both communicating and non-communicating (obstructive) hydrocephalus.
- To be able to recognize the imaging features that distinguish idiopathic normal pressure hydrocephalus from other causes of ventriculomegaly in the adult population.

Key Points
- Neuroimaging (CT and MRI) allows detailed anatomical and physiological information on hydrocephalus and establishes a classification based on its causal mechanism (non-communicating and communicating).

- High-resolution structural and functional MRI sequences provide the best approach to identify the patency of cerebrospinal flow inside the ventricular system and the cause of hydrocephalus.
- Idiopathic normal pressure hydrocephalus (NPH) is a surgically treatable reversible neurological disorder in which neuroimaging plays an essential role in its diagnosis and in predicting surgical response.

2.2.1   Hydrocephalus

Hydrocephalus is currently defined as ventricular dilatation associated with a decrease in extraventricular subarachnoid spaces. The degree of ventricular dilation and the damage produced to brain tissue will depend on various factors, such as the cause and speed of onset of hydrocephalus, and the age of the patient.

With the advent, first of CT and later of MRI, it has been possible to obtain detailed anatomical and physiological information on hydrocephalus and to establish a classification based on its causal mechanism (non-communicating and communicating), a fact that has obvious therapeutic implications (Table 2.2).

Usually brain CT is the first-line imaging procedure, especially in emergency cases with acute hydrocephalus. However, MRI is the method of choice in detailed assessment of this condition. Contrast media injection is not required for the diagnosis unless there is a suspicion of a neoplastic or an inflammatory process. The main purpose of the diagnostic procedures in patient with obstructive hydrocephalus is to find a lesion impeding the cerebrospinal fluid (CSF) flow within the ventricular system and to differentiate this condition from communicating hydrocephalus and other non-hydrocephalic cause of ventricular enlargement such as brain atrophy [38, 39].

In addition to conventional structural MRI sequences, other dedicated sequences should be considered in the assessment of hydrocephalus [40, 41]. Cardiac-gated phase contrast MRI (PC-MRI) is extremely sensitive to CSF flow and has demonstrated value in demonstrating patency of intraventricular CSF circulation (particularly aqueduct patency), but does not offer anatomical information of CSF pathways. Combination of heavily 3D T2-weighted sequences such as CISS (constructive interference steady state) or FIESTA (Fast Imaging Employing Steady-State Acquisition) that offer superb anatomical information, and 3D T2-weighted turbo/fast spin-echo sequences such as SPACE (sampling perfection with application optimized contrast using different flip angle evolutions), VISTA (volume isotropic turbo spin echo acquisition), or CUBE that are

Table 2.2 Causes of hydrocephalus

Non-communicating (obstructive)	Communicating

Any obstacle compressing the foramina from the outside or any intraventricular obstructive lesion at the level of:
1. **Foramen of Monro**: Colloid cyst, tumors (ependymoma, subependymomas, central neurocytoma, glial tumors), adhesions
2. **Cerebral aqueduct**:
  • Non-neoplastic intrinsic lesions (idiopathic/congenital/inflammatory): webs/adhesions/forking, cysts
  • Periaqueductal lesions: pineal gland tumors, tectum glioma, tentorial meningioma, metastasis, infection (meningitis/ventriculitis, abscess), cerebral vascular malformation (vein of Galen aneurysm)
  • Giant cystic mesencephalic Virchow-Robin spaces
3. **Trapped fourth ventricle** (obstruction of all CSF pathways of the fourth ventricle, including foramina of Luschka and Magendie, as well as aqueduct): previous ventricular shunting for hydrocephalus, infection, intraventricular hemorrhage, and post-inflammatory changes after posterior fossa surgery
4. **Fourth ventricular outlets**: cerebellar infarct, posterior fossa tumors (metastasis, meningioma, astrocytoma, medulloblastomas), hemorrhage, meningitis, Dandy–Walker malformation
5. **Foramen magnum:** metabolic diseases, developmental abnormalities, Chiari malformations, osteochondrodysplasia
	With obstruction of CSF absorption:
	  • Subarachnoid hemorrhage
	  • Meningitis—bacterial, aseptic
	  • Leptomeningeal carcinomatosis
	  • Vestibular schwannoma
	Without obstruction of CSF absorption: normal pressure hydrocephalus (NPH)
	  • Secondary (sNPH): subarachnoid hemorrhage, meningitis
	  • Idiopathic (iNPH)

Table 2.3 Protocol recommendations for MRI in suspected hydrocephalus of unknown origin

- 2D/3D sagittal unenhanced T1-weighted (with multiplanar reconstruction)
- 2D axial T2-weighted
- 2D transverse/3D sagittal T2-FLAIR
- 3D sagittal CISS/FIESTA
- 3D sagittal T2-weighted SPACE/VISTA/CUBE
- 2D/3D susceptibility-based sequences

If infectious meningitis or leptomeningeal metastasis suspected add:

- 2D transverse/3D sagittal contrast-enhanced T2-FLAIR
- 2D transverse-coronal/3D sagittal contrast-enhanced T1-weighted

highly sensitive to CSF flow, provides an easy evaluation of CSF pathway and circulation to establish the patency of CSF flow [41]. It has been shown that these sequences provide adequate morphological and similar functional information of CSF patency to cine PC-MRI [42] and should be considered within the imaging strategy for assessing CSF circulation patency in clinical practice (Table 2.3; Fig. 2.4).

2.2.2 Radiological Findings

The typical radiological findings which raise the suspicion of any form of hydrocephalus are as follows:

1. Enlargement of the ventricles that can be quantified by using the Evans' index. The Evans' index is the ratio of maximum width of the frontal horns of the lateral ventricles and maximum internal diameter of skull at the same level measured in axial CT and MRI images. A value of >0.3 is considered abnormal.
2. Dilatation of temporal horns—a very sensitive sign of hydrocephalus. Temporal ventricular horns dilate first due to relatively little resistance of choroidal fissure to expansion and relative bulk of basal ganglia "tamponading" lateral ventricles.
3. Dilatation of the third ventricular recesses.
4. Reduced mamillopontine distance.
5. Upward bowing and thinning of the corpus callosum.
6. Disproportionately narrowed cortical sulci, although they may be normal especially if there was pre-existing widening.

Acute hydrocephalus is an emergency condition requiring urgent treatment because it may lead to severe complications such as cerebral infarction, persistent blindness, herniation, or even death. The most important findings on MRI which enable differentiation between acute and chronic hydrocephalus are hyperintense bands in the periventricular white matter found on T2-weighted or T2-FLAIR images which are compatible with acute interstitial oedema, referred to as transependymal oedema or diapedesis (Fig. 2.5). On CT, these areas appear as low-density regions around the margins of the ventricles.

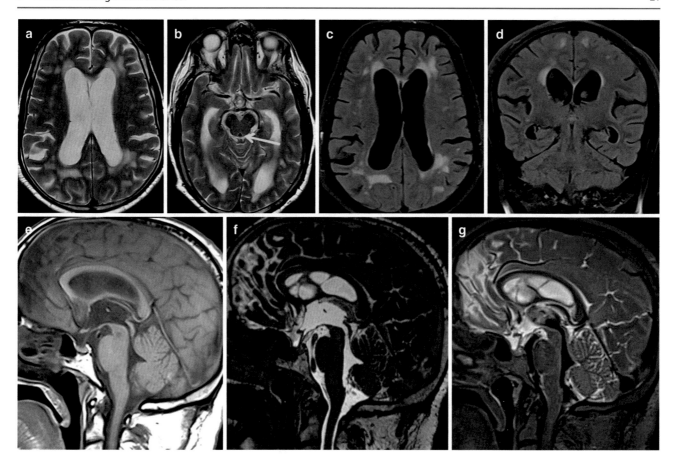

Fig. 2.4 Brain MRI recommended protocol in the diagnostic work-up of hydrocephalus. Axial T2-weighted images (**a**, **b**) show ventriculomegaly associated with the presence of flow void inside the aqueduct (arrow). Transverse and coronal T2-FLAIR images (**c**, **d**) shows mild enlargement of Sylvian fissures associated with blockage of upper convexity CSF spaces. Midsagittal T1-weighted (**e**), 3D CISS (**f**), and 3D SPACE (**g**) images shows a morphological normal aqueduct with marker flow void. These findings indicated the diagnosis of normal pressure hydrocephalus

2.2.3   Non-communicating (Obstructive) Hydrocephalus

Obstructive (non-communicating) hydrocephalus is a complex disorder resulting from an obstruction/blockage of the cerebrospinal fluid circulation along one or more of the narrow apertures connecting the ventricles [40]. This type of hydrocephalus is caused by a variety of conditions including the typical obstruction sites at the level of foramen of Monro, cerebral aqueduct (Fig. 2.6), fourth ventricular outlets (Fig. 2.7), and foramen magnum, produced by either any lesion in the form of space-occupying lesion compressing the foramina from the outside, or any intraventricular obstructive lesion including tumour or haemorrhage [43, 44] (Table 2.2).

Since obstructive hydrocephalus may be a life-threatening condition, this condition requires a prompt and accurate diagnosis in order to offer the most adequate treatment.

2.2.4   Communicating Hydrocephalus

Communicating hydrocephalus is defined as a CSF flow circulation abnormality outside the ventricular system that produces an increase in the ventricular size. Most cases are secondary to obstruction of CSF flow between the basal cisterns and brain convexity and include common conditions such as subarachnoid hemorrhage (SAS), bacterial and aseptic meningitis, and leptomeningeal carcinomatosis. Based on this concept, communicating hydrocephalus is usually associated with CSF absorption impairment, and for that reason this type of hydrocephalus could be better classified as communicating with obstruction, to differentiate them from normal pressure hydrocephalus (NPH), in which there is no objective obstruction of CSF circulation and absorption [45, 46]. Important radiological features that distinguish this type of hydrocephalus from other causes of ventriculomegaly are dilatation of the temporal horns; ballooning of the third ventricular walls, including its anterior recesses; upward bowing

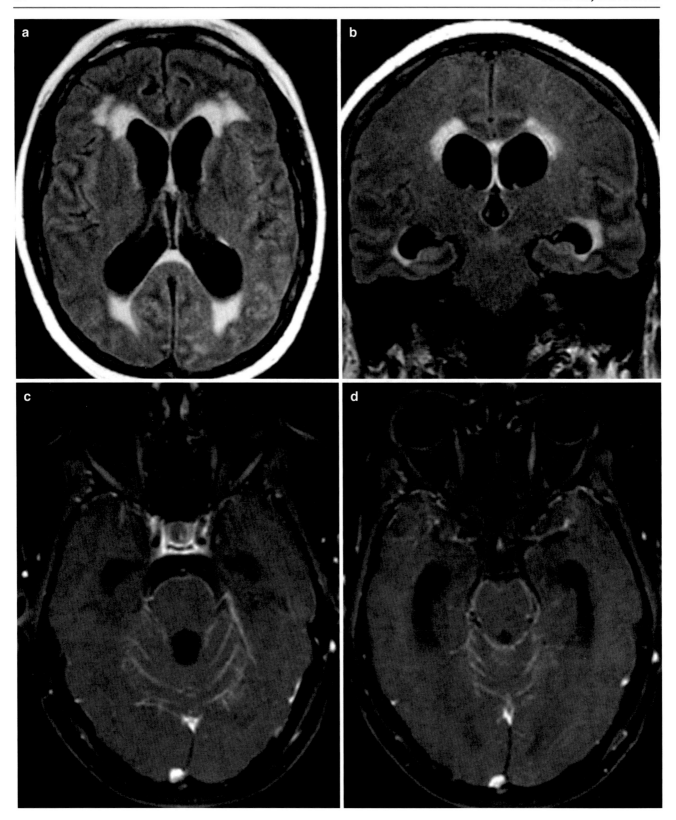

Fig. 2.5 Acute communicating hydrocephalus secondary to leptomeningeal carcinomatosis in a patient previously diagnosis of breast cancer. Transverse (**a**) and coronal (**b**) T2-FLAIR images and contrast-enhanced T1-weighted images (**c**, **d**). Observe the ventriculomegaly associated with periventricular interstitial edema and diffuse leptomeningeal enhancement surrounding the brain stem and cerebellum

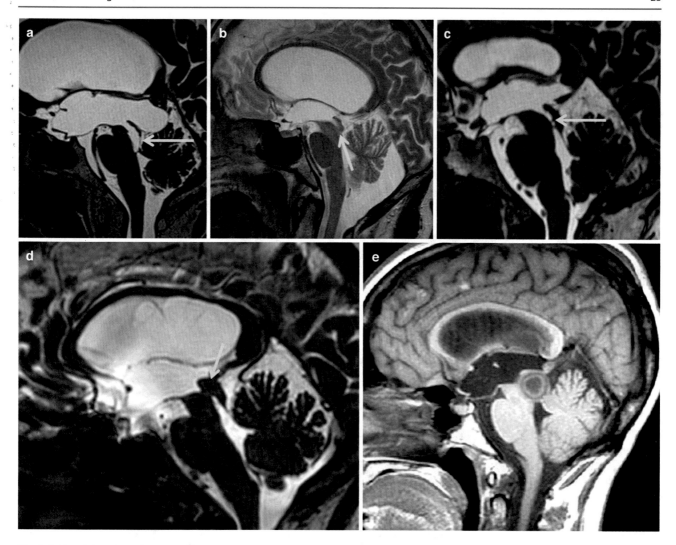

Fig. 2.6 Examples of non-tumoral and tumoral aqueductal stenosis detected on midsagittal MR images. (**a**) Web; (**b**) Adhesion; (**c**) Forking; (**d**) Tectal glioma; (**e**) Abscess

of the corpus callosum; and demonstration of CSF circulation patency inside the ventricular system (Fig. 2.4).

Normal pressure hydrocephalus (NPH) is characterized by the triad of gait disturbance, mental deterioration, and urinary incontinence, which are associated with enlargement of the ventricular system and normal CSF pressure. About 50% of cases with NPH have a known cause (secondary or symptomatic NPH [sNPH]), such as meningitis, subarachnoid haemorrhage, or cranial trauma, while the remaining 50% of cases are idiopathic (iNPH), usually presenting in the seventh decade of life. Typical structural brain changes in iNPH have been grouped under the term "disproportionately enlarged subarachnoid space hydrocephalus" (DESH), which refers to the combination of 1/ventriculomegaly (Evans index >0.3); 2/narrow high-convexity and medial subarachnoid spaces; and 3/Enlarged Sylvian fissures (disproportionate distribution of the CSF between the inferior and superior subarachnoid spaces). Shinoda et al. [47] have proposed the incorporation of two additional radiological features (callosal angle and focal sulcal dilation) [48, 49] to these three components, which in combination have a high positive predictive value in relation to neurological improvement after surgery (Fig. 2.8). Not every patient with possible or probable iNPH will be a candidate for shunt surgery, and the risk to benefit ratio has to be assessed on individual bases. Diagnostic test used for selecting patients for shunt surgery includes those based on surgical invasive procedures (CSF dynamics and intracranial pressure monitoring) [50, 51], and those based on morphological or functional MRI studies [52, 53].

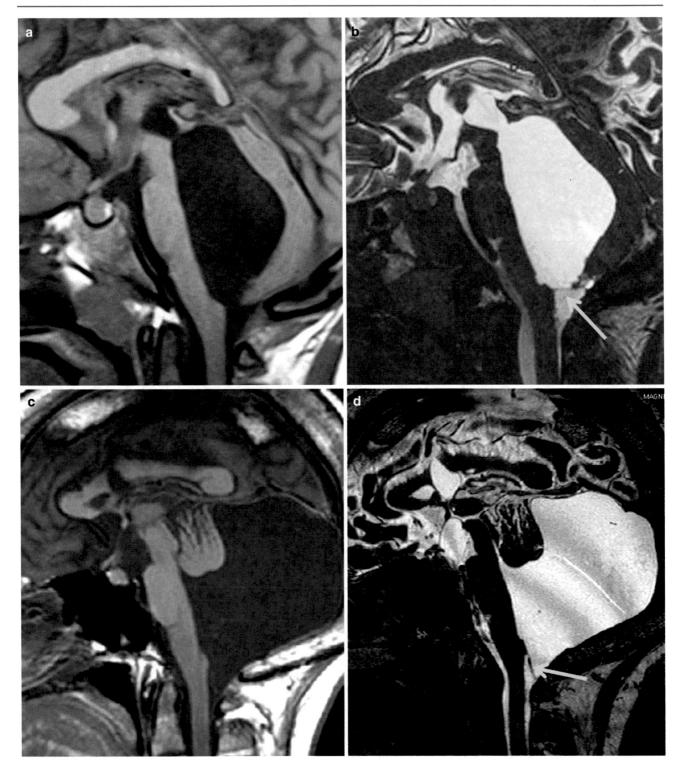

Fig. 2.7 Fourth ventricle hydrocephalus. Non-communicating hydrocephalus secondary to inflammatory obstruction of the fourth ventricle outlets (trapped fourth ventricle) in patients with history of perinatal infection. Sagittal T1-weighted (**a**) shows marked isolated fourth ventricle enlargement. The high-resolution 3D CISS images (**b**) shows thin bands that blocked the CSF pathways of the fourth ventricle, including foramen of Magendie, and aqueduct (arrows). Non-communicating hydrocephalus secondary to obstruction of the fourth ventricle outlets in Dandy–Walker malformation. Sagittal T1-weighted (**c**) shows hypoplasia of the cerebellar vermis and cephalad rotation of the vermian remnant, cystic dilatation of the fourth ventricle extending posteriorly and enlarged posterior fossa. The high-resolution 3D CISS images (**d**) shows a thin band that blocked the foramina of Magendie (arrow)

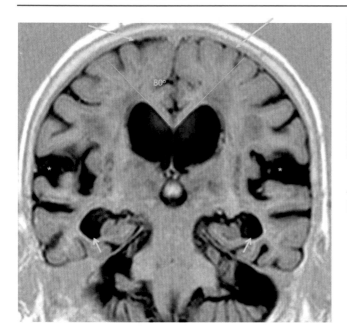

Fig. 2.8 73-year-old man with a diagnosis of idiopathic normal pressure hydrocephalus. All components of DESH are clearly visible on this coronal T1-weighted image. Ventriculomegaly (Evans index >0.3); high-convexity tightness (arrows); enlarged Sylvian fissures (asterisks); reduced callosal angle; and marked dilatation of both temporal horns not explained by hippocampal atrophy (arrows)

2.2.5   Concluding Remarks

Structural and functional MRI play an essential role for understanding the anatomy of the CSF spaces and ventricular system, as well as the hydrodynamics of CSF flow. These principles are important to the comprehension of the different types of hydrocephalus. Combination of heavily 3D T2-weighted sequences such as CISS or FIESTA that offer superb anatomical information, and 3D T2-weighted turbo/fast spin-echo sequences such as SPACE, VISTA, or CUBE that are highly sensitive to CSF flow, provides an easy evaluation of CSF pathway and circulation, and allows an accurate distinction between non-communicating from communicating hydrocephalus and identification of the causative mechanism of these two types of hydrocephalus.

> **Take-Home Messages (3–5)**
> • MRI is the imaging modality of choice in the diagnosis and management of hydrocephalus.
> • Conventional MRI sequences associated with high-resolution 3D T2-weighted sequences seem to be most efficient MRI strategy for assessing CSF pathways and circulation, and consequently in the iden-

tification of the causative mechanism of both communicating and non-communicating hydrocephalus.
• Presence of disproportionately enlarged subarachnoid spaces (DESH) is a useful MRI feature for establishing the diagnosis of idiopathic normal pressure hydrocephalus.

References

1. Vincent M, Wang SJ. Headache Classification Committee of the International Headache Society (IHS) The International Classification of Headache Disorders. Cephalalgia. 2018;38(1):1–211. https://doi.org/10.1177/0333102417738202.
2. Kranz PG, Tanpitukpongse TP, Choudhury KR, Amrhein TJ, Gray L. How common is normal cerebrospinal fluid pressure in spontaneous intracranial hypotension? Cephalalgia. 2016;36(13):1209–17. http://www.ncbi.nlm.nih.gov/pubmed/26682575.
3. Häni L, Fung C, Jesse CM, Ulrich CT, Miesbach T, Cipriani DR, et al. Insights into the natural history of spontaneous intracranial hypotension from infusion testing. Neurology. 2020;95(3):e247–55. http://www.ncbi.nlm.nih.gov/pubmed/32522800.
4. Schievink WI, Maya MM, Moser F, Tourje J, Torbati S. Frequency of spontaneous intracranial hypotension in the emergency department. J Headache Pain. 2007;8(6):325–8.
5. Mokri B, Aksamit A, Atkinson J. Paradoxical postural headaches in cerebrospinal fluid leaks. Cephalalgia. 2004;24(10):883–7. https://doi.org/10.1111/j.1468-2982.2004.00763.x.
6. Yamamoto M, Suehiro T, Nakata H, Nishioka T, Itoh H, Nakamura T, et al. Primary low cerebrospinal fluid pressure syndrome associated with galactorrhea. Intern Med. 1993;32(3):228–31. http://www.ncbi.nlm.nih.gov/pubmed/8329818.
7. Arai S, Takai K, Taniguchi M. The algorithm for diagnosis and management of intracranial hypotension with coma: report of two cases. Surg Neurol Int. 2020;11(267):2–4.
8. Takai K, Niimura M, Hongo H, Umekawa M, Teranishi A, Kayahara T, et al. Disturbed consciousness and coma: diagnosis and management of intracranial hypotension caused by a spinal cerebrospinal fluid leak. World Neurosurg. 2019;121:e700–11. https://linkinghub.elsevier.com/retrieve/pii/S1878875018322484.
9. Kranz PG, Tanpitukpongse TP, Choudhury KR, Amrhein TJ, Gray L. Imaging signs in spontaneous intracranial hypotension: prevalence and relationship to CSF pressure. Am J Neuroradiol. 2016;37(7):1374–8.
10. Dobrocky T, Grunder L, Breiding PS, Branca M, Limacher A, Mosimann PJ, et al. Assessing spinal cerebrospinal fluid leaks in spontaneous intracranial hypotension with a scoring system based on brain magnetic resonance imaging findings. JAMA Neurol. 2019;18:1–8.
11. Schievink WI, Schwartz MS, Maya MM, Moser FG, Rozen TD. Lack of causal association between spontaneous intracranial hypotension and cranial cerebrospinal fluid leaks. J Neurosurg. 2012;116(4):749–54. http://www.ncbi.nlm.nih.gov/pubmed/22264184.
12. Farb RI, Nicholson PJ, Peng PW, Massicotte EM, Lay C, Krings T, et al. Spontaneous intracranial hypotension: a systematic imaging approach for CSF leak localization and management based on MRI and digital subtraction myelography. AJNR Am J Neuroradiol. 2019;40(4):745–53. http://www.ncbi.nlm.nih.gov/pubmed/30923083.

13. Schievink WI, Maya MM, Jean-Pierre S, Nuño M, Prasad RS, Moser FG. A classification system of spontaneous spinal CSF leaks. Neurology. 2016;87(7):673–9. http://www.ncbi.nlm.nih.gov/pubmed/27440149.

14. Kumar N, Diehn FE, Carr CM, Verdoorn JT, Garza I, Luetmer PH, et al. Spinal CSF venous fistula: a treatable etiology for CSF leaks in craniospinal hypovolemia. Neurology. 2016;86(24):2310–2. http://www.ncbi.nlm.nih.gov/pubmed/27178701.

15. Schievink WI, Moser FG, Maya MM. CSF-venous fistula in spontaneous intracranial hypotension. Neurology. 2014;83(5):472–3. http://www.ncbi.nlm.nih.gov/pubmed/24951475.

16. Schievink WI. Spontaneous spinal cerebrospinal fluid and ongoing investigations in this area. JAMA. 2006;295(19):2286–96.

17. Schievink WI, Maya MM. Spinal meningeal diverticula, spontaneous intracranial hypotension, and superficial siderosis. Neurology. 2017;88(9):916–7. http://www.ncbi.nlm.nih.gov/pubmed/28130464.

18. Johnson DR, Carr CM, Luetmer PH, Diehn FE, Lehman VT, Cutsforth-Gregory JK, et al. Diffuse calvarial hyperostosis in patients with spontaneous intracranial hypotension. World Neurosurg. 2021;146:e848–53.

19. Kim DK, Carr CM, Benson JC, Diehn FE, Lehman VT, Liebo GB, et al. Diagnostic yield of lateral decubitus digital subtraction myelogram stratified by brain MRI findings. Neurology. 2021;96(9):e1312–8. https://doi.org/10.1212/WNL.0000000000011522.

20. Brinjikji W, Garza I, Whealy M, Kissoon N, Atkinson JLD, Savastano L, et al. Clinical and imaging outcomes of cerebrospinal fluid-venous fistula embolization. J Neurointerv Surg. 2022;14(10):953–6.

21. Dobrocky T, Häni L, Rohner R, Branca M, Mordasini P, Pilgram-Pastor S, et al. Brain spontaneous intracranial hypotension score for treatment monitoring after surgical closure of the underlying spinal dural leak. Clin Neuroradiol. 2022;32(1):231–8.

22. Kranz PG, Luetmer PH, Diehn FE, Amrhein TJ, Tanpitukpongse TP, Gray L. Myelographic techniques for the detection of spinal CSF leaks in spontaneous intracranial hypotension. AJR Am J Roentgenol. 2016;206(1):8–19. http://www.ncbi.nlm.nih.gov/pubmed/26700332.

23. Watanabe A, Horikoshi T, Uchida M, Koizumi H, Yagishita T, Kinouchi H. Diagnostic value of spinal MR imaging in spontaneous intracranial hypotension syndrome. Am J Neuroradiol. 2009;30(1):147–51.

24. Dobrocky T, Winklehner A, Breiding PS, Grunder L, Peschi G, Häni L, et al. Spine MRI in spontaneous intracranial hypotension for CSF leak detection: nonsuperiority of intrathecal gadolinium to heavily T2-weighted fat-saturated sequences. AJNR Am J Neuroradiol. 2020;41(7):1309–15. https://doi.org/10.3174/ajnr.A6592.

25. Schievink WI, Maya MM, Chu RM, Moser FG. False localizing sign of cervico-thoracic CSF leak in spontaneous intracranial hypotension. Neurology. 2015;84(24):2445–8.

26. Schievink WI, Maya MM, Moser FG, Prasad RS, Cruz RB, Nuño M, et al. Lateral decubitus digital subtraction myelography to identify spinal CSF-venous fistulas in spontaneous intracranial hypotension. J Neurosurg Spine. 2019;31(1):902–5. http://www.ncbi.nlm.nih.gov/pubmed/31518974.

27. Piechowiak EI, Pospieszny K, Haeni L, Jesse CM, Peschi G, Mosimann PJ, et al. Role of conventional dynamic myelography for detection of high-flow cerebrospinal fluid leaks: optimizing the technique. Clin Neuroradiol. 2020;31:633–41. https://doi.org/10.1007/s00062-020-00943-w.

28. Dobrocky T, Mosimann PJ, Zibold F, Mordasini P, Raabe A, Ulrich CT, et al. Cryptogenic cerebrospinal fluid leaks in spontaneous intracranial hypotension: role of dynamic CT myelography. Radiology. 2018;289(3):766–72. http://www.ncbi.nlm.nih.gov/pubmed/30226459.

29. Kim DK, Brinjikji W, Morris PP, Diehn FE, Lehman VT, Liebo GB, et al. Lateral decubitus digital subtraction myelography: tips, tricks, and pitfalls. AJNR Am J Neuroradiol. 2020;41(1):21–8. http://www.ncbi.nlm.nih.gov/pubmed/31857327.

30. Amrhein TJ, Gray L, Malinzak MD, Kranz PG. Respiratory phase affects the conspicuity of CSF-venous fistulas in spontaneous intracranial hypotension. AJNR Am J Neuroradiol. 2020;41(9):1754–6. http://www.ncbi.nlm.nih.gov/pubmed/32675336.

31. Clark MS, Diehn FE, Verdoorn JT, Lehman VT, Liebo GB, Morris JM, et al. Prevalence of hyperdense paraspinal vein sign in patients with spontaneous intracranial hypotension without dural CSF leak on standard CT myelography. Diagn Interv Radiol. 2018;24(1):54–9.

32. Kranz PG, Amrhein TJ, Gray L. CSF venous fistulas in spontaneous intracranial hypotension: imaging characteristics on dynamic and CT myelography. Am J Roentgenol. 2017;209(6):1360–6.

33. Piechowiak EI, Aeschimann B, Häni L, Kaesmacher J, Mordasini P, Jesse CM, et al. Epidural blood patching in spontaneous intracranial hypotension-do we really seal the leak? Clin Neuroradiol. 2023;33(1):211–8.

34. Schievink WI, Morreale VM, Atkinson JLD, Meyer FB, Piepgras DG, Ebersold MJ. Surgical treatment of spontaneous spinal cerebrospinal fluid leaks. J Neurosurg. 1998;88(2):243–6. https://the-jns.org/view/journals/j-neurosurg/88/2/article-p243.xml.

35. Beck J, Ulrich CT, Fung C, Fichtner J, Seidel K, Fiechter M, et al. Diskogenic microspurs as a major cause of intractable spontaneous intracranial hypotension. Neurology. 2016;87(12):1220–6. http://www.ncbi.nlm.nih.gov/pubmed/27566748.

36. Brinjikji W, Savastano LE, Atkinson JLD, Garza I, Farb R, Cutsforth-Gregory JK. A novel endovascular therapy for CSF hypotension secondary to CSF-venous fistulas. AJNR Am J Neuroradiol. 2021;42(5):882–7. http://www.ncbi.nlm.nih.gov/pubmed/33541895.

37. Amrhein TJ, Williams JW, Gray L, Malinzak MD, Cantrell S, Deline CR, et al. Efficacy of epidural blood patching or surgery in spontaneous intracranial hypotension: a systematic review and evidence map. Am J Neuroradiol. 2023;44(6):730–9.

38. Langner S, Fleck S, Baldauf J, et al. Diagnosis and differential diagnosis of hydrocephalus in adults. Fortschr Rontgenstr. 2017;189:728–39.

39. Maller VV, Gray RI. Noncommunicating hydrocephalus. Semin Ultrasound CT MRI. 2016;37:109–19.

40. Kartal MG, Algin O. Evaluation of hydrocephalus and other cerebrospinal fluid disorders with MRI: an update. Insights Imaging. 2014;5:531–41.

41. Rovira A. Communicating hydrocephalus. Normal pressure hydrocephalus. In: Barkhof F, et al., editors. Clinical neuroradiology. Springer Nature Switzerland AG; 2019.

42. Ucar M, Guryildirim M, Tokgoz N, et al. Evaluation of aqueductal patency in patients with hydrocephalus: three-dimensional high-sampling-efficiency technique (SPACE) versus two-dimensional turbo spin echo at 3 Tesla. Korean J Radiol. 2014;15:827–35.

43. Bladowska J, Sasiadek MJ. Obstructive hydrocephalus in adults. In: Barkhof F, et al., editors. Clinical neuroradiology. Springer Nature Switzerland AG; 2019.

44. Barkovich AJ, Newton TH. MR of aqueductal stenosis: evidence of a broad spectrum of tectal distortion. Am J Neuroradiol AJNR. 1989;10:471–6.

45. Hodel J, Rahmouni A, Zins M, et al. Magnetic resonance imaging of noncommunicating hydrocephalus. World Neurosurg. 2013;79(2S):S21.e9–S21.e12.

46. Agarwal A, Bathla G, Kanekar S. Imaging of communicating hydrocephalus. Semin Ultrasound CT MR. 2016;37:100–8.

47. Shinoda N, Hirai O, Hori S, et al. Utility of MRI-based disproportionately enlarged subarachnoid space hydrocephalus scoring for

predicting prognosis after surgery for idiopathic normal pressure hydrocephalus: clinical research. J Neurosurg. 2017;127:1436–42.

48. Ishii K, Kanda T, Harada A, et al. Clinical impact of the callosal angle in the diagnosis of idiopathic normal pressure hydrocephalus. Eur Radiol. 2008;18:2678–83.

49. Virhammar J, Laurell K, Cesarini KG, Larsson EM. Preoperative prognostic value of MRI findings in 108 patients with idiopathic normal pressure hydrocephalus. AJNR Am J Neuroradiol. 2014a;35:2311–8.

50. Williams MA, Malm J. Diagnosis and treatment of idiopathic normal pressure hydrocephalus. Continuum (Minneap Minn). 2016;22(2 Dementia):579–99.

51. Nakajima M, Yamada S, Miyajima M, et al. Guidelines for management of idiopathic normal pressure hydrocephalus (third edition): endorsed by the Japanese Society of Normal Pressure Hydrocephalus. Neurol Med Chir (Tokyo). 2021;61:63–97.

52. Rovira À, Hodel J. Commentary: predictor of shunt response in idiopathic normal pressure hydrocephalus. Neuroradiology. 2022;64:2097–9.

53. Virhammar J, Laurell K, Cesarini KG, Larsson EM. The callosal angle measured on MRI as a predictor of outcome in idiopathic normal-pressure hydrocephalus. J Neurosurg. 2014b;120:178–84.

Stroke and Its Mimics: Diagnosis and Treatment

3

Sarah Power and Achala S. Vagal

Abstract

Imaging is a key step in evaluating the acute stroke patient in order to establish the correct diagnosis and to facilitate fast triage decisions regarding treatment with thrombolysis and endovascular therapy in potentially eligible patients. This chapter explores evidence-based guidelines for stroke imaging, discusses the role of CT and MRI in acute stroke assessment, offers strategies for streamlining imaging workflows, and provides insights into identifying stroke mimics.

Keywords

Stroke · Vessel occlusion · Core · Penumbra · Endovascular thrombectomy · Imaging workflow · Stroke mimics · CT · CTA · MRI

Learning Objectives

- To assess current evidence in treatment of acute ischemic stroke.
- To review the role of multimodal CT and MR imaging including vessel, collateral and perfusion imaging in "FAST positive" or "Code stroke" patients.
- To describe optimal imaging workflows in acute stroke.
- To recognize stroke mimics.

S. Power (✉)
Department of Radiology, Beaumont Hospital, Dublin, Ireland
e-mail: sarahpower@beaumont.ie

A. S. Vagal
Department of Radiology, University of Cincinnati, Cincinnati, OH, USA
e-mail: vagala@ucmail.uc.edu

3.1 Introduction

Imaging is a key step in the evaluation of the acute stroke patient. While imaging strategies may vary between centers, the goal of acute stroke imaging remains the same, establishes the correct diagnosis, and facilitates fast triage decisions regarding treatment with thrombolysis and endovascular therapy in potentially eligible patients. Imaging allows evaluation for the following four critical points:

1. Hemorrhage: Identification of intraparenchymal or subarachnoid hemorrhage is a key differentiator of hemorrhagic from the significantly more common ischemic stroke, both of which have widely different management strategies. In addition, exclusion of any intracranial hemorrhage is important in determining eligibility for thrombolysis.
2. Infarction: Identification of any existing infarction, aging of same as acute, subacute, or chronic, and determining extent of acute infarction is crucial for decision-making regarding both intravenous thrombolysis and endovascular therapy (EVT).
3. Arterial occlusion: Identification of any intracranial arterial occlusion, including large artery, medium and distal occlusions, as well as occlusion of carotid or vertebral arteries in the neck is critical in determining eligibility for EVT.
4. Stroke mimics: A wide range of neurological conditions can present with similar symptoms to acute stroke at the outset and imaging can distinguish between stroke and stroke mimics.

3.2 Imaging in Acute Ischemic Stroke—Evidence-Based Guidelines

Over the years, multiple trials have changed the landscape of acute stroke treatment, it is vital that radiologists are familiar with these paradigm shifting studies. In 2015, five randomized controlled trials (RCTs) (MR CLEAN, ESCAPE,

REVASCAT, SWIFT-PRIME, EXTEND-IA) [1–5] demonstrated benefit for EVT over best medical therapy (BMT) in patients with large vessel occlusion (LVO) of the anterior circulation within 6 h from symptom onset or last known well (LKW). These patients had moderate to severe stroke deficits (National Institutes of Health Score/NIHSS ≥6), absence of widespread established infarction on brain imaging (ASPECT score ≥6 on MRI or CT brain), and occlusion of the carotid terminus or proximal middle cerebral artery (MCA) on either CTA or MRA. As a result, endovascular thrombectomy became standard of care for patients with anterior circulation LVO meeting the above criteria [6, 7].

In 2018, two additional RCTs, DAWN and DEFUSE 3 [8, 9], demonstrated benefit of EVT over BMT in a later time window up to 24 h from onset/LKW. These late window trials used advanced stroke imaging techniques for patient selection, either CT perfusion (CTP) or MRI, and included evaluation of core infarct volume with automated post-processing software (RAPID, iSchemaView). The DAWN trial used clinical-core mismatch as a selection criterion between 6 and 24 h from symptom onset, with variable core volume allowed up to a limit of 51 mL depending on age and severity of stroke symptoms. The DEFUSE 3 trial allowed core volume up to 70 mL for patients from 6 to 16 h from symptom onset, with mismatch ratio >1.8, and mismatch volume >15 mL. These trials provided level 1a evidence for the benefit of EVT in the late time window and changed stroke guidelines, with new recommendations for imaging as well as treatment in delayed time windows [6, 7]. As per guidelines, in adult patients with anterior circulation LVO presenting up to 6 h from onset/LKW, advanced imaging is not necessary for patient selection. However, in patients presenting from 6 to 24 h, advanced imaging with either CT perfusion, diffusion weighted MRI (DW-MRI), or MR perfusion (MRP) is necessary.

Also using advanced imaging techniques, two major trials provided evidence for use of extended window IV thrombolysis beyond 4.5 h. Published in 2018, the WAKE-UP trial [10] randomized IV thrombolysis eligible patients who either awoke with stroke symptoms or had unclear time of onset >4.5 h from LKW. Imaging criteria required mismatch between MR-DWI and fluid-attenuated inversion recovery (FLAIR). The trial demonstrated benefit of IV tPA over placebo in patients with wake up or unknown time of onset stroke, and for whom EVT was not performed. Exclusion criteria included DW-MRI lesions larger than one-third of the MCA territory. Published in 2019, the EXTEND trial [11] evaluated use of IV thrombolysis in patients presenting 4.5–9 h from known stroke onset time, or after awakening with stroke if within 9 h from the midpoint of sleep. Advanced imaging with CTP or MRP was required for patient selection. Inclusion criteria included core infarct volume ≤70 mL and mismatch ratio of >1.2. The study showed better out-

comes for IV tPA versus placebo. Guidelines for the use of IV thrombolysis in extended time window are now published [6, 12], with recommendations for advanced imaging techniques to be used in patient selection.

While EVT is performed for posterior circulation LVO, high level evidence has been lacking. Two recent RCTs have however shown positive results for EVT in basilar occlusion. The BAOCHE trial [13] randomized basilar occlusion patients presenting 6–24 h from onset, with NIHSS >6, and imaging-based inclusion criteria of posterior circulation ASPECTS score (PC-ASPECTS) of ≥6 and pons midbrain index score of ≤2. The ATTENTION trial [14] randomized patients with basilar occlusion presenting within 12 h of onset, with NIHSS >10 and PC-ASPECTS ≥6. It is likely that the benefit of EVT in basilar occlusion demonstrated in these trials will result in updates to the guidelines. Given that both trials included imaging-based selection criteria, the use of a scoring system for acute infarct burden such as PC-ASPECTS may well be incorporated into guideline recommendations.

Most recently, the "large core" trials have garnered significant attention to expand EVT in patients with a large burden of acute infarction. The recent publication of three RCTs has however given level 1 evidence that EVT can improve functional outcome over BMT, with all three trials showing positive effect, even in these severe strokes. RESCUE-Japan LIMIT [15], published in 2022, used predominantly MRI for triage, and included patients with ASPECT score 3–5, carotid terminus or first segment of MCA occlusion (M1), and presenting within 6 h from last known well or within 24 h if there was no early change on FLAIR. In the SELECT2 trial [16], published in 2023, patients had an ICA or M1 occlusion, presented within 24 h of onset, and had large ischemic core volume defined as ASPECT score 3–5 or a core volume of at least 50 mL on CT perfusion or DW-MRI. CT was used for triage in the majority. Published at the same time as SELECT2, the ANGEL-ASPECT trial [17] included patients within 24 h of stroke onset, with intracranial ICA or M1 occlusion. Imaging selection criteria included ASPECT score 3–5 on non-contrast CT with no limitation of infarct-core volume, but also ASPECT score 0–2 with infarct-core volume between 70 and 100 mL. The majority of included patients (85%) had an ASPECT score of 3–5. Together these 3 trials provide evidence that EVT in large core strokes with anterior circulation LVO is safe and more effective than BMT alone. Results from additional large core trials including LASTE (NCT03811769), TESLA (NCT03805308), and TENSION (NCT03094715) are pending. As of this writing, there are no current recommendations in the European and North American guidelines for mechanical thrombectomy in large cores. However, it is reasonable to anticipate future guidelines to incorporate this new evidence.

3.3 Imaging Paradigm

CT is often the workhorse for emergency stroke evaluation due to its speed, availability, fewer contraindications, lower cost, and ease of interpretation, despite MRI's higher sensitivity for early ischemic changes and specific infarct types. MRI imaging times are longer and safety screening can be challenging in the acute stroke situation. Regardless of the modality chosen, a streamlined imaging protocol is essential for effective stroke triage, as discussed in later sections.

3.4 CT: Protocols, Findings, and Pitfalls

A CT-based protocol for acute stroke triage should include a non-contrast CT head (NCCT), CT angiogram (CTA) of both brain and neck vessels, and if available, the option of performing CT perfusion (CTP).

3.4.1 Non-contrast CT Head Imaging

A NCCT head should be performed as the first study to allow exclusion of hemorrhage and facilitate decision-making regarding intravenous thrombolysis in eligible patients. Findings of early infarction on CT include loss of gray white matter differentiation, low attenuation change, and sulcal effacement. In carotid terminus and M1 segment occlusions, the earliest change is frequently seen in the basal ganglia and insula due to lack of collateralization in lenticulostriate perforator territories. However, NCCT can be limited in identification of very early infarcts, and particularly in setting of extensive small vessel disease and older infarcts.

The Alberta stroke program early CT score (ASPECTS) is a widely used scoring system developed to allow objective analysis of the extent of acute infarction in the MCA territory. The MCA territory is segmented into 10 regions: caudate, lentiform, internal capsule, insula, and cortical zones M1–M6. Zones M1–M3 lie at the basal ganglia level, extending anteroposteriorly, while zones M4–M6 are supra-ganglionic and also extend from anterior to posterior. One point is deducted from the original score of 10 for every region involved by acute infarction. Many of the major RCTs providing evidence for the benefit of EVT included ASPECTS as a selection criterion. Higher ASPECT scores are associated with better outcomes following stroke treatment. While the scoring system is objective, there is poor inter-observer reliability and use is limited to MCA territory. The integration of AI in stroke imaging has expanded the capabilities of automated ASPECTS analysis. While these tools are designed to augment, not replace, radiologists, they enhance inter-rater agreement and boost non-expert performance.

A variation of the ASPECT scoring system has been developed for the posterior circulation, PC-ASPECTS. This is also a 10-point scoring system, with points lost for each region affected. Due to the high morbidity associated with brainstem infarction, the score is weighted to a degree for same with pons and midbrain both assigned 2 points each. Other zones include thalami (1 point each), occipital lobes (1 point each), and cerebellar hemispheres (1 point each). A limitation is the relative lack of sensitivity for CT identification of early brainstem infarction.

NCCT can also help identify site of occlusion, as intra-arterial thrombus may appear hyperdense depending on its composition. As well as identifying linear hyperdensity in a proximal artery such as the M1 (hyperdense artery sign), it is helpful to evaluate more distally in the sylvian fissure for a hyperdense "dot" sign which can indicate an M2 occlusion. Other locations of potential hyperdense thrombus include anterior interhemispheric fissure for an anterior cerebral occlusion, prepontine cistern for basilar thrombus, or ambient cistern for posterior cerebral artery occlusion.

3.4.2 CT Angiogram

CTA is quick and highly accurate in identification of LVO. It should be performed from the level of the aortic arch through to vertex, allowing evaluation of extracranial carotid and vertebral arteries for occlusion, stenosis, or dissection which may impact on interventional techniques used and patient outcome. If an extracranial arterial occlusion or stenosis is of an artery in the same territory as the intracranial occlusion, it is termed a tandem lesion.

The term LVO refers to occlusion of the carotid terminus (carotid T), first segment of MCA (M1), intracranial vertebral artery, and basilar artery, and all of these must be scrutinized for patency. There is debate in the literature as to whether occlusion of the second segment of the middle cerebral artery (M2) is a large or medium vessel occlusion (MeVO), particularly given that occlusion of a proximal dominant M2 segment, or more than one proximal M2 segment can behave as an M1 like occlusion in terms of volume of territory at risk of infarction and clinical severity of stroke syndrome. While evidence from RCTs for treatment of M2 occlusion is still lacking, there are many observational studies providing supportive evidence that EVT in M2 occlusions is beneficial and safe [18]. Treatment approaches for symptomatic MeVO (Medium Vessel Occlusions) vary across institutions, some following standard protocols despite limited evidence, while others opt for case-by-case decisions. Ongoing RCTs like ESCAPE-MeVO (NCT05151172) and DISTALS (NCT05152524) aim to establish the efficacy of thrombectomy in MeVO and more distal occlusions.

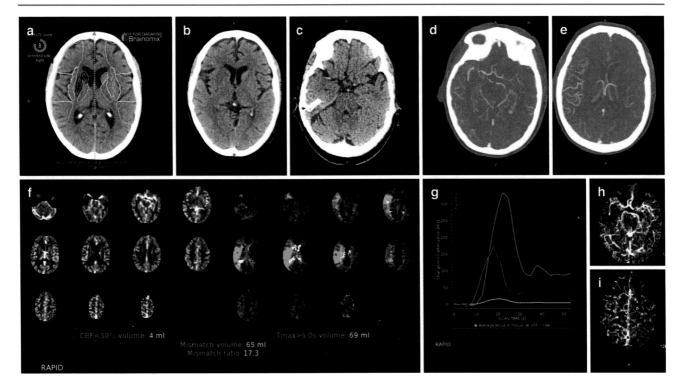

Fig. 3.1 A 77-year-old lady, wake-up stroke, over 12 h from LKW with NIHSS 15. Automated eASPECTS analysis from Brainomix software (**a**), and source images (**b**) ASPECTS 8 with infarction in caudate and lentiform nuclei. Hyperdense right distal M1 segment (**c**) which reflects thrombus and corresponds to site of occlusion on CTA (**d**). Moderate collateral filling on phase 1 (not shown) but good collaterals on phase 2 images with branches filling back to proximal M2 level at distal end of thrombus (**d**, **e**). Perfusion analysis (**f**) using RAPIDAI

software shows small core infarct (purple shading) large territory at risk (green shading), therefore large penumbra with large mismatch ratio 17.3. Technically, adequate CTP study with contrast bolus demonstrating sharp rise and fall in attenuation with clear return to baseline on arterial and venous time density curves (**g**). Location for arterial ROI (**h**, red dot) is correct, usually the ICA terminus, proximal MCA, and ACA are appropriate. The blue dot (**i**) represents the location of venous ROI; superior sagittal sinus or torcula are commonly used sites

As a radiologist, it is important to have a strategy to identify medium and distal occlusions on CTA. The use of thin slice imaging (1 mm or less), multiplanar reconstruction, and maximal intensity projection (MIP) images with a slice thickness of 6–10 mm can all aid in the detection of these occlusions. For example, the sagittal plane is particularly useful for identifying medium and distal M2 occlusions, ACA occlusions, and PCA P2–P3 occlusions, and coronals are useful for proximal M2, proximal ACA and PCA occlusions.

CTA also provides vital insights into collateral pathways, either antegrade via the Circle of Willis (COW) or retrograde through leptomeningeal collaterals. For example, in ICA occlusion below the carotid terminus, collateral supply can come from the anterior communicating artery; if the occlusion is below the posterior communicating artery, it adds another route. However, in M1 or carotid T occlusions, antegrade COW collateralization is unavailable; any collateral supply must be retrograde, typically via leptomeningeal collaterals from ipsilateral ACA or PCA territory.

Numerous studies have shown that good leptomeningeal collateral supply confers benefit in stroke as it sustains brain tissue in the occluded vascular territory for a longer time

with slower infarct growth (slow progressors), smaller final infarct volumes, and improved patient outcomes. Poor collateralization is associated with earlier infarction (fast progressors), larger infarcts, higher rates of hemorrhage, and poor outcomes [19, 20]. While there is no consensus on the type of grading scale, most are restricted to the MCA territory and vary from 2-point (good vs bad) to 5-point scales. The method is usually to compare the extent of arterial opacification in the occluded territory to the contralateral side, with degree of filling expressed as a fraction or percentage. For instance, <50% filling is considered poor, 50–75% moderate, and >75% good. Utilizing thick section MIP images in an axial plane facilitates rapid evaluation of collateral supply (Fig. 3.1).

A pitfall of single-phase CTA is the lack of temporal resolution, which can underscore collateral supply, particularly in cases of poor cardiac output or proximal stenosis. Multiphase CTA with initial arterial phase from arch to vertex, delayed intracranial early venous, and later venous phases can resolve this issue by enabling temporal evaluation of collaterals. More comprehensive grading systems have been developed to facilitate interpretation with evaluation of degree of filling of the occluded territory as well as delay

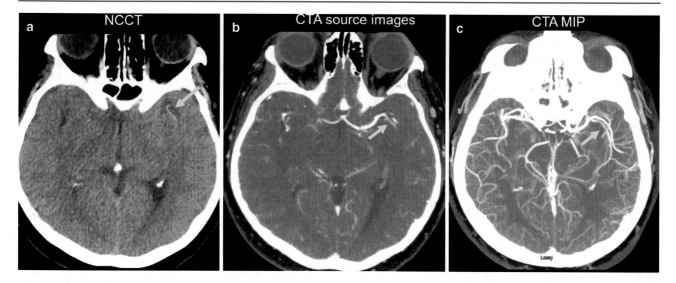

Fig. 3.2 CTA pitfall: false patency of vessel. A 55-year-old female, code stroke, transferred from outside hospital. NCCT in outside institution demonstrates hyperdense M2 (**a**), however this was not available during CTA interpretation. The CTA interpretation overlooked the vessel occlusion as it appears falsely patent (**b, c**). On careful review, there is slightly reduced attenuation on CTA compared to the other vessels (**c**)

across phases [21]. The multiphase evaluation of collaterals can be a valuable tool in triage of LVO patients for thrombectomy, and together with NCCT ASPECTS was the selection criteria in the ESCAPE trial [2]. Multiphase CTA can also provide better depiction of the medium and distal vessel occlusions. Many of the stroke AI solutions include analysis and scoring of collateral supply in MCA territory, as well as automated LVO detection.

Another pitfall of single-phase CTA is pseudo-occlusion, most commonly seen in ICA or vertebral. This occurs with either a severe proximal stenosis or distal occlusion, where a slow flow situation arises with progressively poor contrast opacification of the artery distally giving a "false occlusion" sign, and can overestimate the length of thrombus. Most commonly seen with carotid T occlusion, where the more proximal intracranial and often much of the cervical segment of ICA are not opacified by contrast on a single-phase study, recognition of pseudo-occlusion is important as occlusion length is an important determinant of the efficacy and complication rates of mechanical thrombectomy [22]. Multiphase CTA can overcome this pitfall.

A less common CTA pitfall is the false patency sign, where a particularly hyperdense thrombus can appear isodense to the contrast filled artery, and can be mistaken for contrast opacification of the vessel (Fig. 3.2). Identification of hyperdense thrombus on NCCT is crucial to avoid this pitfall, while widening window settings and levels can also help. A similar problem can be encountered with calcified vessels and can be overcome in the same way.

Key Points: Review CTA Comprehensively to Assess For
- Large vessel occlusion.
- Medium or distal vessel occlusion.
- Extracranial circulation including dissection, plaque, carotid web.
- Access issues such as tortuosity, carotid disease, aneurysms.
- Collateral circulation.

3.4.3 CT Perfusion

CTP is now increasingly incorporated into imaging protocols and allows evaluation of the volume of already infarcted tissue (ischemic core) and volume of tissue that is at risk due to hypoperfusion but not yet irreversibly infarcted (penumbra). It is performed by sequentially imaging a defined section of tissue after administration of a high-flow bolus of iodinated contrast material. Images are then postprocessed using either semi-automated or increasingly fully automated software that utilizes deconvolution algorithms to create perfusion maps, including cerebral blood flow (CBF), cerebral blood volume (CBV), mean transit time (MTT), time to peak (TTP), and time to maximum residue (Tmax).

Many of the AI software solutions include automated post-processing of perfusion data. Generally, reduced CBF <30% of contralateral side is the parameter used to reflect

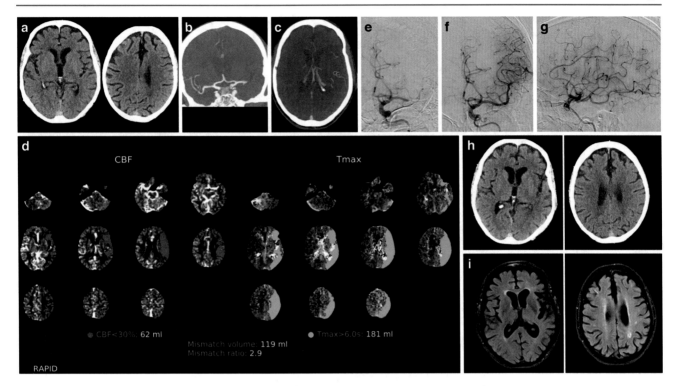

Fig. 3.3 Ghost core. A 76-year-old male, imaging including CTP at 55 min from witnessed stroke onset. No acute infarct on NCCT (**a**). Left M1 occlusion on CTA with poor collaterals on phase 1 (**b**), delayed collateral filling on phase 3 (**c**). CTP shows large volume of CBF <30%, suggesting large core infarct (**d**). Digital subtraction angiogram shows left M1 occlusion (**e**), complete recanalization on frontal (**f**) and lateral (**g**) view after single pass aspiration thrombectomy. No infarction on NCCT at 24 h (**h**), a delayed MRI 6 months later also shows no evidence of established infarction on FLAIR (**i**), confirming overestimation of core by CTP in this very early time window

ischemic core volume. The threshold of Tmax >6 s is the most commonly used to reflect critically hypoperfused territory at risk of infarction. Subtraction of core volume from volume of Tmax >6 s gives penumbra volume. Most software solutions will display a color-coded summary map which provides quantification of core, Tmax >6 s, mismatch and a mismatch ratio (Fig. 3.1). Additional variable thresholds of Tmax as well as CBF are also frequently provided. Further calculations such as the hypoperfusion index ratio (Tmax >10 s volume divided by Tmax >6 s volume) can be performed by automated software. Hypoperfusion index ratio (HIR) can be used to distinguish slow from fast progressors, with higher values in fast progressors, and is a good surrogate of tissue collaterals.

It is important to recognize the multiple pitfalls to automated CT perfusion [23]. There is inherent variation in outputs between different software solutions which can result in different calculations of core volume, territory at risk, penumbra, and mismatch ratio. The variation between different software is usually however not to the extent that it impacts decision-making. An exception can be in analysis of more distal occlusions, where the volumes of rCBF <30% and Tmax >6 s are inherently smaller and even minor variations have a greater impact on mismatch ratio calculation. Secondly, the CBF <30% threshold is not always an accurate

reflection of ischemic core. This is particularly the case for very early presenters, in particular those presenting within 90 min from onset/LSW, where the ischemic core can be overestimated, i.e., ghost core (Fig. 3.3). The additional CBF thresholds can be helpful in this scenario, with recommendation to use CBF <20% threshold in ultra-early windows. Overestimation of core infarct can lead to incorrect exclusion of patients from EVT, potentially missing an opportunity for effective treatment. Poor cardiac output can result in significant delay in arrival of contrast bolus to intracranial vessels, with potential truncation of time density attenuation curves, and inaccuracy of generated perfusion maps. In addition, a chronic carotid occlusion/stenosis can result in a false positive penumbra (Fig. 3.4), while a proximal carotid stenosis can overestimate territory at risk. Use of additional Tmax threshold maps and close correlation with CTA findings aids interpretation in these circumstances.

It is important to check technical adequacy of a CTP before interpretation or decision-making (Fig. 3.1). The arterial input function (AIF) and venous output function (VOF) time density curves should always be inspected as part of the technical checklist of CTP interpretation to ensure they have returned to baseline. Further technical pitfalls include incorrect arterial input and venous output selections, motion artifact, poor signal to noise ratio if contrast bolus is poor, and

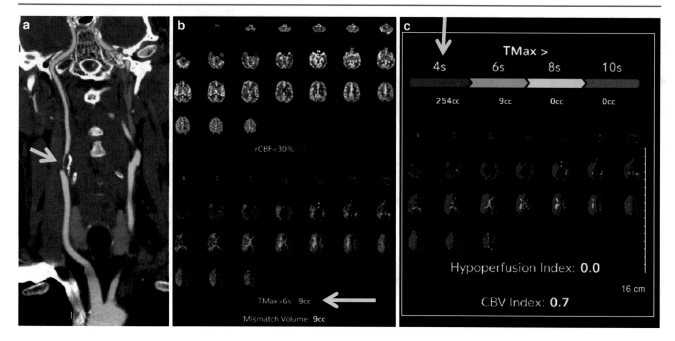

Fig. 3.4 CTP in chronic stenosis false positive penumbra: a 70-year-old male with a known chronic severe stenosis in right ICA (**a**) demonstrates a corresponding perfusion abnormality in the right cerebral hemisphere (**b**, **c**), particularly highlighted with Tmax >4 s (**c**)

limitation with many CT scanners to perform limited coverage perfusion rather than whole brain coverage perfusion.

Despite the above pitfalls, CTP remains key in acute ischemic stroke evaluation, but its role in LVO thrombectomy may change based on upcoming large core infarct trial outcomes. Its importance is growing for detecting at risk medium and distal occlusions, often missed on CTA.

> **Key Points**
> • It is important to recognize technical and diagnostic pitfalls of an automated CTP.
> • Technical pitfalls include truncated time density curve, incorrect selection of arterial or venous input and patient motion.
> • Diagnostic pitfalls include under or overestimation of ischemic core or penumbra.

3.5   MRI: Protocols, Findings, Pitfalls, and Example Cases

An MRI-based paradigm for acute stroke imaging has advantages and disadvantages. A typical protocol for MRI in acute stroke is outlined in Table.

A distinct advantage of MRI is the increased sensitivity of DWI in detection of acute infarcts, particularly impor-

tant in posterior circulation strokes. MRI also meets the criteria of advanced imaging selection in late window patients. Further advantages include the lack of ionizing radiation and ability to perform imaging without use of a contrast agent if needed. The use of MRI for triage may however result in less patients receiving thrombectomy due to detection of greater extent of acute ischemia on DWI [24]. Additional MRI pitfall is the potential reversibility of DWI lesions early in the course of stroke. Several studies have reported partial reversal of DWI after acute reperfusion treatment, with improved outcomes. Complete reperfusion and shorter imaging time to recanalization have been shown to be independently associated with DWI reversal among patients with LVO who received EVT [25].

Disadvantages include potential limited MR availability, and need for patient safety screening prior to scanning, both of which have been identified as a significant source of delay to imaging acquisition [26]. Another potential disadvantage can be longer imaging times, although MRI fast protocols, can be implemented in time frames as little as 6 min [27]. In MRI, as in CT, perfusion analysis automated software that allows fast post-processing is essential to prevent delay in decision-making. Decision-making with MRI for acute stroke includes evaluation for LVO, clinical diffusion mismatch (CDM), FLAIR diffusion mismatch (FDM) (Fig. 3.5), or perfusion diffusion mismatch (PDM).

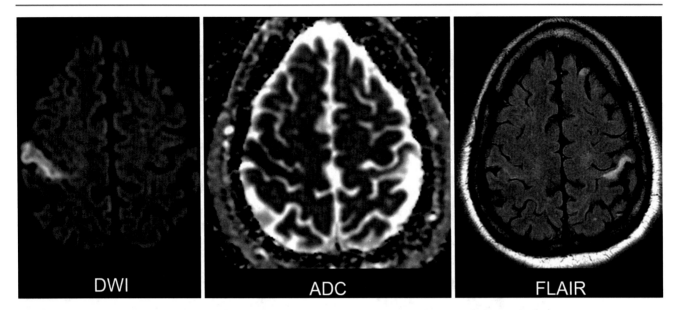

Fig. 3.5 DWI-FLAIR mismatch: a 63-year-old female presented with wake-up stroke. The initial CT workup was negative for early ischemia or vessel occlusion. MRI shows a DWI-FLAIR mismatch in the right post central gyrus. It is important not to heavily window the FLAIR sequences to look for subtle signal changes. A remote infarct is identified in the left post central gyrus

Key Points: MRI Protocol

• DWI	Acute infarcts demonstrate true diffusion restriction with high signal on B1000 images, and low signal on apparent diffusion coefficient (ADC), visible within 20 min of stroke onset
• FLAIR	Acute infarcts appear hyperintense, may take up to 6 h, and indicator of irreversible changes
• MR angiogram	Time of flight (TOF) technique, or contrast-enhanced MRA, requires imaging of COW as minimum, ideally include neck vessels
• GRE/SWI	Evaluate for presence of acute or old hemorrhage, evaluate for blooming sign indicating intra-arterial thrombus similar to hyperdense sign on CT
• MRP	Optional, if advanced imaging desirable or required
• T2 weighted	Optional, preferential for evaluation of posterior fossa

3.6 Approach to Interpreting "Code Stroke" Imaging

Regardless of imaging paradigm used, timely interpretation in the FAST positive/code stroke patient is crucial, whether done on the scanner console, PACS workstation or via AI for immediate triage and treatment decisions. While immediate questions like excluding hemorrhage and identifying LVO need quick answers, imaging must however also be thor-

oughly reviewed for additional and unexpected findings. Mirroring major trauma analogy, imaging interpretation in acute stroke is a two-tiered approach—a fast initial primary survey allowing rapid triage to treatment, followed by a less time pressured secondary definitive survey.

Key Points
- Primary imaging survey
- Hemorrhage: present or not
- Acute infarction: present or not, location, extent, ASPECTS
- Arterial occlusion: intracranial and extracranial sites
- Proximal stenosis: significant or not
- Collateral status: good or bad
- Perfusion defect: core volume, mismatch present or not
- Secondary imaging survey
- Identify additional infarcts including subacute, chronic, and non-MCA territory
- Additional brain findings—e.g., small vessel disease
- Collateral scoring
- Additional arterial occlusions, same vascular territory, different vascular territory
- Atherosclerotic disease, associated stenosis, and degree of same if present
- Consider mechanism of stroke and secondary prevention including artery to artery embolus, cardio-

embolic, soft plaque, carotid web, thrombus in aortic arch or in a vessel proximal to occlusion
- Additional or unexpected perfusion findings, e.g., hyperemia
- Consider additional differentials and stroke mimics
- Incidental findings

3.7 Optimizing Imaging Workflow in Acute Stroke

The ability to do late window thrombectomy up to 24 h from onset/LKW does not negate the need to be fast. From the HERMES collaboration [28] for every 9-min delay in onset to reperfusion, one of every 100 patients will have greater functional disability at 90 days. There is an inverse relationship between in-hospital treatment speeds and functional independence, with reducing rate of good outcome as "door to reperfusion" time increases. Hence, it is critical to establish time efficient imaging workflow in order to reduce key time indicators such as "door to imaging," "door to needle," "door to puncture," and ultimately "door to reperfusion" time. The radiology department is the cornerstone of stroke workflow, and it is important for radiologists to work on optimizing workflow together with imaging technologists, the stroke team, and neurointerventional team. Below are pointers to allow optimization of workflow.

- A pre-alert from EMS to ER, stroke, and imaging teams via a single paging system enables immediate action. On arrival, the patient is met by the stroke team and directly taken to CT/MRI.
- Parenchymal imaging, e.g., NCCT, performed first to allow triage to IV thrombolysis if eligible. Further angiographic and perfusion imaging should not delay administration of thrombolysis which can be given while the patient is in the CT or MRI scanner.
- It is not necessary to delay iodinated contrast administration to check renal function.
- A radiologist should be on standby to review images as patients are scanned, either at the scanner console or a PACS workstation. Automated sending to PACS should be set up, ensuring NCCT or DW-MRI is ready for review as angiograms or perfusion studies are underway.
- AI software solutions with automated ASPECTS, LVO, and perfusion can be very helpful in streamlining workflow, with demonstrated positive impact on key time indicators [29]. Output from most AI software solutions can be viewed on hand-held devices with option for notifications to alert the team and text communication within the team. The current and new generation of radiologists will have to adapt the use of AI in imaging workflow.

3.8 Stroke Mimics

Almost one-third cases of new focal neurological deficits can be stroke mimics [30]. It is important to identify stroke mimics and differentiate from true strokes to avoid inappropriate treatment. MRI has inherent advantages over CT to identify mimics. The more common stroke mimics include seizures, migraines, posterior reversible encephalopathy syndrome, venous thrombosis, and brain tumors.

3.8.1 Seizures

The most frequent stroke mimic is seizures with Todd's paralysis, paresis, or aphasia. The MRI changes are variable, ranging from focal, multifocal, hemispheric, or a diffuse cortical pattern of diffusion hyperintensity with variable ADC levels. Perfusion abnormalities can range from hyperperfusion in ictal phase to hypoperfusion or normal perfusion in the postictal phase. These shifts are due to neuronal activation or inhibition, respectively. Unlike strokes, seizure-related perfusion changes are not confined to a vascular territory, serving as a key clue. Additional distinguishing features of seizures include gyral or leptomeningeal enhancement, and absence of vessel occlusion.

3.8.2 Migraines

Migraine aura without headache can commonly present as a stroke mimic. MR imaging is usually normal, however in a few cases may show reversible restricted diffusion. The differentiating features include prior history of migraine, a non-vascular distribution, and lack of LVO. Perfusion abnormalities are variable with hypoperfusion in acute onset aura and normal or hyperperfusion in prolonged episodes. However, the perfusion abnormality does not usually correspond to a defined vascular territory and can span multiple vascular territories.

3.8.3 Posterior Reversible Encephalopathy Syndrome (PRES)

An acute onset neurological syndrome with vasogenic edema due to loss of auto-regulation and capillary leakage can mimic acute or subacute stroke. The PRES lesions are usually cortical/subcortical with hyperintensity on T2/FLAIR with predilection for parietooccipital lobes and a relatively symmetric pattern. Approximately 10–25% of cases can show restricted diffusion and around 15% have associated parenchymal hemorrhage.

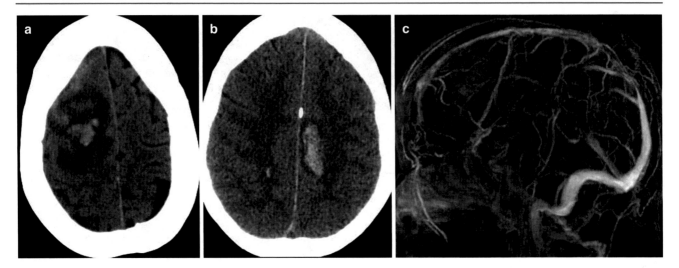

Fig. 3.6 Stroke mimic: bilateral venous infarctions with hemorrhages on NCCT (**a**, **b**). Given the distribution, the possibility of venous thrombosis of superior sagittal sinus needs to be considered. The MR venogram shows a filling defect in the superior sagittal sinus (**c**)

3.8.4 Venous Thrombosis

Both a vasogenic and cytotoxic edema may be present with resultant variable diffusion restriction on DWI. Usually, edema due to venous thrombosis is easy to identify given the lack of arterial territorial distribution, with location of edema dependent on the location of the venous thrombus. T2-GRE with its susceptibility artifact can show abnormal hypointensity and blooming of the venous thrombus. Imaging may demonstrate a flame-shaped hemorrhage due to venous infarction (Fig. 3.6).

3.8.5 Tumors

Brain tumors can mimic code strokes by causing new neurological deficits, requiring prompt differentiation to avoid treatment delays. Small, cortical tumors in an arterial territory can be mistaken for infarcts on the initial imaging. Depending on the cellularity and grade, tumors have variable diffusion hyperintensity and contrast enhancement. Perfusion imaging may be helpful; cerebral blood volume (CBV) in tumors is generally high in tumors but low in acute infarcts.

Additional conditions mimicking stroke include toxic and metabolic etiologies, conversion disorder, infection, peripheral vertigo, syncope, transient global amnesia, and subdural hematoma.

3.9 Concluding Remarks

Efficient, rapid stroke imaging is essential for optimal triage of the acute ischemic stroke patient. The use of artificial intelligence with automated ASPECT score calculation,

automated LVO detection, and automated post-processing of perfusion data is becoming increasingly more widespread. The boundaries of acute stroke treatment continue to expand with lengthening of treatment windows, and EVT in large core as well as distal occlusions. The evolving landscape of stroke imaging and treatment reinforces the radiologist's vital role in translating these changes into practice.

> **Take-Home Messages**
> - Rapidly identify acute infarct, vessel occlusions, and perfusion defects in acute ischemic stroke.
> - Optimize imaging workflows.
> - Differentiate true strokes from stroke mimics.

References

1. Berkhemer OA, Fransen PSS, Beumer D, et al. A randomized trial of Intraarterial treatment for acute ischemic stroke. N Engl J Med. 2014;372(1):11–20.
2. Goyal M, Demchuk AM, Menon BK, et al. Randomized assessment of rapid endovascular treatment of ischemic stroke. N Engl J Med. 2015;372(11):1019–30.
3. Jovin TG, Chamorro A, Cobo E, et al. Thrombectomy within 8 hours after symptom onset in ischemic stroke. N Engl J Med. 2015;372(24):2296–306.
4. Saver JL, Goyal M, Bonafe A, et al. Stent-retriever Thrombectomy after intravenous t-PA vs. t-PA alone in stroke. N Engl J Med. 2015;372(24):2285–95.
5. Campbell BCV, Mitchell PJ, Kleinig TJ, et al. Endovascular therapy for ischemic stroke with perfusion-imaging selection. N Engl J Med. 2015;372(11):1009–18.
6. Powers WJ, Rabinstein AA, Ackerson T, et al. Guidelines for the early Management of Patients with Acute Ischemic Stroke: 2019

update to the 2018 guidelines for the early Management of Acute Ischemic Stroke: a guideline for healthcare professionals from the American Heart Association/American Stroke Association. Stroke. 2019;50(12):e344–418.

7. Turc G, Bhogal P, Fischer U, et al. European stroke organisation (ESO) - European Society for Minimally Invasive Neurological Therapy (ESMINT) guidelines on mechanical Thrombectomy in acute Ischaemic StrokeEndorsed by stroke Alliance for Europe (SAFE). Eur Stroke J. 2019;4(1):6–12.

8. Nogueira RG, Jadhav AP, Haussen DC, et al. Thrombectomy 6 to 24 hours after stroke with a mismatch between deficit and infarct. N Engl J Med. 2017;378(1):11–21.

9. Albers GW, Marks MP, Kemp S, et al. Thrombectomy for stroke at 6 to 16 hours with selection by perfusion imaging. N Engl J Med. 2018;378(8):708–18.

10. Thomalla G, Simonsen CZ, Boutitie F, et al. MRI-guided thrombolysis for stroke with unknown time of onset. N Engl J Med. 2018;379(7):611–22.

11. Ma H, Campbell BCV, Parsons MW, et al. Thrombolysis guided by perfusion imaging up to 9 hours after onset of stroke. N Engl J Med. 2019;380(19):1795–803.

12. Berge E, Whiteley W, Audebert H, et al. European stroke organisation (ESO) guidelines on intravenous thrombolysis for acute ischaemic stroke. Eur Stroke J. 2021;6(1):I-LXII:I.

13. Jovin TG, Li C, Wu L, et al. Trial of thrombectomy 6 to 24 hours after stroke due to basilar-artery occlusion. N Engl J Med. 2022;387(15):1373–84.

14. Tao C, Nogueira RG, Zhu Y, et al. Trial of endovascular treatment of acute basilar-artery occlusion. N Engl J Med. 2022;387(15):1361–72.

15. Yoshimura S, Sakai N, Yamagami H, et al. Endovascular therapy for acute stroke with a large ischemic region. N Engl J Med. 2022;386(14):1303–13.

16. Sarraj A, Hassan AE, Abraham MG, et al. Trial of endovascular thrombectomy for large ischemic strokes. N Engl J Med. 2023;388(14):1259–71.

17. Huo X, Ma G, Tong X, et al. Trial of endovascular therapy for acute ischemic stroke with large infarct. N Engl J Med. 2023;388(14):1272–83.

18. Wang J, Qian J, Fan L, et al. Efficacy and safety of mechanical thrombectomy for M2 segment of middle cerebral artery: a systematic review and meta-analysis. J Neurol. 2021;268(7):2346–54.

19. Sheth SA, Sanossian N, Hao Q, et al. Collateral flow as causative of good outcomes in endovascular stroke therapy. J Neurointerv Surg. 2016;8(1):2–7.

20. Maguida G, Shuaib A. Collateral circulation in ischemic stroke: an updated review. J Stroke. 2023;25(2):179–98.

21. Menon BK, d'Esterre CD, Qazi EM, et al. Multiphase CT angiography: a new tool for the imaging triage of patients with acute ischemic stroke. Radiology. 2015;275(2):510–20.

22. Gralla J, Burkhardt M, Schroth G, et al. Occlusion length is a crucial determinant of efficiency and complication rate in thrombectomy for acute ischemic stroke. AJNR Am J Neuroradiol. 2008;29(2):247–52.

23. Vagal A, Wintermark M, Nael K, et al. Automated CT perfusion imaging for acute ischemic stroke: pearls and pitfalls for real-world use. Neurology. 2019;93(20):888–98.

24. Wisco D, Uchino K, Saqqur M, et al. Addition of hyperacute MRI AIDS in patient selection, decreasing the use of endovascular stroke therapy. Stroke. 2014;45(2):467–72.

25. Yoo J, Choi JW, Lee S-J, et al. Ischemic diffusion lesion reversal after endovascular treatment. Stroke. 2019;50(6):1504–9.

26. Atchaneeyasakul K, Shang T, Haussen D, et al. Impact of MRI selection on triage of endovascular therapy in acute ischemic stroke: the MRI in acute Management of Ischemic Stroke (MIAMIS) registry. Interv Neurol. 2020;8(2–6):135–43.

27. Nael K, Khan R, Choudhary G, et al. Six-minute magnetic resonance imaging protocol for evaluation of acute ischemic stroke: pushing the boundaries. Stroke. 2014;45(7):1985–91.

28. Goyal M, Menon BK, van Zwam WH, et al. Endovascular thrombectomy after large-vessel ischaemic stroke: a meta-analysis of individual patient data from five randomised trials. Lancet. 2016;387(10029):1723–31.

29. Gunda B, Neuhaus A, Sipos I, et al. Improved stroke Care in a Primary Stroke Centre Using AI-decision support. Cerebrovasc Dis Extra. 2022;12(1):28–32.

30. Merino JG, Luby M, Benson RT, et al. Predictors of acute stroke mimics in 8187 patients referred to a stroke service. J Stroke Cerebrovasc Dis. 2013;22(8):e397–403.

Cerebral Neoplasms

4

Girish M. Fatterpekar and Pia C. Sundgren

Abstract

In the past, before 2016, brain tumors were classified into several types, and their respective grades based largely on histology. While this allowed for categorization of tumors, the grading did not always correlate with overall survival. At the same time, neuro-oncology research work demonstrated that tumoral molecular genetics allowed for a better correlation with overall survival. This led to the Revised 2016 WHO classification of brain tumors, which for the first time in neuro-pathology saw the incorporation of mutation profiles applied to classification of brain tumors. Continued development in the field of neuro-oncology meant better categorization of previously described tumors, and the description of newer tumors. This led to another update, the 2021 classification of brain tumors. This chapter provides an overview of these revised brain tumor classification systems, and discusses the imaging profiles of certain select yet important tumor types in detail.

Keywords

Primary brain tumors · WHO classification · IDH · 1p-19q codeletion · TP53 mutation status in adults · BRAF and H3K27 altered tumors in children · Imaging features · Prognosis · Treatment strategies

G. M. Fatterpekar (✉)
Department of Radiology, NYU Grossman School of Medicine, NYU Langone Medical Center, New York, NY, USA
e-mail: Girish.Fatterpekar@nayulangone.org

P. C. Sundgren
Department of Diagnostic Radiology, Institution of Clinical Sciences Lund, Lund University, Lund, Sweden
e-mail: Pia.Sundgren@med.lu.se

Learning Objectives
- To familiarize radiologists with the revised classification of CNS tumors in terms of certain important mutation profiles including IDH mutation, 1p/19q-codeletion status, TP53 mutation, BRAF mutation, and H3K27M-mutation, and their influence on improving diagnostic accuracy, treatment strategies, and overall survival.
- To provide an overview of the imaging phenotypes for the different glioma genotypes.

4.1 Introduction

The World Health Organization (WHO) Classification of Tumors of central nervous system (CNS) provided an update in 2016 nearly 10 years after the 2007 version to help more systematically categorize brain tumors. The revised system for the first time uniquely included molecular and genetic parameters of the individual tumor types, in addition to the always incorporated histological features. Accordingly, each tumor is now identified by both its phenotype (based on histology) and genotype (based on its molecular and genetic parameters) [1]. Subsequently, another update was published in 2021 as the fifth edition of the WHO Classification of tumors of the central nervous system [2]. This focused on further advancing the role of molecular profiling in CNS tumor classification. Also, it emphasized the importance of integrated diagnosis and layered reports. New tumor types and subtypes have been introduced.

4.2 Goals of the Revised Classification

The goals are multi-fold:

1. To resolve some of the confusion created by classifying brain tumors based only on histology

2. Provide greater diagnostic accuracy.
3. Aid better treatment strategies.
4. Allow for an improved assessment of the prognosis based on the specific tumor type.

4.3 Background

A classic example of uncertainty created in the past where tumors were classified based only on histology included the group "oligoastrocytoma." These were tumors which exhibited features of both oligodendroglioma and astrocytoma on histology and were therefore lumped together as oligoastrocytomas [3–5]. Accordingly, their management was not definitive which in turn influenced their prognosis. Categorizing this tumor group based on the underlying 1p/19q codeletion (genetic mutation) status, allows them to be clearly distinguished almost always into either (1p/19q-codeleted) oligodendroglioma or (1p-19q-intact) astrocytoma [6–8]. Only a few tumors cannot be categorized into either group and are known as oligoastrocytoma, NOS (not otherwise specified) [1, 2, 9–11]. This clear distinction allows more accurate diagnosis, which therefore influences more appropriate tumor specific treatment strategies, and a better sense for the overall prognosis. Another perplexing prognostic feature was noted in terms of the overall survival of certain grade 1 low grade gliomas, which surprisingly despite their lower grade performed much worse than grade 3 astrocytomas. This can now be explained based on their IDH mutation status, with IDH-wildtype grade 1 gliomas performing much poorer than IDH-mutant grade 3 astrocytomas [6, 7]. Thus, it is the mutation status which influences the overall prognosis much more than the histology.

Utilizing the background above, the discussion below will mention the salient features of how the revised WHO classification system better classifies infiltrating gliomas in adults, gliomas in children, and certain new tumor types. Please note that a description of all CNS tumor types included in the revised 2016 and 2021 classifications of CNS tumors is beyond the scope of this text.

4.4 Infiltrating Gliomas in Adults

Several mutations have been described associated with infiltrating gliomas in adults. Of these, some of the important ones include IDH mutation, 1p-19q codeletion, and TP53 mutation status [12].

The primary deterministic mutation includes the IDH mutation status—presence suggests IDH-mutant, and absent an IDH-wildtype tumor [12, 13].

4.5 IDH-Mutant Gliomas

There are 2 types of IDH mutation, IDH1 and IDH2 mutated tumors. Most tumors are IDH1 mutated. Hence when a tumor is considered as IDH-mutated, it is the IDH1 status which is considered. Less than 3% of IDH-mutated tumors and exclusively IDH2 mutant tumors [13, 14].

4.5.1 Clinical Relevance and Prognosis

IDH-mutant tumors are seen more commonly in the middle-aged population (30–60 years of age), than IDH-wildtype tumors which are more frequently seen in the older population (>60–65 years of age). The overall survival of IDH-mutant tumors is far better than IDH-wild type tumors. In fact, as mentioned previously low grade (grade 1 by histology), IDH-wild type gliomas have an overall survival close to that of grade 4 IDH-wildtype glioblastomas, but much worse than grade III IDH-mutant gliomas. It is the IDH mutation status which is the driving force in terms of overall prognosis, much more than the histological grade. Furthermore, even among the grade 4 glioblastomas, it has been noted that IDH-mutant glioblastomas have an overall survival much better than IDH-wildtype glioblastomas. Supporting this is the fact that most IDH-mutant glioblastomas are the secondary type, while most IDH-wildtype glioblastomas are the de novo or primary type [15].

It is a known fact in glioma surgery that the wider the resection the better is the overall survival. Knowing preoperatively that the tumor is an IDH-mutant type can influence the surgeon to go for a more complete surgical resection, including the FLAIR signal abnormality surrounding the enhancing mass, especially if the margins of the FLAIR signal abnormality extend into a non-eloquent region of the brain [16].

Key Points
- IDH-mutant tumors, seen more commonly in the middle-aged population (third to sixth decade of life), have a far better overall survival than IDH-wildtype tumors, which are seen more commonly in the older patients (>60–65 years of age).

4.5.2 Radiological Features

Both IDH1 and IDH2 mutations change the role of IDH in the citric acid cycle. This results in accumulation of 2-HG within tumor cells. *2-Hydroxyglutarate (2-HG) can be detected on

MR spectroscopy and is therefore considered to be the imaging hallmark of all IDH-mutant tumors [17]. However, reliable detection is challenging and is possible only at some select centers with special MR spectroscopists on site [17–20].

It has been noted that most IDH-mutated tumors occur in a single lobe, frontal lobe being the most common, followed by temporal, parietal, and occipital lobes [21]. Most such tumors demonstrate a sharp margin and inhomogeneous but mild contrast enhancement. In contrast, IDH-wildtype tumors are frequently multilobar in location, though involvement of only the temporal or frontal lobes is occasionally seen. Preferred site involves the insula with extension into the adjacent temporal, frontal, and parietal lobes [21, 22]. In terms of their morphological appearance, these IDH-wildtype tumors demonstrate ill-defined margins with the adjacent brain especially on FLAIR/T2WI. Necrosis and moderate-to-intense heterogeneous, especially peripheral enhancement are seen (Fig. 4.1). The presence of necrosis, more intense enhancement, and ill-defined margins suggests more oxygen demand, more robust neoangiogenesis, and infiltrative nature of the wildtype tumors than their IDH-mutant counterparts.

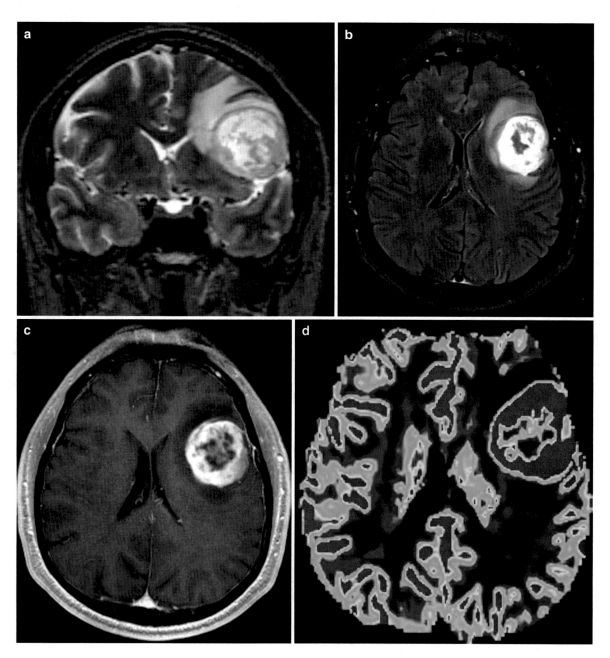

Fig. 4.1 A 69-year-old male with change in mental status. (**a**) Coronal T2WI demonstrates a heterogeneous centrally necrotic mass in the left insular region extending to involve the frontal lobe. (**b**) Axial FLAIR image demonstrates FLAIR signal abnormality surrounding this lesion which shows indistinct margin with the adjacent brain. (**c**) Axial T1 post-contrast image demonstrates heterogeneous but predominantly peripheral intense enhancement. (**d**) Corresponding axial DSC (dynamic susceptibility contrast) perfusion map demonstrates increased relative blood volume from the enhancing component of this lesion. Diagnosis: IDH-wildtype glioblastoma

4.6   1p/19q-Codeletion

IDH-mutant gliomas can subsequently be classified into those which are 1p/19q-codeleted tumors or 1p/19q-intact tumors. Of these, those gliomas which are 1p/19q-codeleted are the oligodendrogliomas, while those which are 1p/19q-intact are astrocytomas [1, 12]. Astrocytomas typically also show TP53 mutation, a mutation which is never seen in oligodendrogliomas, another distinguishing feature that separates these two tumors. As mentioned previously, this 1p/19q-codeleted status and TP53 mutation help clearly separate the confusing oligoastrocytoma group into either oligodendroglioma or astrocytoma (which was not possible based on histological features alone), which helps to better manage these patients.

> **Key Points**
> - 1p/19q-codeletion status in an IDH-mutant tumor is diagnostic of oligodendroglioma;1p/19q-intact status with TP53 mutation is diagnostic of astrocytoma.

4.6.1   Clinical Relevance and Prognosis

It has been shown in two large randomized control trials that chemotherapeutic agents including procarbazine, lomustine, and vincristine (PCV) when added to radiation therapy significantly improve the overall survival in patients with 1p/19q-deleted tumors when compared with radiation therapy alone [23–26]. This therefore is now the standard of care for all 1p/19q-codeleted oligodendrogliomas.

4.6.2   Radiological Features

Frontal lobe is the most common location of 1p/19q-codeleted tumors. Other common sites include the parietal and occipital lobes. In contrast, 1p/19q-intact tumors are seen most often in the temporal lobes and the insular cortex. In terms of their morphological appearance, 1p/19q-codeleted tumors demonstrate a more heterogeneous appearance. Also, calcification is a common feature of such tumors. In fact, presence of florid calcification and enhancement favors a higher grade (grade 3) oligodendroglioma (Fig. 4.2) [14, 21]. An intact margin favors a 1p/19q-intact tumor while ill-defined margins can be seen in both types. T2-FLAIR mismatch sign demonstrates a high positive predictive value for 1p/19q-intact tumors, i.e., mass lesion which appears bright on T2WI and dark of FLAIR sequences (Fig. 4.3).

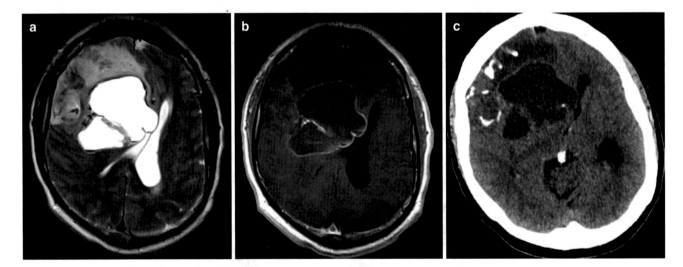

Fig. 4.2 A 48-year-old man with seizures. (**a**) Axial T2WI demonstrates a heterogeneous mass involving the right frontal lobe. (**b**) Corresponding axial T1 post-contrast image demonstrates heterogeneous but minimal enhancement. (**c**) Axial CT scan from the same patient demonstrates multiple arcs of calcification within this mass. Diagnosis: oligodendroglioma, IDH-mutant, 1p/19a codeleted tumor

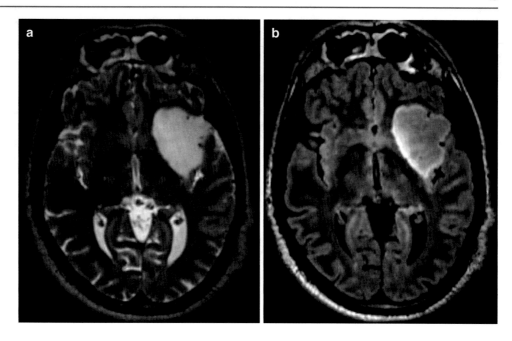

Fig. 4.3 A 34-year-old man with headache. (**a**) Axial T2WI demonstrates a well-defined expansile mass involving the left insula, which appears predominantly bright in its signal intensity when compared to the gray matter. (**b**) Corresponding axial FLAIR image demonstrates the mass to be predominantly hypointense to the gray matter. Diagnosis: diffuse astrocytoma, IDH-mutant, 1p/19q-noncodeleted (intact) tumor

4.7   Gliomatosis Cerebri

Gliomatosis cerebri as a specific tumor subtype was included in the 2007 version of the WHO classification of CNS tumors. This term is deleted from the 2016 update [1]. A diffusely infiltrating non-enhancing tumor extending to involve 3 or more lobes is no longer to be considered as gliomatosis cerebri. It is recognized as a diffuse glioma type, with its subtype dependent on further genetic, molecular testing and histological evaluation [1].

> **Key Points**
> • Gliomatosis cerebri as a tumor term is no longer recognized.

4.8   CNS Tumor Nomenclature, Integrated Diagnosis, and Layered Reports

The term "anaplastic" previously used to describe grade 3 tumors is no longer used. Also, Roman numerals to grading tumors is no longer recommended. It is thought that a typographical error, such as grade II instead of grade III, and similar such mistakes can lead to bad clinical consequences. Hence, Arabic numerals used for other body parts to grade tumors are recommended to describe CNS tumors. It is now recommended that a layered report be used to describe a CNS tumor, which provides histological diagnosis, grade of the tumor, and the mutation status in that order. For example, if oligodendroglioma has to be described, it should be mentioned as oligodendroglioma, grade 3, and IDH-mutant 1p/19q codeleted tumor. Also, the mutation status establishes the grading and not the histology, i.e., if a tumor by histology appears as grade 1, but it carries a TERT-promoter or similar poor prognostic mutation commonly associated with grade 4 tumors, the tumor under consideration in the final report should be read out as a grade 4 tumor [2].

Other terms clearly outlined in the 2021 WHO classification of tumors include NOS (not otherwise specified) and NEC (not elsewhere classified). NOS refers to a tumor which after extensive molecular work-up does not demonstrate a clear molecular signature for it be appropriately classified. NEC refers to a tumor which despite an adequate pathological work-up does not conform to a standard WHO diagnosis [2].

> **Key Points**
> • Arabic and non-Roman numerals are now recommended to be used to describe CNS tumors.
> • Integrated diagnosis, including histology, grade of tumor, molecular profile is the correct way to completely describe a tumor.
> • Molecular profile dictates grade of tumor and not histology.

4.9　Gliomas in Children

Gliomas in children have been known to behave differently than those seen in the adult population. This is related to the fact that mutations seen commonly in gliomas in adults including IDH mutation and 1p/19q-codeletion occur uncommonly in children. The two common mutation types commonly seen in children, include BRAF mutation and histone H3K27 altered [27, 28].

4.10　BRAF Mutation

These tumors are usually well circumscribed and carry an excellent prognosis.

4.10.1　Radiological Features

Cystic lesions with a mural enhancing nodule are common imaging features (Fig. 4.4). This mutation type encompasses pilocytic astrocytoma, pilomyxoid astrocytoma, and ganglioglioma.

> **Key Points**
> - BRAF mutation is one of the most common mutations seen in the pediatric population and includes tumor types such as pilocytic astrocytoma, pilomyxoid astrocytoma, and ganglioglioma.

4.11　Histone H3K27 Altered Tumors

These are diffuse midline gliomas (previously known as diffuse infiltrating pontine glioma) and carry an extremely poor prognosis. Often times they are seen in the brainstem. Location of this tumor type makes it difficult to biopsy these tumors or attempt a surgical resection [28]. They are now known to occur at other sites including the thalami, spinal cord, and sometimes, the cerebral parenchyma. Radiation and chemotherapy are not particularly helpful.

4.11.1　Radiological Features

Brainstem (pons) is the most common location. Other common locations include thalami and spinal cord. As previously described, this is a diffusely infiltrating lesion which results in secondary expansion of the structure involved. Enhancement is variable. Occasionally, heterogeneous enhancement and cyst(s) can be seen. Leptomeningeal dissemination is seen in about one-third of all autopsies.

> **Key Points**
> - H3K27 altered glioma now includes the previously known diffuse infiltrating pontine glioma in its genetic profile of tumors and carries a dismal prognosis.

Fig. 4.4 An 18-year-old boy with seizures. (**a**) Axial T2WI demonstrates a well-defined cystic appearing lesion in the right temporal lobe. (**b**) Corresponding axial T1 post-contrast image demonstrates a mural enhancing nodule along the lateral aspect of this lesion. Diagnosis: pleomorphic xanthoastrocytoma, BRAF-mutant tumor

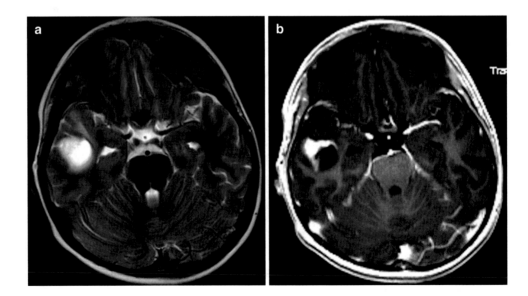

4.12 Solitary Fibrous Tumor (SFT) and Hemangiopericytoma (HPC)

Both these tumors share the same genetic feature which includes genomic inversion at the 12q13 locus, fusing the NAB2 and STAT6 genes. Hence, these 2 previously distinct tumors were combined as SFT/HPC tumor as per the 2016 revised WHO classification of CNS tumors [1]. This was further revised to document these as SFT tumors deleting the term hemangiopericytoma (HPC) to clearly indicate the soft tissue origin of the tumor by the 2021 update on classification of CNS tumors [2]. Three grades have been described with SFT grade 1 a slowly growing tumor carrying excellent prognosis, while SFT grades 2 and 3 have a slightly poor prognosis, carry a high risk to recur following resection, and are associated with metastasis.

Newly recognized tumor types in the revised 2021 WHO classification of CNS tumors diffuse leptomeningeal glioneuronal tumor (first described in 2016).

This is a rare glioneuronal neoplasm mainly seen in children. It is largely localized to the leptomeningeal compartment [1]. Oligodendroglioma-like tumor cells are seen at histology.

4.12.1 Radiological Features

Cluster of diffuse leptomeningeal enhancement is noted. Frequently, the basal cisterns are involved with associated extensive involvement of the subarachnoid space along the surface of the cord. Secondary hydrocephalus is commonly noted. Parenchymal involvement can also be seen. When present, it is seen to involve the spinal cord and the brain stem.

In addition, at least 22 new tumor types have been recognized in the revised 2021 WHO classification of CNS tumors (Table 4.1) [2]. A discussion of all of these is beyond the scope of this text. One of the more common of these entities is the multinodular and vacuolating neuronal tumor as outlined below.

Table 4.1 New glioma tumor types recognized in the revised 2021 WHO classification of CNS tumors

Diffuse astrocytoma, *MYB- or MYBL1 altered*
Polymorphous low-grade neuroepithelial tumor of the young
Diffuse low-grade glioma, MAPK pathway altered
Diffuse hemispheric glioma, H3 G34-mutant
Diffuse pediatric-type high-grade glioma, H3-wildtype and IDH-wildtype
Infant-type hemispheric glioma
High-grade astrocytoma with piloid features
Diffuse glioneuronal tumor with oligodendroglioma-like features
Myxoid glioneuronal tumor
Multinodular and vacuolating neuronal tumor

(Adapted from Table 7—Louis DN, et al. The 2021 WHO classification of the central nervous system: a summary. Neuro-Oncology 2021)

4.13 Multinodular Vacuolating Neuronal Tumor

This rare entity first received mention in the 2016 revised CNS tumor classification. At that time, it was unclear if this was distinct tumor or in the tumor-dysplasia category. In the 2021 revised classification, it has been recognized as a tumor. It carries an excellent prognosis and is believed to be a "Touch-Me-Not" lesion [29].

4.13.1 Radiological Features

It is known to occur anywhere in the brain but commonly in the supratentorial compartment and especially in the frontal and temporal lobes. On morphological appearance, the lesion is seen as a cluster of FLAIR and T2 bright lesions typically in the subcortical white matter. Involvement of the overlying cortex and periventricular white matter has been reported. The lesion appears hypointense on T1WI and does not demonstrate contrast enhancement or diffusion restriction. No susceptibility is seen.

4.14 Conclusion

Concluding Remarks

The revised 2016 and subsequently 2021 classification systems of CNS tumors by including the genetic profile improve diagnostic accuracy of brain tumors. This allows neuro-oncologists and the surgeons to optimize treatment strategies targeted to the specific tumor type, thus allowing for a better prognosis and improved overall survival. The neuroradiologist by identifying the imaging phenotype of the particular glioma genotype plays an important role in guiding the clinical team in their treatment planning.

Take-Home Messages
- IDH-mutated tumors are more solid in their imaging profile and demonstrate less enhancement than IDH-wildtype counterparts.
- 1p/19q-codeleted tumors are more heterogeneous in their imaging appearance and exhibit calcification more frequently than their 1p/19q-intact counterparts.
- BRAF mutant tumors seen more commonly in the pediatric population. These include pilocytic astroc-

tyoma, pilomyxoid astrocytoma, and ganglioglioma in their molecular profile spectrum.
- H3K27 altered tumors are also seen more commonly in the pediatric population. They are more diffuse and aggressive. These mutant tumors encompass the previously described diffuse infiltrating pontine glioma spectrum of tumors.
- New tumor types now recognized have helped us better classify and understand CNS tumors.

References

1. Louis DN, et al. The 2016 World Health Organization classification of tumors of the central nervous system. Acta Neuropathol. 2016;131(6):803–20.
2. Louis DN, et al. The 2021 WHO classification of the central nervous system: a summary. Neuro-Oncology. 2021;23(8):1231–51.
3. Louis DN, et al. The 2007 WHO classification of tumours of the central nervous system. Acta Neuropathol. 2007;114(2):97–109.
4. Giannini C, et al. Oligodendrogliomas: reproducibility and prognostic value of histologic diagnosis and grading. J Neuropathol Exp Neurol. 2001;60:248–62.
5. van den Bent MJ. Interobserver variation of the histopathological diagnosis in clinical trials on glioma: a clinician's perspective. Acta Neuropathol. 2010;120:297–304.
6. Cancer Genome Atlas Research Network, Brat DJ, et al. Comprehensive integrative genomic analysis of diffuse lower-grade gliomas. N Engl J Med. 2015;372:2481–98.
7. Metellus P, et al. Absence of IDH mutation identifies a novel radiologic and molecular subtype of WHO grade II gliomas with dismal prognosis. Acta Neuropathol. 2010;120(6):719–29.
8. Sahm F, et al. Farewell to oligoastrocytoma: in situ molecular genetics favor classification as either oligodendroglioma or astrocytoma. Acta Neuropathol. 2014;128:551–9.
9. Wiestler B, et al. Integrated DNA methylation and copy-number profiling identify three clinically and biologically relevant groups of anaplastic glioma. Acta Neuropathol. 2014;128:561–71.
10. Huse JT, et al. Mixed glioma with molecular features of composite oligodendroglioma and astrocytoma: a true "oligoastrocytoma"? Acta Neuropathol. 2015;129:151–3.
11. Wilcox P, et al. Oligoastrocytomas: throwing the baby out with the bathwater? Acta Neuropathol. 2015;129:147–9.
12. Appin CL, et al. Molecular pathways in gliomagenesis and their relevance to neuropathologic diagnosis. Adv Anat Pathol. 2015;22(1):50–8.
13. Cohen AL, et al. IDH1 and IDH2 mutations in gliomas. Curr Neurol Neurosci Rep. 2013;13(5):345.
14. Smits M, et al. Imaging correlates of adult glioma genotypes. Radiology. 2017;284:316–31.
15. Yan H, et al. IDH1 and IDH2 mutations in gliomas. N Engl J Med. 2009;360(8):765–73.
16. Beiko J, et al. IDH1 mutant malignant astrocytomas are more amenable to surgical resection and have a survival benefit associated with maximal surgical resection. Neuro-Oncology. 2014;16(1):81–91.
17. Esmaeili M, et al. 2-hydroxyglutarate as a magnetic resonance biomarker for glioma subtyping. Transl Oncol. 2013;6(2):92–8.
18. Andronesi OC, et al. Detection of 2-hydroxyglutarate in IDH-mutated glioma patients by in vivo spectral-editing and 2D correlation magnetic resonance spectroscopy. Sci Transl Med. 2012;4(116):116ra4.
19. Bertolino N, et al. Accuracy of 2-hydroxyglutarate quantification by short-echo proton-MRS at 3T: a phantom study. Phys Med. 2014;30(6):702–7.
20. Pope WB, et al. Non-invasive detection of 2-hydroxyglutarate and other metabolites in IDH1 mutant glioma patients using magnetic resonance spectroscopy. J Neurosci. 2012;107(1):197–205.
21. Khalid L, et al. Imaging characteristics of oligodendrogliomas that predict grade. AJNR Am J Neuroradiol. 2012;33(5):852–7.
22. Willman M, et al. Update for astrocytomas: medical and surgical management considerations. Explor Neurosci. 2023;2:1–26.
23. Weller J, et al. PCV chemotherapy alone for WHO grade 2 oligodendroglioma: prolonged disease control with low risk of malignant progression. J Neuro-Oncol. 2021;153:283–91.
24. Cairncross G, et al. Phase III trial of chemoradiotherapy for anaplastic oligodendroglioma: long-term results of RTOG 9402. J Clin Oncol. 2013;31:337–43.
25. van den Bent MJ, et al. Adjuvant procarbazine, lomustine, and vincristine chemotherapy in newly diagnosed anaplastic oligodendroglioma: long-term follow-up of EORTC brain tumor group study 26951. J Clin Oncol. 2013;31:344–50.
26. Patel SH, et al. T2-FLAIR mismatch, an imaging biomarker for IDH and 1p/19q status in lower-grade gliomas: a TCGA/TCIA project. Clin Cancer Res. 2017;23:6078–85.
27. Tan JY, et al. Paediatric gliomas: BRAF and histone H3 as biomarkers, therapy and perspective of liquid biopsies. Cancers (Basel). 2021;13:607.
28. Nunes RH, et al. Multinodular and vacuolating neuronal tumor of the cerebrum: a new "leave me alone" lesion with a characteristic imaging pattern. AJNR Am J Neuroradiol. 2017;38:1899. https://doi.org/10.3174/ajnr.A5281.
29. Louis DN, Perry A, Wesseling P, et al. The 2021 WHO classification of tumors of the central nervous system: a summary. Neuro Oncol. 2021;23(8):1231–51.

Nontraumatic Intracranial Hemorrhage

5

Pamela W. Schaefer and Myriam Edjlali

Abstract

Spontaneous ICH is usually intraparenchymal or subarachnoid in location. Intraparenchymal hemorrhages, encompassing lobar or centrally located hematomas, have diverse underlying causes, with cerebral amyloid angiopathy, characterized by lobar hemorrhage, being the most common. Hypertension is the second most common cause with a predilection for the basal ganglia, pons, and cerebellum. Subarachnoid hemorrhage is linked to aneurysm rupture in 85% of cases. Other relatively common causes of spontaneous intracranial hemorrhage include hemorrhagic conversion of ischemic infarction, cerebral arteriovenous malformations, dural arteriovenous fistulas, venous sinus thrombosis, cavernous malformations, reversible cerebral vasoconstriction syndrome, coagulopathy, and underlying tumors.

Computed tomography followed by CT angiography is used for initial assessment of spontaneous ICH. However, MRI is more sensitive than CT for the detection of ICH and plays an important role in their etiology characterization. In this paper, the authors present a logical approach to imaging spontaneous intracranial hemorrhage including identifying prognostic factors, determining etiology, and establishing treatment.

Keywords

Intracranial hemorrhage · Intraparenchymal hemorrhage Subarachnoid hemorrhage · Microhemorrhage · Lobar hemorrhage · Basal ganglia hemorrhage cerebral amyloid angiopathy · Hypertensive hemorrhage Leptomeningeal hemosiderosis · Cerebral venous sinus thrombosis · Cerebral arteriovenous malformation

Learning Objectives
- To know the CT and MRI protocols used to detect and characterize intracranial hemorrhage.
- To understand the key imaging features of intracranial hemorrhage on CT and MRI including signs that determine prognosis.
- To know the differential diagnosis of nontraumatic ICH based on hemorrhage location and patient demographics.
- To understand the key imaging characteristics of the major causes of nontraumatic intracranial hemorrhage.
- To know how to triage patients with nontraumatic intracranial hemorrhage for further imaging and treatment.

5.1 Introduction and Imaging Protocol

Nontraumatic intracranial hemorrhage accounts for up to 15% of all strokes and has an incidence of 10–30/100,000. Morbidity and mortality are higher for hemorrhagic stroke compared to ischemic stroke with a 1-year survival of approximately 30%. The incidence increases with age and is higher in males than females. The most common risk factor is hypertension. Other factors such as diabetes, anticoagulant therapy, dyslipidemia, and alcohol abuse also play an impor-

P. W. Schaefer
Radiology Department, Massachusetts General Hospital,
Boston, MA, USA
e-mail: pschaefer@partners.org; pschaefer@mgh.harvard.edu

M. Edjlali (✉)
Radiology Department, Garches and Ambroise Paré Hospital,
BioMaps, Paris Saclay University, Paris, France
e-mail: myriam.edjlali@aphp.fr

J. Hodler et al. (eds.), *Diseases of the Brain, Head and Neck, Spine 2024-2027*, IDKD Springer Series,
https://doi.org/10.1007/978-3-031-50675-8_5

tant role. Prognosis depends on the severity of risk factors as well as complications of ICH such as the development of hydrocephalus, brain herniation, or vasospasm.

The initial radiological assessment typically includes a CT scan followed by CT angiography to detect acute hemorrhages and their causes. While MRI is less common in the acute phase, it offers high sensitivity, particularly when performed shortly after symptom onset (<24 h).

When investigating intracranial bleeding causes after excluding intracranial aneurysms with CT angiography, MRI proves valuable for identifying the underlying factors. The imaging protocol should encompass DWI for the detection of associated ischemia, ideally 3D FLAIR to minimize CSF artifact for detection of edema and subarachnoid hemorrhage, SWI imaging for chronic microbleeds and hemosiderosis from amyloid angiopathy, time-of-flight MRA (possibly with gadolinium enhancement for distal arterial stenosis), and dynamic MRA to assess arteriovenous shunts. An arterial spin labeling sequence (ASL) is highly useful for detecting increased cerebral blood flow (CBF), which may indicate tumors or vascular shunts. ASL, being insensitive to blood components, is the preferred perfusion sequence for analyzing hemorrhagic components. 3D T1-weighted sequences with and without contrast to assess for an underlying mass lesion should also be obtained.

5.2 Subarachnoid Hemorrhage

5.2.1 Overview

Subarachnoid hemorrhage (SAH) is the third most common subtype of stroke. The incidence of SAH has decreased over the past few decades, possibly due to factors like lifestyle changes, such as quitting smoking and better management of hypertension. Around a quarter of SAH patients don't survive before they can be admitted to the hospital. However, the overall outcomes are better for those who make it to the hospital, although they still face an increased risk of long-term neuropsychiatric issues like depression. This condition continues to have a significant impact on public health, as the average age of onset is in the mid-50 s, leading to many years of reduced quality of life [1]. Subarachnoid hemorrhage (SAH) is defined as blood in the cerebrospinal fluid contained in the basal cisterns and the subarachnoid spaces of the cerebral hemispheres, located between the arachnoid mater and the pia mater. Nontraumatic subarachnoid hemorrhage (SAH) has an annual incidence of 9 per 100,000 individuals. It is a rare yet serious event, with an estimated mortality rate of 40% within the first 48 h. In 85% of cases, it is associated with the rupture of an intracranial aneurysm (Fig. 5.1). If SAH is suspected, cerebral imaging should be

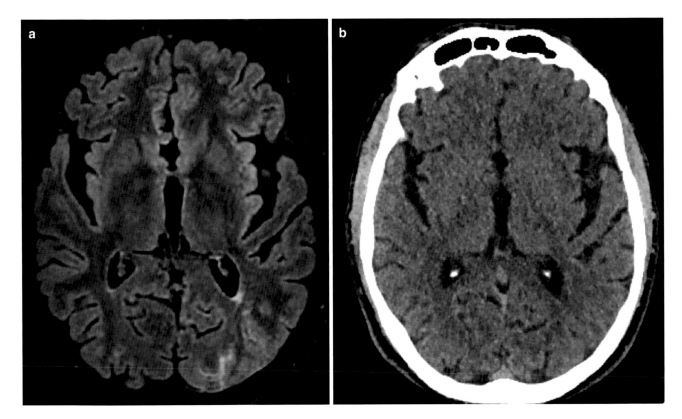

Fig. 5.1 Enhanced FLAIR sensitivity (**a**) in detecting subarachnoid hemorrhage compared to a negative CT scan (**b**) acquired on the same day, 5 days after the onset of severe headaches in a 45-year-old male

performed urgently to confirm the diagnosis, identify any complications, and investigate its cause. During the early phase, within the first 24 h, a CT scan of the brain combined with CT angiography of the circle of Willis is the recommended examination for a positive SAH diagnosis and for etiological diagnosis to detect an intracranial aneurysm. A diagnosis of subarachnoid hemorrhage (SAH) can be established through a CT scan when an unenhanced hyperdensity is observed within the subarachnoid spaces, typically involving the basal cisterns, interhemispheric sulci, and lateral sulci. If the patient's clinical condition allows, cerebral MRI may be considered. The FLAIR sequence is more sensitive than a CT scan in demonstrating subarachnoid hemorrhage (Fig. 5.2), especially after 48 h from symptom onset, and has

a higher sensitivity for the etiological diagnosis of sulcal hemorrhages. In addition, combining FLAIR and SWI represents the most effective protocol for detecting subarachnoid hemorrhage (SAH) in the acute, subacute, or late phases of the hemorrhage. If these examinations yield normal results but clinical suspicion remains high, a lumbar puncture should be performed.

5.2.1.1 Main Etiologies of a SAH

Subarachnoid hemorrhage (SAH) [1] can result from various underlying causes, with the primary etiologies falling into several categories [2]:

1. **Aneurysm** [3]: Aneurysms, which are weakened and bulging areas in the walls of blood vessels, are a leading cause of SAH. When an aneurysm ruptures, it releases blood into the subarachnoid space, leading to SAH. The most common aneurysms associated with SAH are saccular aneurysms found in the circle of Willis.
2. **Dural AVF (Arteriovenous Fistula) or cortical venous thrombosis** [4]: Abnormal connections between arteries and veins within the dura mater (the membrane surrounding the brain) known as dural arteriovenous fistulas or cortical venous thrombosis can also result in SAH. These conditions disrupt normal blood flow, increasing the risk of hemorrhage.
3. **RCVS (Reversible Cerebral Vasoconstriction Syndrome)** [5]: RCVS is a relatively rare but important cause of SAH. It involves the sudden narrowing of cerebral blood vessels, which can lead to severe headaches and, in some cases, SAH. The vasoconstriction is typically reversible with time.
4. **Other**: Nontraumatic subarachnoid hemorrhage (SAH) can also stem from less typical sources, including endocarditis leading to mycotic aneurysm formation, vasculitides, amyloid angiopathy [6], tumors, arteriovenous malformations, bleeding disorders, and infections (Fig. 5.3). In certain instances, pinpointing the exact underlying cause may pose a diagnostic challenge, necessitating a comprehensive evaluation. Understanding the underlying etiology of SAH is crucial for appropriate management and treatment decisions, as each cause may necessitate distinct diagnostic workup and therapeutic approaches.

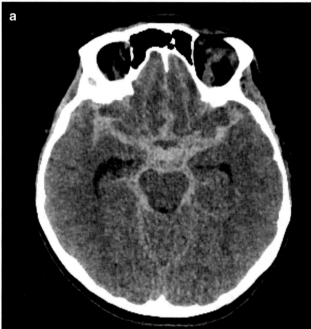

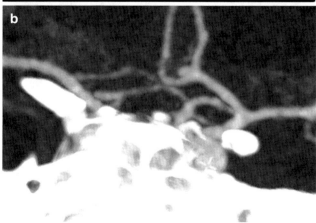

Fig. 5.2 A 62-year-old female with severe headaches. Noncontrast CT (**a**) reveals spontaneous hyperdensity in the subarachnoid spaces, indicative of an acute subarachnoid hemorrhage, along with initial ventricular dilation suggesting the onset of hydrocephalus. CT Angiography (**b**) identifies the source of the bleeding as a ruptured aneurysm of the anterior communicating artery

5.2.1.2 How Can I Determine Which of the Multiple Intracranial Aneurysms Has Bled During a SAH Assessment?

In cases where multiple intracranial aneurysms are present, accounting for 15 to 20% of cases, it is essential to prioritize treatment for the ruptured aneurysm before addressing the others. While the distribution of the SAH may provide some clues about the ruptured aneurysm, it is often insufficient for a definitive conclusion.

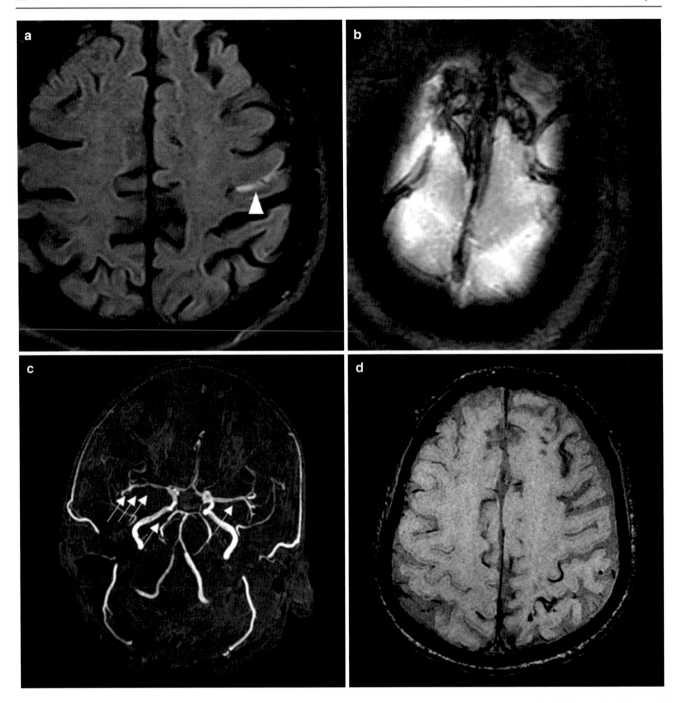

Fig. 5.3 Spontaneous subarachnoid hemorrhage at the vertex (**a**, head arrow) and various non-aneurysmal causes, including cerebral sinus and cortical vein thrombosis (**b**), reversible cerebral vasoconstriction syndrome (**c**), and amyloid angiopathy (**d**)

One indicator to consider is the irregular, scalloped "blister-like" appearance of the aneurysm wall, which suggests fissuring or rupture. Other indicators are size over 6 mm, interval grow from a prior scan.

Furthermore, on 3 Tesla MRI with 3D T1-weighted FSE sequences and gadolinium enhancement, circumferential enhancement of the aneurysm wall is believed to be a sign favoring unstable aneurysms (Fig. 5.4). These are more commonly observed in cases of aneurysms that have ruptured

compared to aneurysms within the same patient that have not yet ruptured [7].

5.2.1.3 When Dealing with a Cisternal SAH and a Negative CT Angiogram, Three Possibilities Should Be Considered

1. **Undetected arterial abnormality**: It is possible that an arterial abnormality exists but has not been detected.

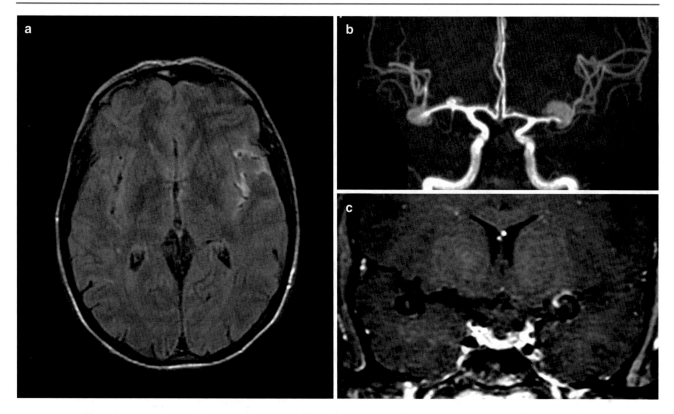

Fig. 5.4 Spontaneous subarachnoid hemorrhage (**a**) resulting from a ruptured aneurysm in a 50-year-old female with multiple aneurysms (angioMR 3D time-of-flight, **b**). The ruptured aneurysm is the only one exhibiting arterial wall enhancement in vessel wall imaging (**c**), confirming its association with the site of bleeding as seen in the FLAIR image

Small intracranial aneurysms in the posterior circulation can be challenging to identify on standard imaging. Sometimes, a small aneurysm may not be visible due to overlapping with normal branches of the circle of Willis. Analyzing vessels individually, aided by volume rendering techniques, can be helpful in detecting such aneurysms. Additionally, there is the possibility of a "blister" type of aneurysm [8], which represents a local intracranial dissection without a distinct sac. In such cases, irregularities in the arterial wall should be closely examined, particularly near the subarachnoid spaces where the hemorrhage is most significant, as well as in the walls of specific arterial segments.

2. **Intracranial dissection**: Another possibility is a dissecting intracranial arterial abnormality, especially in the V4 segment of the vertebral arteries. Intracranial dissections, particularly those affecting the posterior circulation, can lead to subarachnoid hemorrhage and account for 5% of SAH cases. These dissections are characterized by thinner arterial walls and a lack of an external elastic limiting layer, making them prone to rupture and causing SAH. Detecting intracranial dissections is crucial, as they require specific treatment.

3. **No arterial lesion**: Perimesencephalic hemorrhages (Fig. 5.5), accounting for 5–10% of nontraumatic subarachnoid hemorrhages (SAH) [9], result from venous bleeding that leads to subarachnoid hemorrhage situated in the interpeduncular and peripontine cisterns. The bleeding, while it may extend slightly, remains confined primarily to the suprasellar cisterns and the basal regions of the motor cortex or interhemispheric sulci. Occasionally, a subtle blood presence can be observed in the occipital horns without actual intraventricular hemorrhage. Patients typically present with stable clinical conditions and unimpaired consciousness. Diagnosing perimesencephalic hemorrhage relies on the clinical and radiological criteria mentioned earlier, coupled with the absence of an aneurysmal structure evident in CT angiography or MRA or on the cerebral arteriography of the circle of Willis. The initial clinical manifestations, as well as the long-term outcomes and prognosis, are considerably more favorable compared to SAH caused by aneurysms. Most medical teams opt for a secondary non-invasive investigation into the underlying cause, typically conducted a few weeks after the initial event.

5.3 Intraparenchymal Hemorrhage

5.3.1 Overview

Intraparenchymal hemorrhage accounts for approximately 15% of all strokes [10]. In older adults, the most common etiologies are hypertension, cerebral amyloid angiopathy, anticoagulation, hemorrhagic transformation of acute ischemic strokes, and underlying primary or secondary tumors. In younger adults and children, common vascular malformations such as arteriovenous malformations, cavernous malformations, and cerebral venous sinus thrombosis and rarer lesions such as moyamoya and dural arteriovenous fistulas

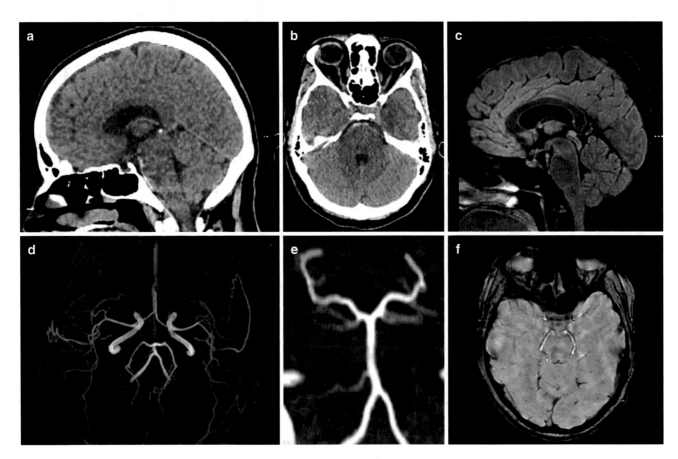

Fig. 5.5 Perimesencephalic hemorrhage is observed on noncontrast CT anterior to the pons (**a**, **b**) and on the FLAIR image (**c**), with no arterial abnormalities detected on angioMR time-of-flight (**d**, **e**) and no lesions detected on susceptibility-weighted imaging (SWI, **f**)

should be considered. Additional rarer causes of IPH include Reversible Cerebral Vasoconstrictive Syndrome (RCVS), posterior reversible encephalopathy syndrome (PRES), vasculitis, drug toxicity, and infections such as mucormycosis and aspergillosis.

5.3.2 Key Imaging Features of Intraparenchymal Hemorrhage

Acute intraparenchymal hemorrhage typically demonstrates homogeneous hyperdensity due to high protein content on NCCT, measuring approximately 40–80 HU. The presence of fluid fluid levels or foci of hypoattenuation (the swirl sign) may represent hyperacute (unclotted) hemorrhage, a coagulation disorder, and/or active bleeding. As the IPH breaks down, it usually becomes isodense to brain at 1–2 weeks and hypodense approaching the attenuation of cerebrospinal fluid at 1–2 months. On MRI in the first few hours, an intracerebral hematoma consists of intact red blood cells containing mainly oxyhemoglobin that is isointense on T1 and hyperintense on T2-weighted images. Over time changes begin at the periphery and extend inward. From 1 to 3 days, the hemorrhage is characterized predominantly by deoxyhemoglobin which is isointense on T1 and hypointense on T2WI. In the early subacute phase (3–7 days), deoxyhemoglobin converts to intracellular methemoglobin which is hyperintense on T1 and hypointense on T2WI. Subsequently at 1–4 weeks, the red blood cells lyse. The extracellular methemoglobin is hyperintense on both T1 and T2WI. After 4 weeks, the resultant cavity shrinks to become slit like and contains mainly hemosiderin laden macrophages with hypointensity on T1 and T2WI (Table 5.1). Oxyhemoglobin and extracellular methemoglobin do not exhibit susceptibility effects, while deoxyhemoglobin, intracellular methemoglobin, and hemosiderin do exhibit susceptibility effects. After the first few hours, since hematomas contain a combination of blood products, they nearly always show blooming on SWI images. Surrounding edema increases for the first 2 weeks and resolves by approximately 1 month. From 1 week to 1 month, following the injection of intravenous gadolinium, there is a smooth rim of enhancement due to an inflammatory response and breakdown of the blood brain barrier.

> **Key Points # 2**
> - The timing of IPH can be determined by its CT and MR appearance.
> - Imaging features of IPH (swirl sign, intraventricular extension, contrast extravasation, volume, and infratentorial location) can be used to predict hematoma expansion and determine prognosis.

5.3.3 Prognostic Factors

A number of factors should be included when describing hematomas because they predict higher mortality and may require neurosurgical intervention. These include findings that predict hematoma expansion such as areas of hypodensity within a hematoma on noncontrast CT, irregular margin or shape, contrast extravasation on CTA, intraventricular extension, and hematoma size which can be measured using the ABC/2 formula. Brain herniation suggesting the need for hemicraniectomy, and hydrocephalus suggesting the need for shunt placement are also important. Age and Glasgow coma score are key clinical factors that predict mortality. The ICH score incorporates many of these factors and allows an early rapid estimation of patient prognosis [11]. A score of 4 or higher predicts a 97% mortality rate.

5.3.4 Entities with Underlying Vascular Abnormality on CTA or MRA

When a patient presents to the emergency room with a lobar hemorrhage, they typically undergo CT angiography scanning (Table 5.2). Approximately 15% have an underlying large or medium vessel vascular abnormality visualized on CTA. The most common underlying vascular abnormalities in one large study were arteriovenous malformation (43%), aneurysm (24%), and venous sinus thrombosis (19%). Rarer causes include moyamoya syndrome, vasculitis, and reversible cerebral vasoconstriction syndrome [12].

Table 5.1 CT and MR characteristics of intracranial hemorrhage

Time	NCCT	CECT	T1	T2	T2*
Hyperacute (<6 h)	Hyperdense		Isointense	Hyperintense	
Acute (6 h – 3 days)	Hyperdense		Isointense	Hypointense	Hypointense
Early subacute (3–7 days)	Hyper/isodense		Hyperintense rim Isointense center	Hypointense	Hypointense center
Late subacute (1–4 weeks)	Iso/hypodense	Rim enhancement	Hyperintense	Hyperintense	Hypointense
Chronic (months – years)	Hypodense		Hypointense	Hypointense	Hypointense

Density/Intensity compared to normal brain parenchyma. *NCCT* noncontrast CT, *CECT* contrast enhanced CT

Table 5.2 Most common etiologies of intraparenchymal hemorrhage with or without underlying vascular abnormality on CTA

Entity	Clinical	Key imaging features in addition to parenchymal hematoma
Underlying vascular abnormality on CTA		
Arteriovenous malformation	• Age—Children, young adults • Risk factors—Older age, larger size, deep venous drainage, venous stenosis, feeding artery, or intranidal aneurysm • Syndromes—HHT, Wyburn-Mason, RASA • Symptoms—Seizure, headache, acute neurologic deficit • Etiology—Congenital	• Hemorrhage location—Lobar or deep gray nuclei • NCCT—Hyperdense vessels, Ca+ • CTA/MRA—Arterial phase opacification of feeding arteries, nidus, draining veins • T2WI—Flow voids, pulsation artifact • FLAIR—Gliosis, edema
Cerebral venous sinus thrombosis	• Age—Children, young and older adults • Risk factors—Prothrombosis, pregnancy, oral contraceptives, dehydration, infections • Symptoms—Headache, seizure, encephalopathy, acute neurologic deficit • Etiology—Hypercoagulability	• Hemorrhage location—Lobar (superior sagittal, transverse, sigmoid sinus) or deep gray nuclei (ICV, VOG, straight sinus) • NCCT—Hyperdense vein (cord sign), hyperdense sinus (triangle sign) • T2 WI—Absence of flow void • FLAIR—Edema • DWI—Facilitated or restricted diffusion • SWI—Blooming in clotted vessel/vein • CTV, CE MRV, CE MPRAGE, and T2 SPACE all highly sensitive and specific for thrombosis detection
Hemorrhagic transformation of ischemic stroke	• Age—Older adults > young adults and children • Risk factors—Reperfusion therapy, larger stroke size, older age, hypertension, hyperglycemia • Timing—1–4 days • Etiology—Reperfusion into ischemic tissue	• Hemorrhage location—Peripheral petechial > parenchymal (in basal ganglia with MCA M1 strokes) • CTA—Recanalization or persistent clot when reperfusion from collaterals causes hemorrhage • SWI is superior to NCCT for hemorrhage detection
Aneurysm	• Age—Young > older adults • Risk factors—Aneurysm size >5 mm, lobulation, growth between scans • Symptoms—Severe headache, focal neurologic deficit • Etiology—Congenital	• Hemorrhage location—Basal ganglia (M1 segment aneurysm), anterior temporal lobe (MCA bifurcation aneurysm), inferior frontal lobe (anterior communicating artery aneurysm), other (mycotic aneurysms); usually has associated subarachnoid hemorrhage • NCCT—Aneurysm is less hyperdense than clot • T2 WI—Flow void with lamellated appearance • CTA and CE MRA—>90% sensitive and specific for aneurysm detection
Moyamoya	• Age—Children and young adults • Symptoms—Acute neurologic deficits • Associations—Radiation, NF1, Down's syndrome, atherosclerosis • Etiology—Idiopathic	• Hemorrhage location—Basal ganglia • FLAIR—"ivy sign" – Sulcal hyperintensity from slow blood flow in collateral vessels • T2 W1—Flow voids in collateral network and absence of flow voids in distal ICAs and proximal • Strokes of variable ages in anterior circulation and border zone distributions • CTA/MRA—Severe narrowing or occlusion of distal ICAs, proximal MCAs and ACAs with circle of Willis and pial collaterals from posterior circulation • MCAs and ACAs
Reversible cerebral vasoconstriction syndrome	• Age—Young to middle age females • Risk factors—Pregnancy, migraines, vasoactive drugs • Symptoms—Recurrent thunderclap headaches, focal neurologic deficit • Etiology—Reversible vasospasm	• Hemorrhage location—Lobar parenchymal plus cerebral convexity subarachnoid hemorrhage • CTA/MRA—Multifocal stenoses in first and second order branches • DWI—Border zone infarctions • FLAIR—Cortical and subcortical vasogenic edema • Vessel wall imaging—Uniformly thickened walls without enhancement
Primary CNS vasculitis	• Age—Middle age males • Symptoms—Headache, encephalopathy, stroke, seizure • Etiology—T-cell mediated inflammation	• Hemorrhage location—Lobar plus subarachnoid at the cerebral convexities • CTA/MRA—Proximal and/or distal circle of Willis vessel stenoses • DWI/FLAIR—Strokes of different ages in different vascular distributions • CE T1—Leptomeningeal enhancement • Vessel wall imaging—Concentric enhancement

Table 5.2 (continued)

Entity	Clinical	Key imaging features in addition to parenchymal hematoma
Dural AV fistula	• Age—Middle age to older adult • Risk factors—Prior sinus thrombosis, cortical venous drainage • Symptoms—Pulsatile tinnitus, cranial nerve palsies, orbital symptoms, strokes • Etiology—Idiopathic or resulting from trauma, surgery, VST, tumor, infection	• Hemorrhage location—Lobar - cerebellum, medial temporal and occipital lobes; subarachnoid at the cerebral convexities • Time resolved CTA/MRA—Enlarged feeding arteries (ICA, ECA, MMA), direct connection(s) to enlarged draining veins or abnormal venous sinuses with channels and arterialized flow • T2 WI—Abnormal flow voids
Posterior reversible encephalopathy syndrome	• Age—Young adults • Symptoms—Headache, seizure, encephalopathy, visual changes • Etiology—Loss of autoregulation due to acute blood pressure change, neurotoxins	• Hemorrhage location—Lobar hemorrhages in 20% • FLAIR—Edema/ischemia in parietal and occipital subcortical white matter or in border zone distribution • CTA/MRA—Posterior circulation vasoconstriction and/or vasodilatation with beading
Infections	• Age—Any age • Risk factors—Immunocompromised • Etiology—*Mucormycosis/aspergillosis*— Spread from sinonasal cavity to the skull base and circle of Willis *bacterial endocarditis*—Hematogenous spread to distal MCA, ACA, PCA branches	• *Mucormycosis/aspergillosis*—Circle of Willis vascular narrowing and/or pseudoaneurysm formation with basal ganglia hemorrhages, infarctions, abscesses, and edema • *Bacterial endocarditis*—Distal pseudoaneurysms with lobar hemorrhages, abscesses, infarctions, edema
No underlying vascular abnormality on CTA		
Cerebral amyloid angiopathy	• Age—Over 65 • Symptoms—Cognitive impairment, focal neurologic deficits, seizures • Etiology—Deposition of cerebral amyloid- β peptide in walls of small leptomeningeal and cortical vessels	• Hemorrhage location—Lobar • Microhemorrhages at gray–white matter junctions • Leptomeningeal hemorrhage/hemosiderosis • Periventricular leukoencephalopathy • Cortical/subcortical lacunes • Prominent perivascular spaces • Leptomeningeal enhancement (inflammatory CAA) • Vasogenic edema (inflammatory CAA)
Hypertensive vasculopathy	• Age—Older adults • Symptoms—Acute neurologic deficits • Etiology—Poorly controlled hypertension	• Hemorrhage location—Basal ganglia, thalami, brainstem, cerebellum • Microhemorrhages • Lacunar infarctions • Diffuse leukoaraiosis
Cavernous malformation	• Age—40–60 • Risk factors—Radiation • Symptoms—Acute neurologic deficits, seizures • Etiology—Hyalinized thin-walled capillaries with surrounding hemosiderin	• Central "popcorn" appearance with T1 hyperintense foci • Complete hemosiderin rim • Enhancement due to central leakage of contrast • Edema if recent bleeding • Numerous additional lesions seen only on SWI in familial forms
Tumoral hemorrhage	• Age—Older adults • Risk factors—Chemotherapy, radiation, hypertension, anticoagulation • Symptoms—Acute neurologic deficits, seizures • Etiology—Rupture of tumoral blood vessels, tumoral invasion of parenchymal arteries or veins	• Enhancing tissue • Delayed evolution of products of hemorrhage • Incomplete hemosiderin rim • Fluid fluid levels or blood cystic-necrotic levels • Disproportionately large amount of edema
Hemorrhagic encephalitis	• Age—Any age • Symptoms—Fever, encephalopathy, seizures • Etiology—Herpes virus, flaviviruses, Epstein–Barr virus	• FLAIR/T2 hyperintense expansile lesions with hemorrhage involving cortex and subcortical white matter • Herpes simplex virus—Limbic system • Flaviviruses, Epstein–Barr virus—Basal ganglia, thalami, brainstem

5.3.4.1 Arteriovenous Malformation

An arteriovenous malformation is composed of large feeding arteries, a central nidus through which arteriovenous shunting occurs and enlarged draining veins. AVMs are most commonly intraparenchymal but may be intraventricular or located in the subarachnoid space [13]. Eighty-five percent of AVMs are supratentorial, and approximately 65% of supratentorial AVMs are superficial (lobar). They are typically sporadic but may be associated with syndromes such as hereditary hemorrhagic telangiectasia, Wyburn-Mason syndrome, or the RASA 1 mutation. AVMs are typically diagnosed in childhood or young adulthood. Risk of rupture increases with age, presence of a feeding artery or intranidal aneurysm, venous stenosis, or deep venous drainage.

AVMs are typically classified according to the Spetzler Martin grading system in order to predict the risk of surgical complication based on size, presence of deep venous drainage, and eloquence of location. The hemorrhagic risk is higher for AVMs that are infratentorial, have a deep location and/or deep venous drainage, or have previously bled. AVMs may have calcifications and appear mildly hyperdense on noncontrast CT, enhance during the arterial phase on CTA and dynamic contrast-enhanced MRA, and have prominent flow voids and pulsation artifact on T2-weighted MRI images. Additional features may include edema or gliosis (best identified on FLAIR images) and acute or chronic hemorrhage (best identified on SWI images) in the surrounding brain parenchyma. Digital subtraction angiography remains the gold standard for diagnosing and assessing AVMs.

5.3.4.2 Cerebral Venous Sinus Thrombosis

Cerebral venous sinus thrombosis refers to the formation and propagation of clot leading to occlusion of intracranial venous sinuses and veins. Important risk factors are prothrombotic conditions, pregnancy, oral contraceptives, dehydration, infectious and inflammatory conditions, and malignancy. Symptoms and imaging findings vary by location [14]. The most common symptoms are headache, seizure, encephalopathy, and focal neurologic deficits. Lobar hemorrhages are typically caused by thrombosis of the superior sagittal, transverse and sigmoid sinuses, and/or of cortical veins (Fig. 5.6). Basal ganglia and thalamic hemorrhages

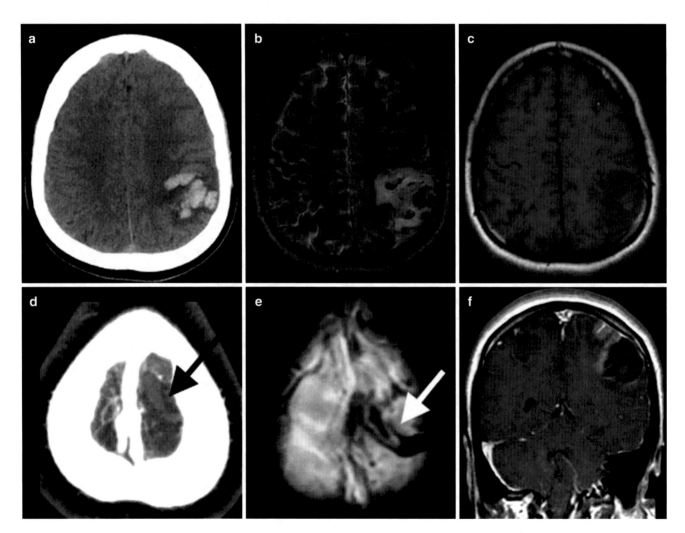

Fig. 5.6 A 36-year-old female with severe headache, right-sided weakness, and cortical vein thrombosis. Noncontrast CT (**a**) shows a left parietal parenchymal hematoma. The hematoma has areas that are hypointense on T2-weighted images (**b**) and isointense on T1-weighted images (**c**), consistent with deoxyhemoglobin and areas that are hyperintense on T2-weighted images and isointense on T1-weighted images, consistent with oxyhemoglobin. CTA source images (**d**) show nonopacification of a cortical vein, consistent with thrombosis (black arrow). There is blooming of the vein on the gradient echo images (**e**), confirming thrombosis. Coronal contrast-enhanced T1-weighted images (**f**) show gyriform enhancement, typical of subacute ischemic lesions

are typically caused by thrombosis of the internal cerebral veins, vein of Galen, or straight sinus. Findings on NCCT include hyperdensity in the thrombosed vein (cord sign) or sinus (dense triangle sign), present in approximately 30% of cases, as well as parenchymal hemorrhage in a nonarterial distribution and/or vasogenic edema and mass effect. CT venography is over 90% sensitive and specific for the detection of CVT. Findings on MRI include absence of a normal flow void on T2 weighted images. The clot and parenchymal hematoma are typically characterized by T1 isointensity and T2 hypointensity in the acute stage, by T1 hyperintensity and T2 hypointensity in early subacute stage and by T1 and T2 hyperintensity in the late subacute stage. Edema is typically best visualized on the FLAIR images and is characterized by restricted and/or facilitated diffusion. Contrast-enhanced MR venography, contrast-enhanced volumetric T1-weighted images, and T2 volumetric SPACE sequences demonstrate higher than 90% sensitivity and specificity for detection of CVT.

5.3.4.3 Hemorrhagic Transformation of Ischemic Stroke

Hemorrhagic transformation of acute ischemic stroke has been variably reported. Risk factors include reperfusion therapy with intravenous thrombolytic agents and/or thrombectomy, larger stroke size, older age, hypertension, and hyperglycemia [15]. Most hemorrhagic transformation manifests as petechial hemorrhage with small isodense or hyperdense peripheral foci on CT that bloom on SWI and is asymptomatic. A minority results in parenchymal hematoma which is typically in the basal ganglia in large anterior circulation strokes. In patients who receive IVtPA, hemorrhagic transformation typically occurs in the first 24 h and is symptomatic in 6%. Spontaneous hemorrhage occurs up to 4 days after stroke onset and is symptomatic in 3%. Following reperfusion therapy, dual-energy CT can be used to distinguish between contrast blush and hemorrhage.

5.3.4.4 Aneurysm

Aneurysms typically present with subarachnoid hemorrhage but can present with isolated IPH when they are located at the M1 segment and point superiorly into the basal ganglia, at the MCA bifurcation and point posteriorly into the temporal lobe, or at the anterior communicating artery and point superolaterally into the inferior frontal lobe. Peripheral mycotic aneurysms can also rupture into adjacent brain parenchyma (Fig. 5.7). Proximal aneurysms that cause isolated IPH are typically greater than 12 mm [16]. On NCCT, they are less hyperdense than the adjacent hematoma, but may have a partially thrombosed hyperdense wall similar in density to the adjacent hematoma. On MRI, aneurysms show a flow void on T2WI with a lamellated appearance with signal intensity depending on the stage of hemorrhage if there is

partial thrombosis. Aneurysms may be associated with pulsation artifact. CTA and contrast-enhanced MRA are greater than 90% sensitive and specific for identifying aneurysms.

5.3.4.5 Moyamoya Syndrome

Moyamoya disease is an idiopathic, non-arteriosclerotic, noninflammatory arterio-occlusive syndrome that occurs in young children and young adults. It is characterized predominantly by progressive occlusion of the distal internal carotid arteries and of the proximal anterior and middle cerebral arteries, although the posterior circulation can be involved in up to 50% [17]. As a compensatory mechanism, multiple collateral vessels form in the region of the circle of Willis and involve the lenticulostriate and thalamoperforating arteries as well as leptomeningeal and dural arteries. Pial collaterals, typically from the posterior circulation, also form. Children typically present with borderzone and subcortical white matter infarctions, while young adults more commonly present with basal ganglia hemorrhage due to rupture of collateral vessels (Fig. 5.7). CTA and MRA are highly sensitive for identifying the large vessel occlusions and stenoses and larger collateral vessels, but digital angiography remains the gold standard for delineating the extent of collateral vessels. Findings on MRI include abnormal flow voids on T2 WI, the ivy sign (sulcal FLAIR hyperintensity due to slow flow in collateral vessels), acute ischemic strokes, and intraparenchymal hemorrhage including microhemorrhages in the basal ganglia and deep white matter. Moyamoya syndrome refers to a number of conditions that mimic MMD on imaging. These include atherosclerosis, hematologic disorders such as sickle cell disease, inflammatory and infectious etiologies, and radiation therapy. Treatment includes surgical direct revascularization options such as MCA to STA bypass or indirect revascularization options such as EDAS (encephaloduroarteriosynangiosis).

5.3.4.6 Reversible Cerebral Vasoconstriction Syndrome

Reversible cerebral vasoconstriction syndrome is characterized by rapid onset of frequently recurrent thunderclap headaches and cerebral vasospasm that resolves by 12 weeks. The syndrome occurs most frequently in young to middle age adult females and is associated with pregnancy, migraines, and the use of vasoactive drugs such as triptans, amphetamines, selective serotonin reuptake inhibitors, and cocaine. CTA, MRA, and DSA show smooth, tapered narrowing of large- to medium-sized arteries (first- and second-order branches) followed by abnormally dilated segments or a beaded appearance distal to the stenoses (Fig. 5.7). Lobar hemorrhages occur in up to 20%, subarachnoid hemorrhage at the cerebral convexity in up to 35%, border zone infarctions in nearly 30%, and cortical and subcortical vasogenic edema in nearly 40% [18]. Of note, FLAIR identifies the extent of edema, DWI readily dif-

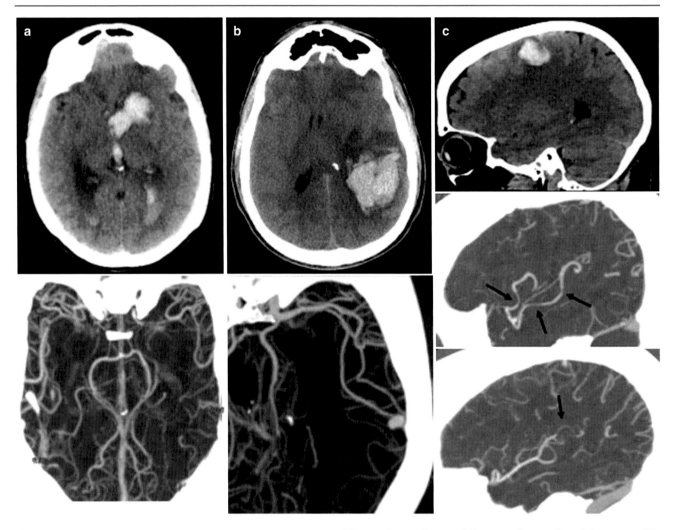

Fig. 5.7 Multiple entities with parenchymal hematomas and underlying vascular lesion on CTA or MRA Patient 1 with moyamoya, Column **a**—The top image shows left caudate head hemorrhage with extension into the lateral and third ventricles. The lower image shows severe attenuation of the bilateral M1 and A1 segments with collateral vessels. Patient 2 IV drug abuser with mycotic pseudoaneurysm, Column **b**— The top image shows a left temporal parenchymal hematoma. The lower image shows an underlying distal MCA mycotic pseudoaneurysm. Patient 3 with reversible cerebral vasoconstrictive syndrome, Column **c**—The top image shows right posterior frontal intraparenchymal and subarachnoid hemorrhage. The middle and lower images show stenoses (arrows) in bilateral MCA branches

ferentiates between vasogenic and cytotoxic edema, FLAIR sulcal hyperintensity can reflect subarachnoid hemorrhage or slow flow in collateral vessels and SWI can delineate the extent of hemorrhage. Vessel wall imaging typically shows uniformly thickened wall that does not enhance. Treatment includes calcium channel blockers and 90% of patients recover without persistent neurologic deficits.

5.3.4.7 Miscellaneous

Infections

Intracranial infections can lead to intraparenchymal hemorrhage due to arterial invasion with mycotic aneurysm forma-

tion and rupture. Mucormycosis and aspergillosis are angioinvasive fungal infections that occur in the sinonasal cavity. They can directly invade the skull base with spread to the circle of Willis leading to basilar meningitis, pseudoaneurysm formation, basal ganglia hemorrhages, infarctions, and abscesses. Bacterial organisms associated with infectious endocarditis can spread hematogenously to gray–white matter junctions where infection leads to peripheral pseudoaneurysm formation, lobar hemorrhages, infarctions, and abscesses. While varicella vasculopathy is typically associated with vascular narrowing and ischemic infarctions, aneurysms can form and result in intraparenchymal or subarachnoid hemorrhage.

Primary CNS Vasculitis

Primary CNS vasculitis occurs most frequently in middle age males and is thought to result from T-cell mediated inflammation of medium and small brain parenchymal and leptomeningeal arteries. Common presenting symptoms are headache, encephalopathy, strokes, and seizures. Common imaging findings include proximal and/or distal stenoses in 60%, parenchymal hemorrhages and hemorrhagic infarctions, strokes of different ages in different vascular distributions, leptomeningeal enhancement, subarachnoid hemorrhage at the cerebral convexities, and concentric vessel wall enhancement [19]. Treatment is with steroids and cytotoxic agents. Systemic vasculitides can have similar CNS findings but are distinguished by their involvement of multiple organ systems.

Dural AV Fistula

Dural arteriovenous fistulas (dAVFs) are acquired vascular malformations in which there are abnormal connections between arteries that typically supply the meninges and the dural venous sinuses. Symptoms depend on the fistula location and whether or not there is brain edema or hemorrhage and include pulsatile tinnitus, cranial nerve palsies, orbital symptoms (cavernous carotid fistulas), and focal neurologic deficits. In one large study, approximately 24% of patients had intracranial hemorrhage with 52% having isolated intraparenchymal hemorrhage, 22% having isolated SAH, and 23% having both [20]. The fistula involved the tentorium, petrosal sinuses, torcular, transverse sinuses, and/or foramen magnum in 66%. The IPH was usually located near the point of fistulization in the cerebellum or medial temporal or occipital lobes. The risk of hemorrhage is higher when there is cortical venous drainage, and nearly all patients with dural AVF and intracranial hemorrhage have cortical venous reflux. Time-resolved CTA and MRA are over 90% sensitive for detecting dural AVF [21]. CTA and MRA findings include enlarged internal carotid, external carotid or meningeal arteries, enlarged transosseous vessels, an abnormal dural venous sinus (abnormal channels, early filling, and arterialized flow), and dilated cortical and meningeal veins. These abnormal vessels can also be visualized as abnormal flow voids on T2WI. SWI images may show intraparenchymal, subarachnoid, intraventricular, or subdural hemorrhage. Brain parenchymal edema (best seen on FLAIR images) may also be present. The Cognard and Borden scales address the type of venous drainage which predict the future risk of hemorrhage.

Pres

Posterior Reversible Encephalopathy Syndrome is a neurotoxic state characterized by loss of autoregulation and disruption of the blood–brain barrier due to acute changes in blood pressure and/or circulating toxins. Typical presenting symptoms are headache, seizures, encephalopathy, and visual changes. Key imaging findings are FLAIR/T2 hyperintense edema in the parietal and occipital subcortical white matter and cortex and/or in a borderzone distribution. Affected regions can have parenchymal hemorrhages in up to 15% and infarctions characterized by restricted diffusion in 10–25% [22]. CTA, MRA, and DSA can show foci of vasoconstriction, vasodilation, or both (a beaded appearance).

5.3.5 Entities with No Underlying Vascular Abnormality on CTA or MRA

When a patient presents to the emergency room with a lobar hemorrhage, they typically undergo CT angiography scanning. In approximately 85%, the CTA or MRA does not demonstrate a causative vascular lesion. The most common intraparenchymal hemorrhages in this situation result from hypertension, cerebral amyloid angiopathy, coagulopathy, or underlying tumor.

5.3.5.1 Cerebral Amyloid Angiopathy

Cerebral amyloid angiopathy is a cerebrovascular disease that results from deposition of cerebral amyloid-β peptide in the walls of small leptomeningeal and cortical vessels. CAA is the cause of up to 50% of spontaneous intracerebral hemorrhages in patients older than 65 years of age, and the incidence increases with age. For example, approximately 5–9% of people between ages 60 and 69 have amyloid deposition at autopsy while 43–58% of people over 90 years of age have amyloid deposition at autopsy [23]. Common presentations are headache, focal neurologic deficits, seizures, and cognitive impairment. The Boston criteria 2.0 (Table 5.3) combine clinical, radiographical, and pathological criteria to determine the probability of diagnosis [24]. Key imaging features are lobar hemorrhage, microhemorrhages at gray–white matter junctions, leptomeningeal hemorrhage and hemosiderosis, periventricular leukoencephalopathy, cortical/subcortical lacunes, and prominent perivascular spaces (Fig. 5.8). Inflammatory CAA has additional findings of leptomeningeal enhancement and vasogenic edema and tends to present at a

Table 5.3 Boston Criteria 2.0 for sporadic cerebral amyloid angiopathy

1. Definite CAA	Full post-mortem examination demonstrating: • Presentation with spontaneous ICH, TFNEs, cSAH, or CI/dementia • Severe CAA with vasculopathy • Absence of other diagnostic lesion
2. Probable CAA with supporting pathology	Clinical data and pathologic tissue (evacuated hematoma or cortical biopsy) demonstrating: • Presentation with spontaneous ICH, TFNEs, cSAH, or CI/dementia • Some degree of CAA in specimen • Absence of other diagnostic lesion
3. Probable CAA	Clinical data and MRI demonstrating • Age ≥ 50 years • Presentation with spontaneous ICH, TFNEs, or CI/dementia • ≥2 of the following strictly lobar hemorrhagic lesions on T2* weighted MRI, in any combination – ICH, CMB, cSS/cSAH foci OR • 1 lobar hemorrhagic lesion +1 white matter feature (severe CSO-PVS or WMH-MS) • Absence of any deep hemorrhagic lesions (ICH, CMB) on T2*- weighted MR • Absence of other cause of hemorrhagic lesions • Hemorrhagic lesion in cerebellum not counted in either lobar or deep hemorrhagic lesion
Possible CAA	Clinical data and MRI demonstrating • Age ≥ 50 years • Presentation with spontaneous ICH, TFNEs, or CI/dementia • Absence of other cause of hemorrhage • 1 strictly lobar hemorrhagic lesion on T2* weighted MRI: ICH, CMB, cSS/cSAH focus OR • 1 white matter feature (severe CSO-PVS or WMH-MS) • Absence of any deep hemorrhagic lesions (ICH, CMB) on T2*- weighted MR • Absence of other cause of hemorrhagic lesions • Hemorrhagic lesion in cerebellum not counted in either lobar or deep hemorrhagic lesion

ICH intracranial hemorrhage, *TFNE* transient focal neurologic episode, *cSAH* convexity subarachnoid hemorrhage, *CI* cognitive impairment, *CMB* cerebral microbleed, *cSS* cortical superficial siderosis, *CSO-PVS* visible centrum semiovale perivascular spaces, *WMH-MS* white matter hyperintensities in a multispot pattern

slightly younger age. CAA is most commonly sporadic but numerous rare hereditary types, that are typically autosomal dominant and present in middle age, have also been described.

5.3.5.2 Hypertensive Hemorrhage

Long standing, poorly controlled hypertension is the most common cause of intracranial hemorrhage. Patients develop hypertensive vasculopathy characterized by lipohyalinosis in small- and medium-sized vessels such as the lenticulostriate, thalamoperforating, and pontine perforating arteries as well as cerebellar arterioles. Hemorrhages result from the rupture of microaneurysms with a rebleed rate of 2% per year, and most frequently occur in the basal ganglia (35–40%), thalami (10–20%), pons (5–10%), and cerebellum (5–10%) [25] (Fig. 5.9). Hemorrhages occasionally occur in the subcortical white matter (1–2%). Presenting symptoms vary depending upon the hemorrhage location. Microhemorrhages and lacunar infarctions in the deep gray nuclei, brainstem and cerebellum, and diffuse leukoaraiosis support the diagnosis.

5.3.5.3 Cavernous Malformation

Cavernous malformations are composed of clusters of hyalinized thin-walled capillaries with surrounding hemo-siderin. The majority are sporadic and remain asymptomatic. Symptomatic lesions typically present between ages 40 and 60 with headache, seizures, or focal neurologic deficits. Ten to thirty percent are multiple and seen in association with familial multiple cavernous malformation syndrome for which mutations in the KRIT1, CCM2, and PDCD10 genes have been identified. Cavernous malformations can also develop after radiation therapy. On CT, cavernous malformations are usually mildly hyperdense with foci of calcification in 40–60%. On MRI, they have a variable appearance depending on the stage of internal blood products with a central "popcorn appearance," characterized by foci of T1 hyperintensity and isointensity and T2 hyperintensity and hypointensity [26] (Fig. 5.10). They typically have a smooth, complete hemosiderin rim that is hypointense on T2 WI. Lesions show marked blooming on SWI images. In addition, SWI images detect small lesions that are not seen on other MRI sequences. Cavernous malformations may enhance due to leakage of contrast into them and may have surrounding edema if they have recently bled. Cavernous malformations are occasionally associated with developmental venous anomalies.

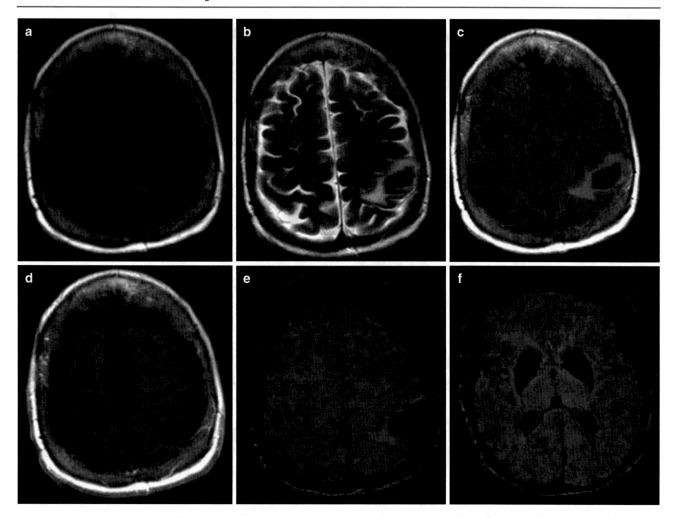

Fig. 5.8 A 70-year-old female with right-sided weakness and amyloid angiopathy. There is an acute parenchymal hematoma in the left parietal lobe that isointense on T1-weighted images (**a**), hypointense on T2 (**b**), and FLAIR (**c**) weighted images, does not show and underlying lesion on gadolinium-enhanced T1-weighted images (**d**) and blooms on SWI (**e**). SWI images (**e** and **f**) show microhemorrhages at gray–white matter junctions as well as hemosiderosis in left frontal sulci

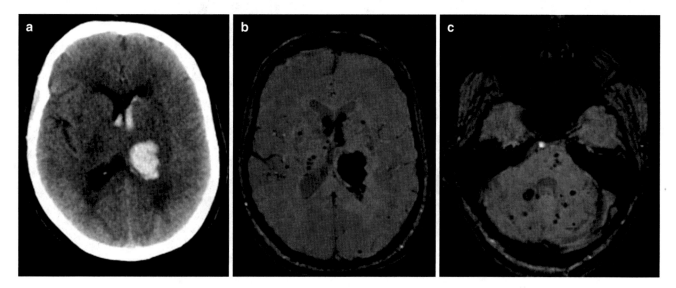

Fig. 5.9 A 53-year-old female with unsteady gait, confusion, and hypertensive hemorrhages. Noncontrast CT (**a**) shows acute hemorrhage in the left thalamus with intraventricular extension. SWI images (**b** and **c**) confirm hemorrhage in the left thalamus and ventricles and show microhemorrhages in the cerebellum, pons, and deep gray nuclei

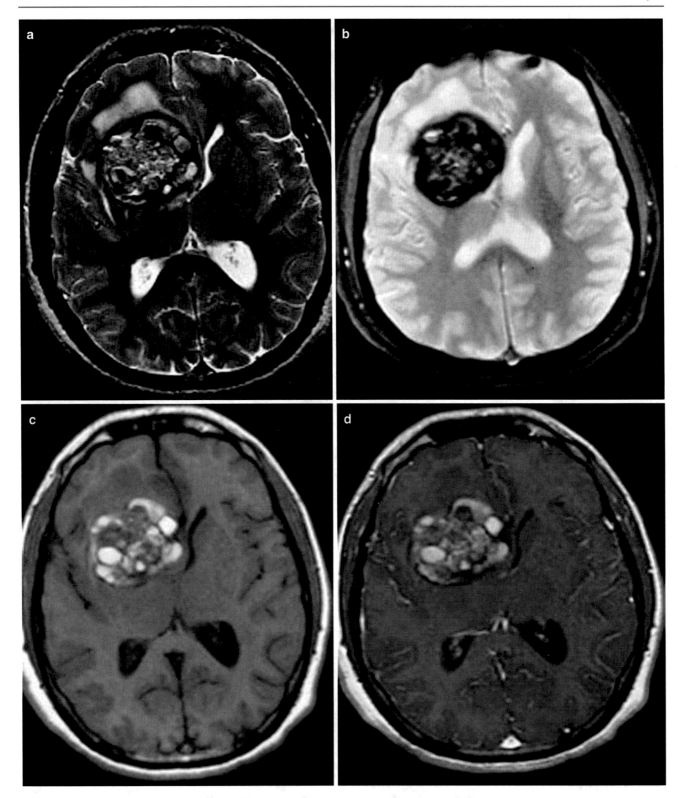

Fig. 5.10 A 50-year-old male with left-sided weakness and a cavernous malformation with a "popcorn" appearance. There is a hemorrhagic mass in the right basal ganglia and right frontal lobe characterized by heterogeneous signal on T2 (**a**) and T1 (**c**) weighted images with foci of T1 hyperintensity consistent with methemoglobin. There is blooming on the GRE images (**b**) due to the subacute and chronic products of hemorrhage. A smooth, complete hemosiderin rim is seen on T2 and GRE (**b**) images. There is no enhancement on gadolinium-enhanced T1-weighted images (**d**)

5.3.5.4 Tumoral Hemorrhage

Approximately 5% of intraparenchymal hemorrhages are secondary to intratumoral or peritumoral hemorrhage. Intratumoral hemorrhage may result from rupture of tumoral blood vessels, tumoral invasion of parenchymal blood vessels, and tumor necrosis. Intratumoral or peritumoral hemorrhage can also result from radiation therapy or chemotherapy. Other risk factors include hypertension, anticoagulation, and advanced age. Tumors most commonly associated with intratumoral hemorrhage are high grade primary tumors such as high grade glial neoplasms, and metastases, most commonly from breast carcinoma, melanoma, renal cell car-

cinoma, thyroid carcinoma, and choriocarcinoma. Thrombotic tumor emboli from atrial myxoma, thrombotic coagulopathy, and venous sinus thrombosis from tumor invasion or malignancy induced coagulopathy may also result in intraparenchymal hemorrhage in cancer patients. Imaging findings that suggest an underlying tumor include: (1) enhancing tissue, (2) delayed evolution of the products of hemorrhage, (3) an incomplete hemosiderin rim, (4) the presence of multiple foci of susceptibility, (5) the presence of fluid fluid levels or blood-cystic necrotic levels, and (6) the presence of a disproportionately large amount of edema (Fig. 5.11).

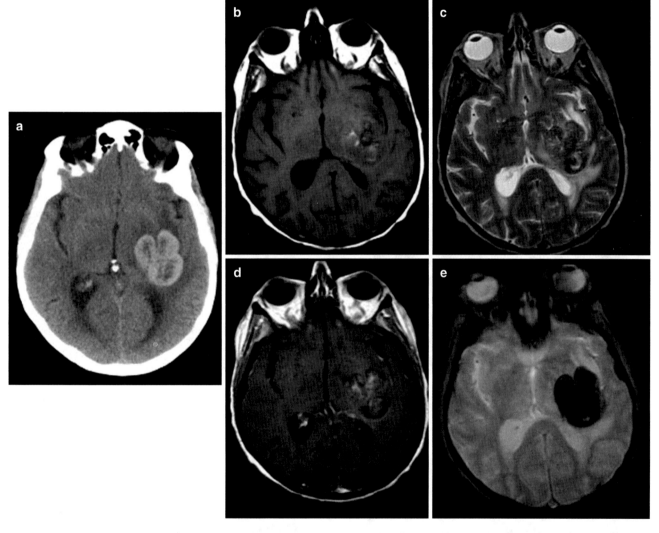

Fig. 5.11 A 65-year-old female with acute right-sided weakness and a hemorrhagic breast carcinoma metastasis. Noncontrast CT (**a**) shows parenchymal hemorrhage in the left basal ganglia and external capsule with surrounding edema. The hemorrhage is heterogenous with hyperintense foci on T1-weighted images (**b**) consistent with methemoglobin and hypointense foci on T2-weighted images, consistent with deoxyhemoglobin or intracellular methemoglobin (**c**). Following the administration of gadolinium (**d**), there is patchy enhancement confirming the presence of an underlying mass. GRE images (**e**) show blooming consistent with hemorrhage

5.3.5.5 Coagulopathy

Approximately, 0.3–0.6 percent of patients on oral antico-agulant therapy have intracranial hemorrhage, most commonly in an intraparenchymal lobar or cerebellar location [27]. Large or multiple synchronous hemorrhages, the presence fluid-fluid levels, and intraventricular extension are characteristic features of both congenital and acquired coagulation disorders. In addition, hemorrhages due to coagulopathy have an increased incidence of ongoing bleeding.

5.3.5.6 Hemorrhagic Encephalitis

Herpes simplex virus is a necrotizing meningoencephalitis that occurs due to latent reactivation in the case of immunosuppression or other stress. It typically involves the limbic system in a bilateral asymmetric distribution. Typical imaging findings include FLAIR/T2 hyperintense edema in the medial temporal lobes, insula, and cingulate gyri with areas of restricted diffusion due to cytotoxic edema, and blooming on SWI due to hemorrhage. Gyriform enhancement is present in the subacute stage. Other viruses that may cause hemorrhagic encephalitis include the flaviviruses (dengue, Japanese, Murray Valley, Powassan, St Louis, Rocio, and West Nile) and Epstein–Barr virus that typically involve the basal ganglia, thalami, and brainstem in varying patterns.

Key Points #3
- Common causes of lobar IPH without underlying vascular abnormality on CTA are amyloid angiopathy, coagulopathy, and underlying tumor and cavernous malformations in younger patients. The presence of microhemorrhages, underlying enhancement or a "popcorn appearance" can help differentiate these entities.
- Deep gray nuclei, brainstem, and cerebellar intraparenchymal hemorrhages without underlying vascular abnormality on CTA are most commonly caused by hypertension. Associated microhemorrhages and lacunar infarcts are common.

Key Points #4
- Common causes of IPH with underlying vascular abnormality on CTA are AVM, cerebral venous sinus thrombosis, and hemorrhagic transformation of acute ischemic stroke.
- AVMs have abnormal flow voids on T2W1 as well as a feeding artery, nidus, and early venous opacification on CTA.

- Cerebral venous sinus thrombosis is characterized by hyperdense vein or sinus on CT, and lack of flow void on T2WI. CTA and MRV are highly accurate for detection.
- Hemorrhagic transformation of ischemic stroke occurs in a vascular territory and is associated with large vessel occlusion.

5.4 Other Hemorrhage

5.4.1 Microhemorrhage

Microhemorrhages are punctate brain hemorrhages which result from rupture of tiny vessels measuring less than 200 μm in diameter and are best seen on SWI images. As mentioned above, they are most commonly seen in a peripheral distribution in association with amyloid angiopathy or concentrated in the deep gray nuclei, brainstem, and cerebellum in association with hypertension. Multiple microhemorrhages are also seen in patients with familial cavernous malformations, CADASIL in 25–70% of cases, history of cardiac bypass surgery, cerebral vasculitis, hemorrhagic micrometastases, fat emboli, septic emboli, and radiation induced cerebral vasculopathy. Microhemorrhages have also been reported in critically ill patients with acute respiratory distress syndrome, high altitude sickness, and Covid 19 who have coagulation impairment and thrombotic microangiopathy.

5.4.2 Subdural and Epidural Hemorrhage

Subdural and epidural hemorrhage are usually associated with head trauma. However, they may occur spontaneously in patients who are receiving anticoagulants or antiplatelet therapy. They can also occur in patients with coagulopathies, dural and osteodural arteriovenous fistulas, intracranial hypotension, and dural or calvarial metastases.

5.5 Blood Mimics

5.5.1 On CT

Distinguishing between acute hemorrhage and hyperattenuating mimics poses a common challenge on CT in neuroradiology. Certain materials with high atomic numbers, such as iodine, calcium, and silicone oil, can exhibit similar attenuation levels to acute blood components, depending on their concentration. Dual-energy CT offers a solution to differentiate between hemorrhage and these high atomic number materials due to their distinct absorption patterns of X-ray photons at different incident energy levels.

5.5.2 On MR

Fat and blood both appear hyperintense on T1W and T2W FSE sequences. Relying solely on these conventional sequences to distinguish between the two is insufficient. However, fat-suppressed sequences can help determine the correct diagnosis. The Gradient Echo (GRE) and susceptibility-weighted imaging (SWI) sequences, utilizing T2*W-based contrast, are typically employed for the detection of hemorrhage, calcification, and iron accumulation in different tissue types. Since these entities all show low signal on GRE and SWI., differentiating between them can be a genuine challenge. SWI filtered phase images can be useful since hemosiderin and deoxyhemoglobin (both paramagnetic) have signal that is opposite to that of calcium (diamagnetic). Additionally, it is worth noting that two other etiologies, proteinaceous cysts (e.g., colloid cysts) and dense cell packing (lymphoma), can be hyperintense on T1-weighted images and mimic methemoglobin.

5.6 Conclusion

Neuroimaging plays an essential role in management of intracranial hemorrhage. It allows the identification and characterization of intracranial hemorrhage according to location, volume, extent, and age. In conjunction with patient demographics, neuroimaging allows the determination of underlying etiology and is a cornerstone for determining prognosis and appropriate treatment.

> **Take-Home Messages**
> - The imaging characteristics of intracranial hemorrhages vary predictably over time for both CT and MRI.
> - For SAH, the etiology can be determined by location and findings on CTA. FLAIR is more sensitive than NCCT. The Modified Fisher Grade predicts the risk of vasospasm.
> - For IPH without an underlying vascular abnormality on CTA or MRA, amyloid angiopathy (with lobar IPH, peripheral microhemorrhages, and hemosiderosis) and hypertension (with deep gray nuclei, brainstem, or cerebellar IPH and microhemorrhages) are common etiologies.

- For IPH with abnormal vessels on CTA, common etiologies are AVM (with feeding artery, nidus and arterialized vein), cerebral venous sinus thrombosis (with hyperdense vein or sinus that doesn't opacify on CTA), hemorrhagic transformation of ischemic stroke (with large vessel occlusion), dural AVF (with a direct connection between feeding artery and vein), and moyamoya (with severe stenosis of the distal ICAs and proximal ACAs and MCAS) are relatively common etiologies.
- Calcification and other materials with high atomic numbers can mimic hemorrhage on NCCT. Dual energy CT can help differentiate these entities. Calcification, proteinaceous material, melanin, iron, and dense cell packing can mimic hemorrhage on MRI. SWI-filtered phase images can sometimes help differentiate calcification from hemorrhage.

References

1. Claassen J, Park S. Spontaneous subarachnoid haemorrhage. Lancet. 2022;400:846–62.
2. Edjlali M, Rodriguez-Régent C, Hodel J, et al. Subarachnoid hemorrhage in ten questions. Diagn Interv Imaging. 2015;96:657–66.
3. Etminan N, Chang H-S, Hackenberg K, et al. Worldwide incidence of aneurysmal subarachnoid hemorrhage according to region, time period, blood pressure, and smoking prevalence in the population: a systematic review and meta-analysis. JAMA Neurol. 2019;76:588–97.
4. Kumar H, Ali S, Kumar J, et al. Dural venous sinus thrombosis leading to subarachnoid hemorrhage. Cureus. 2021;13:e13497.
5. Perillo T, Paolella C, Perrotta G, et al. Reversible cerebral vasoconstriction syndrome: review of neuroimaging findings. Radiol Med. 2022;127:981–90.
6. Viguier A, Raposo N, Patsoura S, et al. Subarachnoid and subdural hemorrhages in lobar intracerebral hemorrhage associated with cerebral amyloid angiopathy. Stroke. 2019;50:1567–9.
7. Edjlali M, Guédon A, Ben Hassen W, et al. Circumferential thick enhancement at Vessel Wall MRI has high specificity for intracranial aneurysm instability. Radiology. 2018;289:181–7.
8. Tateoka T, Yoshioka H, Kanemaru K, et al. Blood blister-like aneurysms at the junction of the internal carotid and posterior communicating artery: characteristics and treatment strategies. World Neurosurg. 2023;170:e645–51.
9. Hou K, Yu J. Current status of perimesencephalic non-aneurysmal subarachnoid hemorrhage. Front Neurol. 2022;13:960702.
10. Sacco S, Marini C, Toni D, et al. Incidence and 10-year survival of intracerebral hemorrhage in a population-based registry. Stroke. 2009;40:394–9.
11. Hemphill JC, Bonovich DC, Besmertis L, et al. The ICH score: a simple, reliable grading scale for intracerebral hemorrhage. Stroke. 2001;32:891–7.
12. Romero JM, Artunduaga M, Forero NP, et al. Accuracy of CT angiography for the diagnosis of vascular abnormalities causing intraparenchymal hemorrhage in young patients. Emerg Radiol. 2009;16:195–201.

13. Tranvinh E, Heit JJ, Hacein-Bey L, et al. Contemporary imaging of cerebral arteriovenous malformations. AJR Am J Roentgenol. 2017;208:1320–30.

14. Canedo-Antelo M, Baleato-González S, Mosqueira AJ, et al. Radiologic clues to cerebral venous thrombosis. Radiographics. 2019;39:1611–28.

15. Álvarez-Sabín J, Maisterra O, Santamarina E, et al. Factors influencing haemorrhagic transformation in ischaemic stroke. Lancet Neurol. 2013;12:689–705.

16. Jabbarli R, Reinhard M, Roelz R, et al. Intracerebral hematoma due to aneurysm rupture: are there risk factors beyond aneurysm location? Neurosurgery. 2016;78:813–20.

17. Li J, Jin M, Sun X, et al. Imaging of moyamoya disease and moyamoya syndrome: current status. J Comput Assist Tomogr. 2019;43:257–63.

18. Singhal AB, Hajj-Ali RA, Topcuoglu MA, et al. Reversible cerebral vasoconstriction syndromes: analysis of 139 cases. Arch Neurol. 2011;68:1005–12.

19. Abdel Razek AAK, Alvarez H, Bagg S, et al. Imaging spectrum of CNS vasculitis. Radiographics. 2014;34:873–94.

20. Koch MJ, Stapleton CJ, Guniganti R, et al. Outcome following hemorrhage from cranial dural arteriovenous fistulae: analysis of the multicenter international CONDOR registry. Stroke. 2021;52:e610–3.

21. in't Veld M, Fronczek R, Dos Santos MP, et al. High sensitivity and specificity of 4D-CTA in the detection of cranial arteriovenous shunts. Eur Radiol. 2019;29:5961–70.

22. Hefzy HM, Bartynski WS, Boardman JF, et al. Hemorrhage in posterior reversible encephalopathy syndrome: imaging and clinical features. AJNR Am J Neuroradiol. 2009;30:1371–9.

23. Walker DA, Broderick DF, Kotsenas AL, et al. Routine use of gradient-echo MRI to screen for cerebral amyloid angiopathy in elderly patients. AJR Am J Roentgenol. 2004;182:1547–50.

24. Charidimou A, Boulouis G, Frosch MP, et al. The Boston criteria version 2.0 for cerebral amyloid angiopathy: a multicentre, retrospective, MRI-neuropathology diagnostic accuracy study. Lancet Neurol. 2022;21:714–25.

25. Kranz PG, Malinzak MD, Amrhein TJ. Approach to imaging in patients with spontaneous intracranial hemorrhage. Neuroimaging Clin N Am. 2018;28:353–74.

26. Kuroedov D, Cunha B, Pamplona J, et al. Cerebral cavernous malformations: typical and atypical imaging characteristics. J Neuroimaging. 2023;33:202–17.

27. Steiner T, Weitz JI, Veltkamp R. Anticoagulant-associated intracranial hemorrhage in the era of reversal agents. Stroke. 2017;48:1432–7.

Intracranial Infection and Inflammation

6

Tchoyoson Lim and Majda M. Thurnher

Abstract

Although uncommon compared to traumatic and cerebrovascular disease, radiologists should recognize the typical imaging features of meningitis, abscess, and encephalitis; and be aware of autoimmune mimics. DWI, SWI, and vessel wall imaging are useful advanced MRI techniques for problem-solving.

Keywords

Meningitis · Abscess · Encephalitis · Virus · Bacteria
Tuberculosis · HIV · Parasite · Autoimmune encephalitis

Learning Objectives
- To review basic cranial MRI features of common CNS infections.
- To recognize typical imaging patterns of meningitis, abscess, and encephalitis.
- To apply imaging features that may differentiate different infections and non-infectious mimics.
- To identify imaging findings in autoimmune brain diseases.
- To evaluate the role of radiologists and the importance of multidisciplinary teams.

Key Points
- DWI, SWI, and vessel wall imaging are useful advanced pulse sequences, whilst MR perfusion and spectroscopy may be used judiciously for problem-solving.
- Meningeal enhancement and subarachnoid pus collections are typical of infectious meningitis.
- Ring enhancing lesions with restricted diffusion on DWI are characteristic of untreated pyogenic abscess.
- Hippocampal swelling and increased signal may be caused by herpes simplex virus type 1 encephalitis or LGI1-antibody encephalitis.

6.1 Approach to CNS Infection

CNS infections are uncommon diseases (compared to trauma, cerebrovascular disease) in the casemix of a typical modern metropolitan hospital or university radiology practice. Radiologists infrequently receive imaging requests to rule out or to assess complications in patients with the classic clinical triad of fever, nuchal rigidity, and altered mental status characteristic of meningism. Often, CNS infection is an unexpected differential diagnosis or missed diagnosis in unsuspected patients being investigated for cortical swelling, abnormal ring, or meningeal enhancement, where the clinical diagnosis is stroke, tumour, or other diseases. Finally, in some instances, typical imaging features characteristic of CNS infection may be caused by unexpected non-infectious diseases, such as LGI1 autoimmune encephalitis being mistaken for herpes simplex virus type 1 (HSV-1) encephalitis.

Hence, radiologists should have a good grasp of typical features and differential diagnosis of CNS infections; although infections can be classified by taxonomy of causative organism (viral, bacterial, fungal), this chapter will

T. Lim (✉)
Neuroradiology, Radiological Sciences Academic Clinical Program, National Neuroscience Institute, Duke-NUS Medical School, Singapore, Singapore
e-mail: Tchoyoson.lim@singhealth.com.sg

M. M. Thurnher
Section of Neuroradiology and Musculoskeletal Radiology, Department of Biomedical Imaging and Image-guided Therapy, University Hospital Vienna, Vienna, Austria
e-mail: majda.thurnher@meduniwien.ac.at

J. Hodler et al. (eds.), *Diseases of the Brain, Head and Neck, Spine 2024-2027*, IDKD Springer Series,
https://doi.org/10.1007/978-3-031-50675-8_6

focus on imaging patterns on CT and MRI. This broad sweep is not exhaustive and includes a section on inflammatory diseases, especially as they pertain to differential diagnosis of infections. With the worldwide trends of warming temperatures, travel and migration, outbreaks of pandemic COVID-19 and other organisms, we are reminded of the importance of this topic.

6.2   MRI Technique

CT yields limited information, and MRI is more sensitive and specific for features of CNS infection. Contrast injection should be routine in suspected infection if there are no contraindications, and DWI (with high lesion to normal contrast and sensitivity) can be routinely added to conventional T1-, T2-weighted images, and FLAIR. High-resolution, thin-section 3D sequences such as constructive interference in steady state (CISS), fast imaging employing steady state acquisition (FIESTA), and FLAIR images allow visualization of small structures such as parasitic scolex, cranial nerves, and capsule wall details. MR angiography and venography can be included to assess ischemic and thrombotic complications. More recently, during the COVID-19 pandemic, susceptibility-weighted imaging (SWI) has been helpful to detect tiny focal microhaemorrhages.

Advanced MRI techniques including perfusion-weighted images (using DSC or ASL techniques) and MR spectroscopy may be helpful in problem-solving if used judiciously, especially since patients that are recalled after an initially ambiguous study can be hemodynamically unstable and require sedation or monitoring in the MRI suite. Point-of-care MRI using low-field scanners has shown promise. Radionuclide studies and PET have not been widely used in clinical practice although ^{18}F-fluorodeoxyglucose (^{18}F-FDG) typically reveals that infections generally have lower metabolic activity than tumours.

6.3   Meningitis

6.3.1   Imaging Features of Meningitis

In patients with suspected meningitis, CSF analysis after lumbar puncture (LP) is necessary to diagnose the responsible pathogen(s) and determine antimicrobial sensitivity for bacterial meningitis; imaging is adjunctive, but does not replace LP. Typical pyogenic bacteria result in neutrophilic pleocytosis, elevated protein, and low glucose (fungi cause very high opening pressure but normal glucose), and viruses usually cause lymphocytic pleocytosis and normal glucose. Acute lymphocytic meningitis of viral origin is usually benign and self-limited. Eosinophilic meningitis, defined by >10% eosinophil or >10 eosinophils per cubic millimetre of CSF, is typically a marker of helminthic parasite disease. Often, CT request to rule out raised intracranial pressure before an LP is the result of an abundance of caution, but this can also lead to a false sense of security.

CT typically shows diffuse cereal swelling, effaced subarachnoid spaces (especially basal cisterns), and dilated ventricles. Unenhanced MRI more sensitively shows the corresponding abnormal signal from elevated protein in infectious exudates as increased signal on FLAIR images or DWI (Fig. 6.1) [1, 2]. Sometimes, DWI may be the only images that detect subtle, tiny amounts of pus within the subarachnoid space and ventricles.

Gadolinium contrast extravasation into the subarachnoid space due to increased permeability of the blood–brain barrier, resulting in characteristic leptomeningeal enhancement in meningitis. This is visible particularly in the depth of cerebral sulci and cisterns, sometimes extending to the larger cranial nerve surfaces as either thin, linear serpentine enhancement (over cerebral convexity in typical viral/pyogenic bacterial meningitis) or thicker, irregular, nodular enhancement (often involving the basilar cisterns in tuberculous meningitis). The difference between leptomeningeal (extending into the sulcal depths and filling the subarachnoid spaces and cisterns) and pachymeningeal (thick "felt-tip pen" enhancement limited to the outer, dural surface either focally or diffusely) features can be seen in Fig. 6.2. Leptomeningeal enhancement is often better demonstrated using post-contrast 3D T2-FLAIR than conventional T1-weighted sequences (Fig. 6.3) [3].

6.3.2   Differential Diagnosis of Meningitis

On MRI, with its multiple different tissue characterisation on different pulse sequences, differential diagnosis can sometimes be difficult. Mimics of leptomeningitis include subarachnoid haemorrhage (which typically shows high signal on T1-weighted images and low signal on gradient-recalled echo/SWI), leptomeningeal carcinomatosis, administration of oxygen and drugs. Differentials for pachymeningeal enhancement include post-surgery and post-LP states, spontaneous intracranial hypotension, non-infectious granulomatous diseases, and tumours.

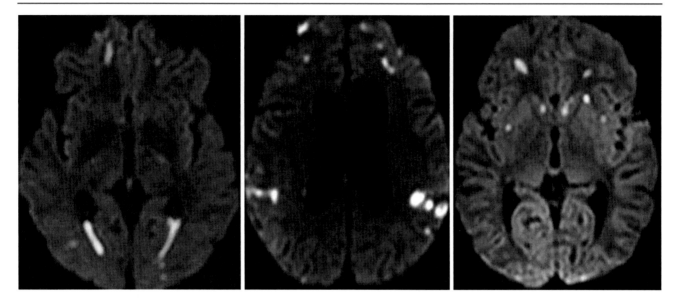

Fig. 6.1 Diffusion-weighted MRI abnormalities in meningitis. (Reprinted with permission from Thurnher, M.M., Sundgren, P.C. (2020). Intracranial Infection and Inflammation. In: Hodler, J., Kubik-Huch, R., von Schulthess, G. (eds) Diseases of the Brain, Head and Neck, Spine 2020–2023. IDKD Springer Series. Springer, Cham)

Key Points

- Post-contrast 3D T2-FLAIR is very sensitive for infectious leptomeningitis.
- Leptomeningitis and pachymeningitis show different enhancement patterns.
- Hyperintensity on DWI is sensitive to tiny amounts of pus and is characteristic in untreated pyogenic abscess.
- Radiologists should search for causes and complications of meningitis; MRA and MRV may be helpful.

6.3.3   Causes and Complications of Meningitis

On MRI, features of causes and complications of meningitis should be sought. Of the main routes of infectious spread, direct inoculation from traumatic or iatrogenic injury/surgical interventions is often visible. Local extension into the cranium from adjacent sinusitis, otitis media/mastoiditis, dental, head and neck infection should be included in the radiological search pattern, as well as along cranial nerves. However, the most common source of spread is via hematogenous route, and a high index of suspicion is needed in patients with a clinical history of immunosuppression, diabetes, alcoholism, congenital heart disease, pulmonary arteriovenous malformation or abscess, intravenous drug use, or bacterial endocarditis.

The most important complication of meningitis is cerebral abscess (see Sect. 6.4.1), which represents an important change in management often resulting in surgical referral for drainage for large lesions. Extra-axial fluid collections may also be seen, representing sterile subdural effusions or purulent empyema (which demonstrate diffusion restriction like cerebral abscess); empyema can be life-threatening and should be surgically drained. Hydrocephalus can result from disturbed CSF resorption or mass lesions compressing normal drainage pathways and if severe, can lead to brain herniation; this is especially important in tuberculous meningitis. Vascular complications including venous sinus thrombosis, vasculitic occlusion, and subsequent infarction, typically result from syphilis, tuberculosis, and angioinvasive aspergillosis (see Sect. 6.6.3).

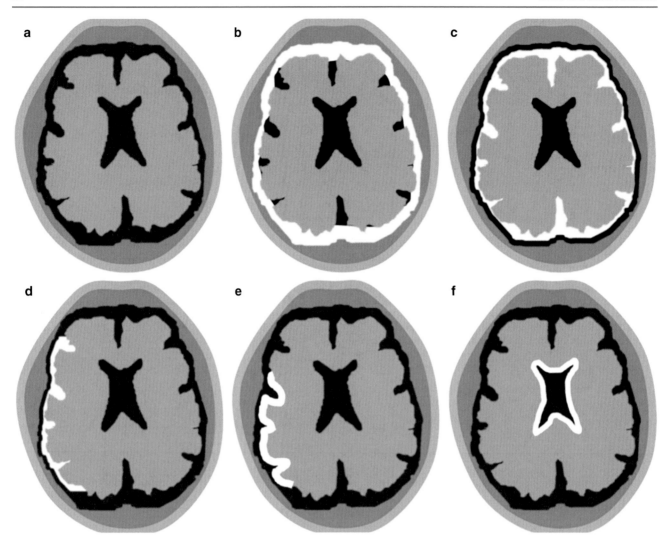

Fig. 6.2 Patterns of meningeal contrast enhancement (white outlines). Normal meninges (**a**). Diffuse pachymeningeal (**b**). Diffuse leptomeningeal (**c**) and localized leptomeningeal (**d**). Gyriform cortical (**e**). Ependymal (**f**). (Reprinted with permission from Duong MT, Rudie JD, Mohan S. Neuroimaging Patterns of Intracranial Infections: Meningitis, Cerebritis, and Their Complications. Neuroimaging Clin N Am. 2023 Feb;33(1):11–41)

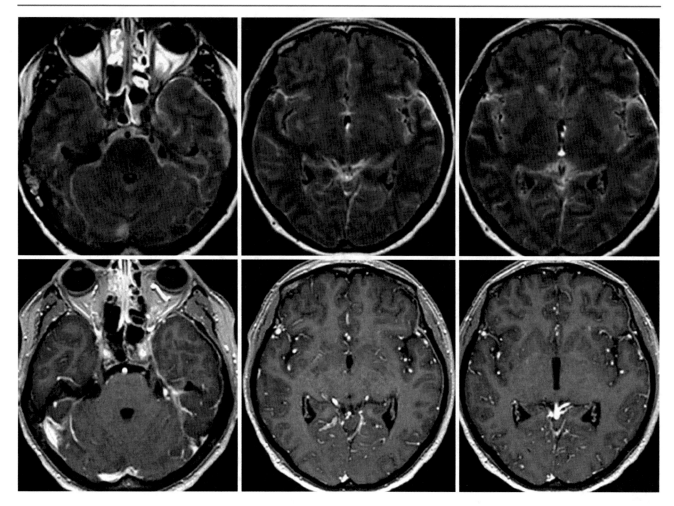

Fig. 6.3 Superiority of post-contrast 3D T2-FLAIR (top row) to post-contrast T1WI (bottom row) in the detection of leptomeningeal enhancement. (Reprinted with permission from Thurnher, M.M., Sundgren, P.C. (2020). Intracranial Infection and Inflammation. In: Hodler, J., Kubik-Huch, R., von Schulthess, G. (eds) Diseases of the Brain, Head and Neck, Spine 2020–2023. IDKD Springer Series. Springer, Cham)

6.4 Brain Abscess

6.4.1 MRI Features of Diagnosis of Brain Abscess

Mature pyogenic brain abscesses have a characteristic MRI appearance. There is typically central high signal with a smooth, thin, circumferential low-signal capsule on T2-weighted images (central low signal with high-signal rim on T1-weighted images), and prominent ring-like enhancement with surrounding white matter T2 prolongation from vasogenic oedema. If cerebral abscesses are introduced via hematogenous spread, they are typically located at the grey–white junction within middle cerebral artery territories bilaterally. Although abscess is preceded by cerebritis (poorly defined brain inflammation with increased vascular permeability but without capsular neovascularization or angiogenesis), this is rarely detected by imaging studies. Left untreated, a vascularized, collagenous capsule forms and is accompanied by a central abscess cavity of purulent exudate and surrounding vasogenic oedema.

On DWI, diffusion restriction is the hallmark feature of untreated pyogenic abscesses: proteinaceous, purulent debris comprising bacterial and inflammatory exudate have high viscosity, showing high signal on DWI and low signal on ADC maps (this feature can be useful to distinguish abscess from necrotic high-grade glioma, which typically do not show diffusion restriction) (Fig. 6.4). This feature becomes less prominent after antibiotic treatment. Usually, the medial or ventricular wall is thinner than the lateral wall due to poorer blood supply, and predisposes to rupture into the ventricle, causing ventriculitis. SWI sometimes shows the "dual rim sign" of concentric circles (hypointense outer layer and hyperintense inner layer), which may be incomplete.

MR spectroscopic profile of pyogenic abscess includes peaks representing branched chain amino acids valine, leucine, isoleucine (at 0.9 ppm), and succinate (2.4 ppm). In anaerobic abscesses, elevated acetate (1.9 ppm) is often seen (Fig. 6.5).

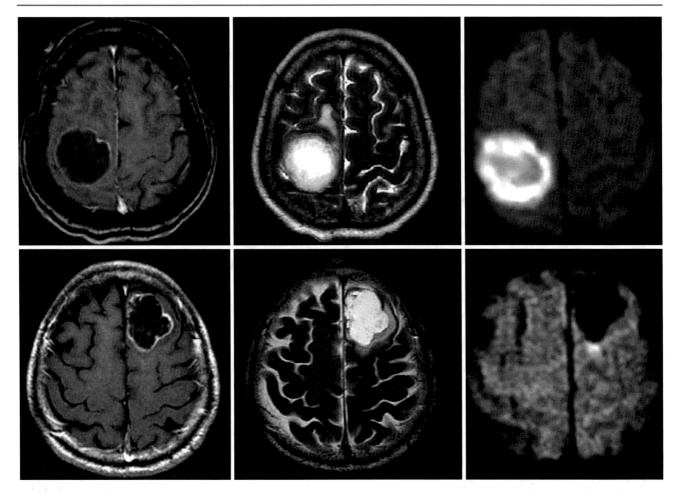

Fig. 6.4 DWI in cerebral abscess. Post-contrast T1-weighted and T2-weighted images are similar in a patient with cerebral abscess (top row) and another patient with metastatic cancer (bottom row). On DWI, high signal in the abscess cavity is distinguishable from low signal in metastasis

6.4.2 Differential Diagnosis of Ring Enhancing Lesions

Problem-solving in the assessment of ring enhancing lesions can benefit from history (immunocompromise, endemic/travel history, primary cancer), physical examination (fever), imaging features (incomplete ring, multiplicity, shape, and location), and advanced MRI techniques. Although MR spectroscopy can show elevated choline (at 3.2 pm) in neoplasms, necrotic tumours with predominant lipid and lactate peaks (at 1.3 ppm) may not be easily distinguishable. Decreased perfusion is usually seen in the central cavity and capsule; rarely, high rCBV may be seen in the vascularized abscess capsule, mimicking neoplasia; especially in granulomatous disease, which can mimic neoplasia on advanced MRI techniques. A combined approach with multidisciplinary team conference would be most helpful for management decision-making.

Key Points
- Differential diagnosis of ring enhancing lesions.
  - Pyogenic abscess.
  - Tuberculoma/tuberculous abscess.
  - Fungal abscess.
  - Toxoplasmosis.
  - Parasites (especially neurocysticercosis, see Sect. 6.5.1).
  - Metastatic tumour.
  - Primary glioma, lymphoma.
  - Subacute infarct.
  - Contusion/hematoma.
  - Demyelination.

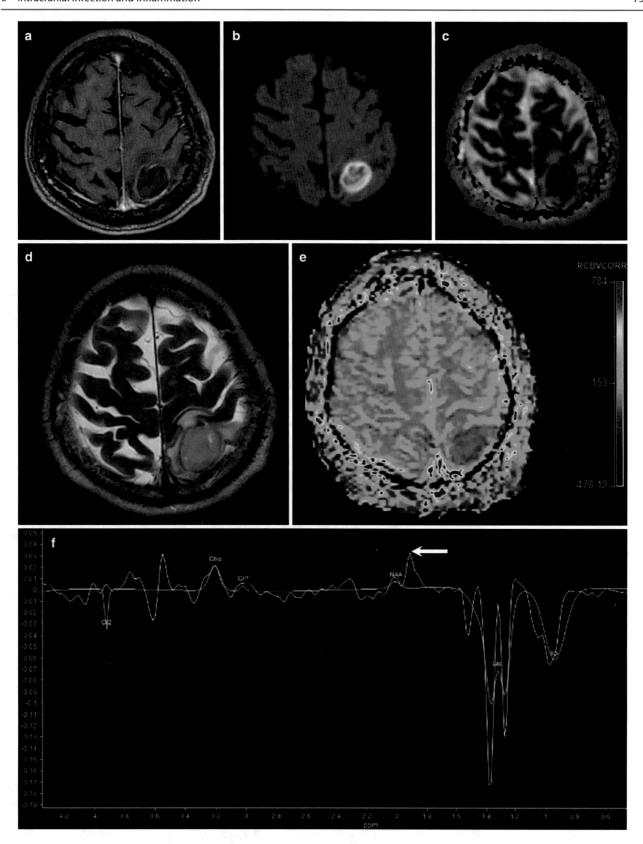

Fig. 6.5 Advanced MRI in cerebral abscess. Post-contrast T1-weighted image shows typical ring enhancement (**a**), with increased signal on DWI (**b**) and decreased ADC (**c**) and mixed increased signal on T2-weighted images (**d**). Perfusion MRI (blue in **e**) shows decreased relative cerebral volume in both the cavity and walls. MR spectroscopy (**f**) with long echo time of 144 ms shows low choline (Cho, 3.2 ppm), creatine (Cr, 3.0 ppm), N-acetyl aspartate (NAA, 2.0 ppm), and a large inverted W lactate (Lac, 1.4 ppm) and lipid (0.9 ppm) peaks. Note the acetate peak (arrow) at 1.9 ppm which is the anaerobic breakdown product of NAA

6.5 Parasitic Diseases

Although unicellular (amoeba, toxoplasmosis, see Sect. 6.6.1) and multicellular (helminths such as schistosomiasis) parasites are uncommon in the developed world, these are important diseases in endemic areas and can be seen with increasing frequency due to travel and migration. Common features of helminthic infection include eosinophilia and differing features according to parasite life cycle.

6.5.1 Neurocysticercosis

Cysticercal infection is endemic in many parts of Asia, Africa, and Central/South America, and CNS cysticercosis is the commonest cause of seizures and CSF eosinophilia worldwide. Four classic stages can be seen; the vesicular stage typically shows a non-enhancing cyst which is iso-signal to CSF, with a T2 hypointense, FLAIR hyperintense, and enhancing scolex visible on high-resolution thin-section 3D MRI FLAIR/CISS sequences. The vesicular-colloidal stage (Fig. 6.6) results in complex increased cyst signal on T1-weighted and FLAIR images with ring enhancement and surrounding oedema (often mimicking abscess or metastasis, unless concomitant non-enhancing vesicular cysts or non-enhancing calcific nodular stages are recognized during visual search). The cyst becomes smaller during the granular nodular stages with signal changes from calcification; the final non-enhancing calcific nodular stage shows mineralization without surrounding oedema (Fig. 6.7).

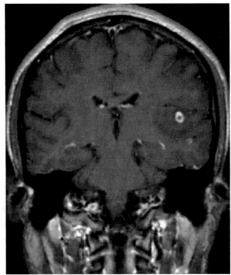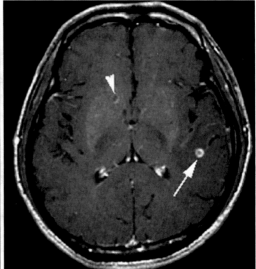

Fig. 6.6 Neurocysticercosis: Post-contrast T1-weighted images shows a ring enhancing left temporal lobe vesicular-colloidal cyst with surrounding vasogenic oedema (arrow). A second, non-enhancing vesicular lesion without oedema is seen in the right basal ganglia (arrowhead)

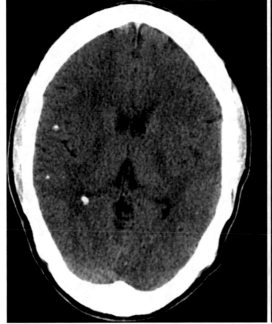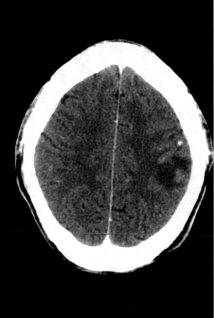

Fig. 6.7 Unenhanced CT shows an isodense left frontal lobe lesion surrounded by vasogenic oedema. Multiple concomitant chronic calcific nodular lesions are seen in the rest of the brain, consistent with neurocysticercosis infection in different stages

6.6   HIV Infection and Specific Organisms

HIV positive patients can present with a wide range of complications, including opportunistic infections, lymphoma, progressive multifocal leukoencephalopathy (PML, see Sect. 6.7.3), CD8 encephalitis, and immune reconstitution inflammatory syndrome (IRIS) [4]. IRIS is caused by an intense, dysregulated inflammatory immune response in situations with a combination of successful antiretroviral therapy (ART), improving CD4 and decreasing viral load. There is paradoxical worsening of clinical and imaging features, accompanied by florid enhancement on MRI. The clinical course of IRIS is usually self-limiting, but radiologists should first rule out new opportunistic infection, drug toxicity, and other complications.

> **Key Points**
> - Patients living with HIV can present with opportunistic infections, primary HIV infection, inflammatory reactions, and treatment effects.
> - Opportunistic infectious agents include toxoplasma, JC virus (PML), cryptococcus, cytomegalovirus, tuberculosis, and varicella zoster virus.
> - Primary HIV infection can result in acute meningoencephalitis, acute inflammatory demyelinating polyneuropathy (AIDP), chronic inflammatory demyelinating polyneuropathy (CIDP), HIV-associated neurocognitive disorder (HAND), myelitis, and cerebrovascular disease.

6.6.1   Toxoplasmosis

Toxoplasmosis is the most frequent opportunistic infection in patients with HIV. MRI typically shows multifocal enhancing nodules in the basal ganglia or frontoparietal regions with vasogenic oedema and sometimes haemorrhage. Although the "eccentric target sign" has high specificity (but can also be seen in tuberculoma and metastasis), unfortunately it is not very sensitive (Fig. 6.8).

6.6.2   Aspergillosis

Immunocompromised patients (not only in HIV infection but also in transplantation etc) are prone to angioinvasive aspergillosis, which can occlude the perforating arteries and result in basal ganglia, thalamic or brainstem infarction, sometimes with blood products.

6.6.3   Tuberculosis

CNS tuberculosis (TB) can affect patients with and without HIV infection: TB remains one of the major causes of mortality and morbidity worldwide and is an especially important health threat for people living with HIV. TB meningitis results in especially florid enhancement with infection especially often involving the basilar cisterns (Fig. 6.9) and can be associated with dural thickening and enhancement from concomitant pachymeningitis (TB is more common than syphilis or Lyme disease in causing both leptomeningeal and pachymeningeal infection). TB vasculitis can occlude the

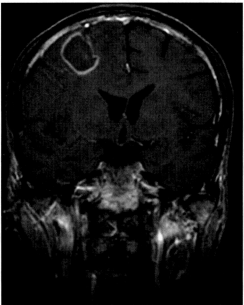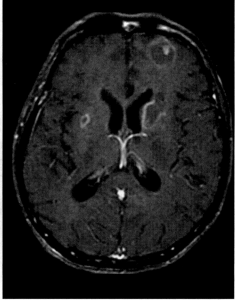

Fig. 6.8 Toxoplasmosis: Post-contrast T1-weighted images showing characteristic eccentric target sign of enhancement

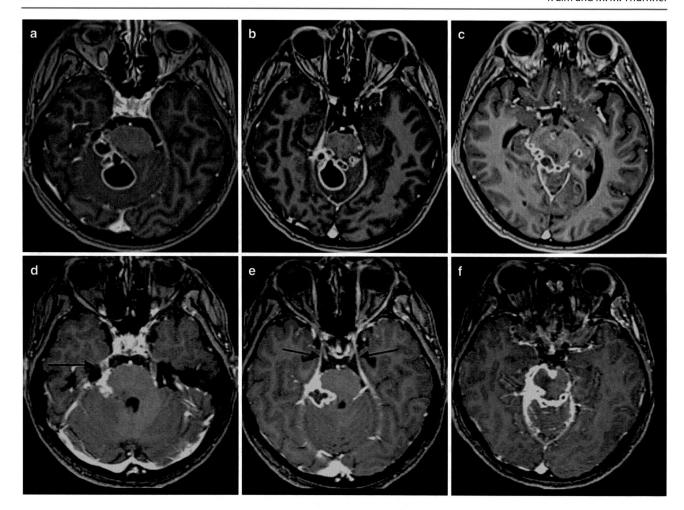

Fig. 6.9 Proven tuberculous meningitis with multiple ring enhancing tuberculomas in the basal cistern (**a–c**). With disease progression, there was perineural spread with thickened and enhancing cranial nerves (**d–f**, red arrows) (Reprinted with permission from Thurnher, M.M., Sundgren, P.C. (2020). Intracranial Infection and Inflammation. In: Hodler, J., Kubik-Huch, R., von Schulthess, G. (eds) Diseases of the Brain, Head and Neck, Spine 2020–2023. IDKD Springer Series. Springer, Cham)

small medial lenticulostriate and thalamo-perforating branches, resulting in basal ganglia and thalamus infarctions. These can be sensitively demonstrated using DWI, and MRA or black blood, high-resolution, thin-section 3D black blood, black CSF vessel wall imaging (VWI) (Fig. 6.10) sequences can reveal narrowed enhancing vasculitic vessels (other infectious causes of vasculitis include aspergillosis and varicella zoster virus (VZV) infection).

Tuberculoma is the most common parenchymal form of CNS; imaging appearances depend on the different stages of infection; and tuberculomas heal by resolving or calcifying. Early, non-caseating tuberculomas show homogenous, nodular enhancement with low signal on T1-weighted images and high signal on T2-weighted images, and surrounding oedema. Solid caseating tuberculomas show variable signal intensity due to paramagnetic free radicals. Liquifying caseating tuberculomas resemble pyogenic abscess in signal and enhancing characteristics but are typically smaller with less surrounding oedema. Tuberculous abscesses are rarer, larger, multilocu-

lated and are often indistinguishable from pyogenic abscess. Miliary TB with innumerable small enhancing lesions at the grey-white matter junction typically occurs in immunocompromised patients with widespread extracranial disease. Spinal cord/meningeal TB, including osteomyelitis/disc infection, and psoas abscess, should also be sought.

Key Points
- Characteristic complications of tuberculosis.
  - Thick leptomeningeal enhancement affecting basal cisterns.
  - Hydrocephalus.
  - Tuberculomas.
  - Tuberculous abscesses.
  - Vasculitic stenosis/beading and infarction (especially basal ganglia/thalamus).
  - Cranial nerve enhancement and pachymeningitis.

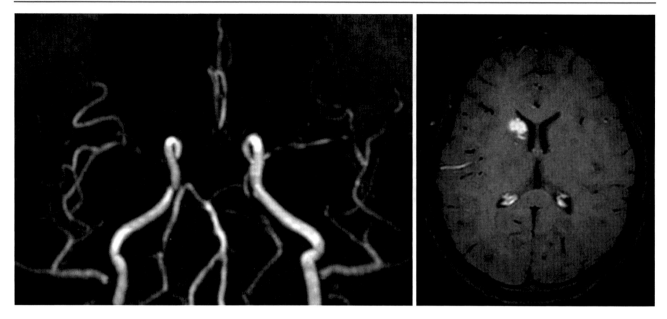

Fig. 6.10 Tuberculous vasculitis: Time-of-flight MR angiography shows signal dropout in the right worse than left middle cerebral artery (MCA). Contrast-enhanced black blood, black CSF vessel wall imag- ing shows linear enhancing vessel wall from vasculitis of the MCA branch artery, and enhancing subacute infarction of the right caudate nucleus

6.7 Viral Infections

6.7.1 Herpes Simplex Virus

HSV-1 is the commonest cause of acute encephalitis syndrome, comprising 10–20% of identifiable viruses. Typical findings include unilateral or bilateral asymmetric swelling and hyperintensity on T2-weighted/FLAIR images, affecting hippocampus, anterior and medial temporal lobes and insular cortex (but often sparing the basal ganglia) (Fig. 6.11). There is sometimes haemorrhage, DWI restriction, and contrast enhancement (compared to autoimmune encephalitis, see Sect. 6.8.1).

> **Key Points**
> - Many viral causes of encephalitis have yet to be identified.
> - HSV-1 is the commonest virus and affects the hippocampus/temporal lobe.
> - LGI1 antibody limbic encephalitis often mimics HSV-1 infection.
> - Many arboviruses affect the thalamus bilaterally, sometimes with blood products.
> - Varicella zoster virus is a major cause of vasculopathy and stroke in children.

6.7.2 Arboviruses and Other Viruses

Arthropod-borne pathogens are spread by mosquitos, ticks, or other vectors. They include Japanese encephalitis virus (JEV), dengue virus (DENV), and Zika viruses and typically have geographic and seasonal variability. In patients with bilateral thalamic involvement (especially with haemorrhage), JEV and influenza-associated encephalitis (IAE) should be considered (Fig. 6.12). IAE is most common in children under 5 years of age, the elderly, and patients with co-morbidities. Enterovirus and rabies virus infections can involve the brainstem; VZV infection is a major cause of vasculopathy and ischemic stroke in children.

6.7.3 Progressive Multifocal Leukoencephalopathy

Progressive multifocal leukoencephalopathy (PML) is a demyelinating disease caused by reactivation of JC virus (a polyomavirus) infection in immunocompromised patients, especially people living with HIV. Typical features are bilateral asymmetric frontal or/and parietooccipital subcortical U fibre white matter involvement (very rarely is periventricular white matter affected first); the middle cerebellar peduncle, pons, peri-dentate white matter may also be affected, but isolated spinal cord lesions are rare. Classic PML is typically hyperintense on T2-weighted and FLAIR images, low or iso-

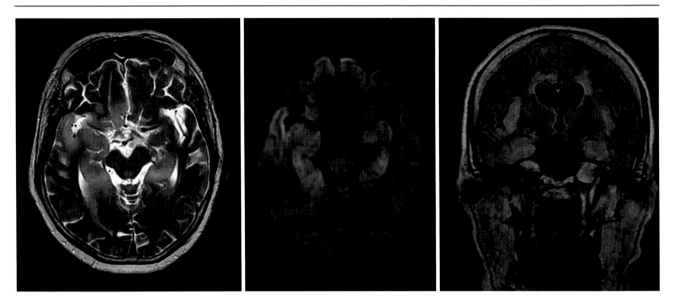

Fig. 6.11 Herpes simplex virus type 1: bilateral asymmetric (worse on the right) swelling and increased signal on T2-weighted, DWI, and FLAIR images involving the medial temporal lobe (especially the hippocampus) and insula cortex (see Fig. 6.15 for comparison)

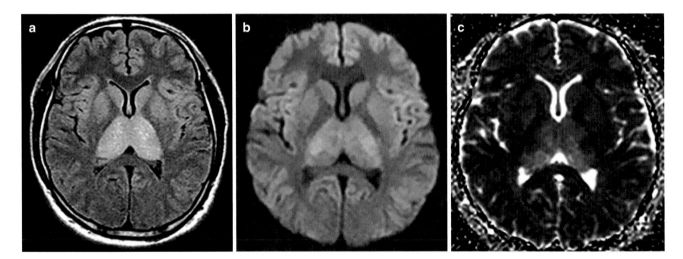

Fig. 6.12 Japanese encephalitis (**a**) FLAIR image shows bilateral symmetric high-signal lesions in the thalamus. (**b**, **c**). Most of the lesions show high signal on DWI and mixed ADC values. (Reprinted with permission from Ramli NM, Bae YJ. Structured Imaging Approach for Viral Encephalitis. Neuroimaging Clin N Am. 2023 Feb;33(1):43–56)

signal on T1-weighted images, without enhancement, vasogenic oedema, or mass effect (Fig. 6.13). DWI appearances vary according to stage of disease, with restricted diffusion in newer lesions or the advancing edge of active infection/ demyelination. Inflammatory PML (with enhancement, vasogenic oedema, and mass effect) is a less common presenting phenotype or may be visualized in IRIS.

Fig. 6.13 Progressive multifocal leukoencephalopathy: T2-weighted images before (left) and after (right) antiretroviral therapy showing reduced extent of high signal in the subcortical white matter

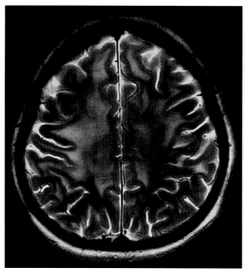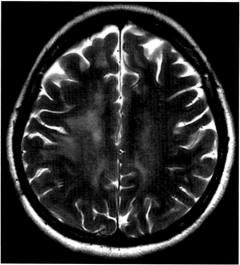

6.8   Inflammatory Diseases of the CNS

Immune-mediated inflammatory diseases of the CNS (Fig. 6.14) may be encountered by radiologists in patients with known cancer (paraneoplastic syndromes), in patients with known rheumatological diseases (e.g. systemic lupus erythematosus SLE, Sjogren's disease), in patients after a viral infection (e.g. acute disseminated encephalomyelitis or ADEM), and finally as mimics of infection based on typical MRI patterns [5, 6]. Many of the imaging patterns of leptomeningitis, pachymeningitis, encephalitis, or vascular disease, described in the preceding sections of this chapter may also be caused by non-infectious inflammation. Familiarity with these inflammatory mimics may help diminish morbidity and future disability by facilitating appropriate treatments early, avoiding invasive brain biopsy, and triggering appropriate CT of the chest, abdomen, and pelvis to screen for underlying cancer or sarcoidosis.

6.8.1   Autoimmune and Limbic Encephalitis: LGI1 Antibody Encephalitis

The cause of acute encephalitis syndrome can be either infective or noninfective. Clinically, limbic encephalitis often presents with anterograde memory loss, seizures, behavioural or psychiatric symptoms, with MRI abnormalities affecting the hippocampus and medial temporal lobes bilaterally. Leucine-rich glioma inactivated 1 (LGI1) antibody is the commonest cause of limbic encephalitis mimicking HSV-1 infection (Fig. 6.15). Fever, a fulminant clinical course, unilateral involvement, absence of basal ganglia involvement, DWI restriction, and contrast enhancement, all favour HSV-1. Other autoimmune encephalitis is less consistent in their imaging appearance; MRI in NMDA receptor encephalitis is more often normal, white matter abnormalities in MS, ADEM and MOG may mimic PML, and bilateral caudate and putamen abnormalities may be seen in anti-CV2/collapsin response mediator protein 5 (CRMP5) antibodies in occult small cell lung cancer. Brainstem, cerebellar, and spinal cord lesions are also associated with multiple autoimmune pathologies.

6.8.2   Leptomeningeal Enhancement: Neurosarcoidosis

This multisystem inflammatory granulomatous disease has a predilection to affect the leptomeninges (50%, especially basal meninges, mimicking TB), pituitary gland, optic and facial cranial nerves, and spinal meninges (Fig. 6.16). Differentiation of neurosarcoidosis from TB can be difficult or impossible by imaging alone.

> **Key Points**
> - Neurosarcoidosis can affect different brain/spine compartments and mimics tuberculosis.
> - Focal pachymeningeal disease can be caused by TB, syphilis, Lyme disease, sarcoidosis, IgG4-related disease, antineutrophil cytoplasmic antibody associated (ANCA), and tumours such as meningioma or metastasis.
> - Autoimmune CNS vasculitis has variable, often nonspecific imaging findings.
> - Many antibodies in paraneoplastic and immune-mediated inflammatory diseases have yet to be identified.

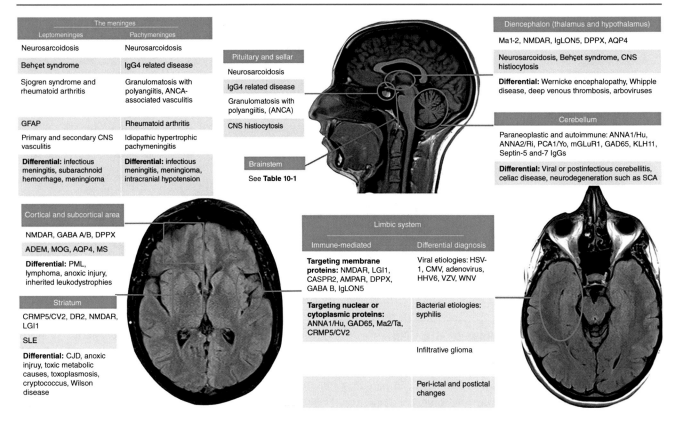

Fig. 6.14 Autoimmune and inflammatory central nervous system (CNS) disorders and radiographic differential diagnoses based on typical location. (Reprinted with permission from Wahed LA, Cho TA. Imaging of Central Nervous System Autoimmune, Paraneoplastic, and Neuro-rheumatologic Disorders. Continuum (Minneap Minn). 2023 Feb 1;29(1):255–291)

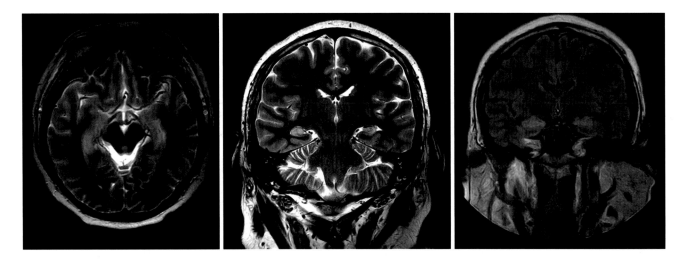

Fig. 6.15 LGI1 antibody encephalitis. Axial and coronal T2-weighted and FLAIR images showing bilateral symmetrical swelling and increased signal in the hippocampus (see Fig. 6.11 for comparison)

6.8.3 Pachymeningeal Enhancement: IgG4-Related Diseases

IgG4-related disease is a multisystem chronic progressive fibroinflammatory autoimmune disease; as the disease definition is updated, some conditions are now felt to overlap with IgG4 related spectrum of disease, including orbital pseudotumor. Commonly, IgG4 disease affects the pancreas, biliary tract, kidneys, retroperitoneum/aorta, and thorax. In the head and neck (second commonest site of presentation after the pancreas), the salivary (especially submandibular), lacrimal, and pituitary glands may be affected, and localized

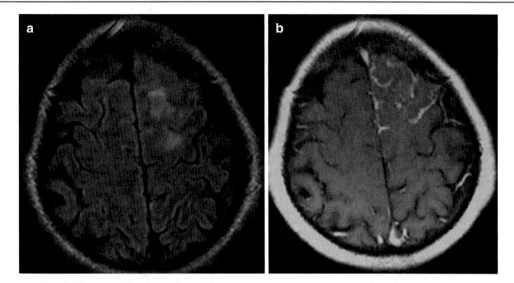

Fig. 6.16 Axial FLAIR (**a**) and T1-weighted post-contrast administration (**b**) demonstrate diffuse, focal, increased FLAIR signal in the underlying brain parenchyma and focal left-sided leptomeningeal enhancement in a patient with neurosarcoidosis. (Reprinted with permission from Thurnher, M.M., Sundgren, P.C. (2020). Intracranial Infection and Inflammation. In: Hodler, J., Kubik-Huch, R., von Schulthess, G. (eds) Diseases of the Brain, Head and Neck, Spine 2020–2023. IDKD Springer Series. Springer, Cham)

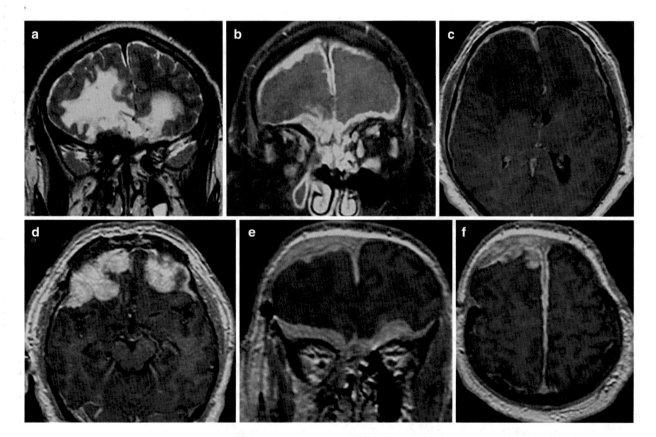

Fig. 6.17 Thick, dural enhancement is observed bilaterally frontally and along the falx (**b–f**). T2-high-signal intensity is also seen in the parenchyma of both frontal lobes, reflecting compression of the brain parenchyma (**a**) (Reprinted with permission from Thurnher, M.M., Sundgren, P.C. (2020). Intracranial Infection and Inflammation. In: Hodler, J., Kubik-Huch, R., von Schulthess, G. (eds) Diseases of the Brain, Head and Neck, Spine 2020–2023. IDKD Springer Series. Springer, Cham)

or diffuse pachymeningeal thickening and enhancement can be seen (Fig. 6.17). Tissue biopsy is the gold standard for diagnosis but MRI typically shows low signal on both T1- and T2-weighted images, with homogeneous enhancement; remission after steroid therapy (in almost 90%) can be a helpful feature.

6.8.4 Autoimmune CNS Vasculitis

Cerebral vessel walls are inflamed in CNS vasculitis, which can be caused by primary angiitis of the CNS, or can be secondary to underlying systemic vasculitis (such as SLE, rheumatoid arthritis, and Sjogren's disease), or secondary to infections (such as TB, VZV, or syphilis). MRI is nearly always abnormal, and a normal study can exclude vasculitis. Typical findings include infarcts of different ages in different arterial territories (Fig. 6.18), sometimes accompanied by parenchymal or subarachnoid blood. DSA is more sensitive than MRA and CTA in detecting "beading"; alternating stenosis and dilatation in at least two separate vascular distributions, but findings often not specific for the cause. Concentric wall thickening favours vasculitis over atherosclerosis (which tends to show eccentric thickening) on VWI but is also not specific for the type of vasculitis. Diagnosis often depends on biopsy.

6.8.4.1 Autoimmune CNS Vasculitis

Granulomatosis with polyangiitis (GPA)(previously called Wegener's granulomatosis) is a systemic vasculitis of small and medium vessels and can rarely affect the CNS, characterized by high mortality. MRI typically shows focal granulomas spreading from the frontal sinus, leptomeningeal contrast enhancement, and white matter hyperintensities (Fig. 6.19).

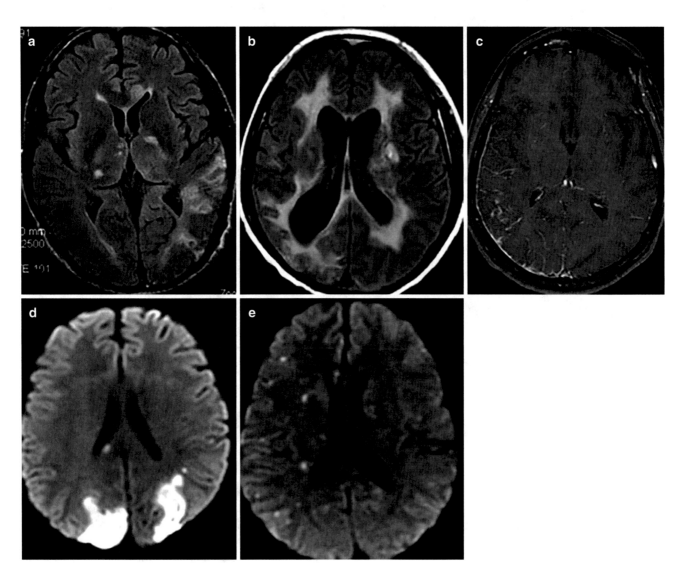

Fig. 6.18 Different imaging findings in patients with known vasculitis; (**a**) hyperintense FLAIR lesions, (**b**) confluent white matter signal abnormalities, (**c**) leptomeningeal contrast enhancement, (**d**) cortical infracts, (**e**) multiple acute lacunar infarcts (Reprinted with permission from Thurnher, M.M., Sundgren, P.C. (2020). Intracranial Infection and Inflammation. In: Hodler, J., Kubik-Huch, R., von Schulthess, G. (eds) Diseases of the Brain, Head and Neck, Spine 2020–2023. IDKD Springer Series. Springer, Cham)

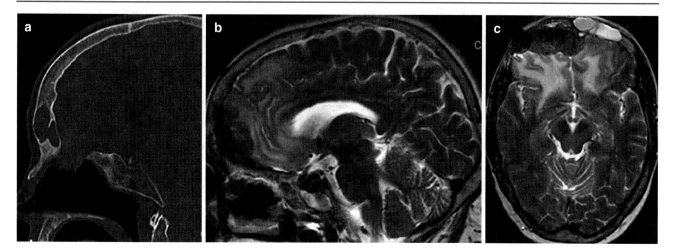

Fig. 6.19 (**a**) Sagittal CT (bone window) demonstrates opacification of the frontal sinus. (**b**, **c**) Granuloma extension into the frontal lobes bilaterally with surrounding oedema and gliosis (Reprinted with permission from Thurnher, M.M., Sundgren, P.C. (2020). Intracranial Infection and Inflammation. In: Hodler, J., Kubik-Huch, R., von Schulthess, G. (eds) Diseases of the Brain, Head and Neck, Spine 2020–2023. IDKD Springer Series. Springer, Cham)

6.9 Concluding Remarks

Radiologists should be aware of the three characteristic imaging patterns in meningitis, abscess, and encephalitis. Clinical problem-solving based on MRI pattern recognition remains a fundamental skillset: our knowledge of typical features and their anatomical distribution enables us to process new data in novel infectious/inflammatory agents considering past differential diagnosis. Conventional and advanced MRI techniques and new point-of-care scanners have the potential to improve diagnostic performance in CNS infections, especially in future outbreaks and pandemics (Fig. 6.20) [7]. Future advances in PCR technology, machine learning, and new MRI biomarkers hold great promise for elucidating the pathogen and immune-mediated mechanisms of neuronal damage and complications. The role and value of radiologists are enhanced by multidisciplinary team discussions, because "No man is an island"; we do not work in isolation, all of us are an essential part of the healthcare teams.

Take-Home Messages
- Multimodal MRI, including post-contrast 3D T2-FLAIR, DWI, SWI, and vessel wall imaging is useful for problem-solving.
- Although CNS infection typically presents with characteristic patterns of meningitis, abscess, HSV-1 encephalitis, it is important to remember their mimics and differentiating features.
- Restricted diffusion on DWI has high sensitivity and specificity for meningitis and pyogenic abscess, respectively.
- HSV-1 infection and LGI1-antibody encephalitis can both cause medial temporal and hippocampal abnormalities.
- Specific infectious agents including HIV and TB may have characteristic MRI appearances and complications.

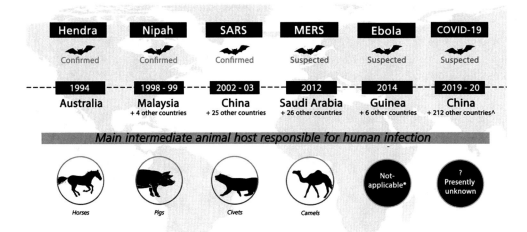

Fig. 6.20 Summary of major emerging zoonotic outbreaks related to bats, 1994–2019. Confirmed bat-borne viruses include Hendra, Nipah, and SARS-CoV-1 viruses; bats are also suspected to be viral reservoirs for MERS, Ebola, and SARS-CoV-2 (cause of the current COVID-19 pandemic) viruses. Years when outbreaks occurred and confirmed or suspected intermediate hosts involved in virus spillover are also shown. *Indicates that although the 2014 Ebola outbreak was believed to have started with direct bat-to-human transmission, nonhuman primates have been implicated in previous Ebola outbreaks. ^Data accurate as of May 11, 2020. (Reprinted with permission of Duke-NUS Medical School)

References

1. Thurnher MM, Sundgren PC. Intracranial infection and inflammation. In: Hodler J, Kubik-Huch R, von Schulthess G, editors. Diseases of the brain, head and neck, spine 2020–2023, IDKD Springer Series. Cham: Springer; 2020.
2. Thurnher MM. Bacterial infections. In: Barkhof F, Jäger R, Thurnher M, Rovira A, editors. Clinical neuroradiology. Berlin: Springer; 2019.
3. Duong MT, Rudie JD, Mohan S. Neuroimaging patterns of intracranial infections: meningitis, cerebritis, and their complications. Neuroimaging Clin N Am. 2023;33(1):11–41.
4. Thurnher MM. Infections in immunocompromised patients. In: Barkhof F, Jäger R, Thurnher M, Rovira A, editors. Clinical neuroradiology. Berlin: Springer; 2019.
5. Graus F, Titulaer MJ, Balu R, et al. A clinical approach to diagnosis of autoimmune encephalitis. Lancet Neurol. 2016;15:391–404.
6. Wahed LA, Cho TA. Imaging of central nervous system autoimmune, paraneoplastic, and neuro-rheumatologic disorders. Continuum (Minneap Minn). 2023;29(1):255–91.
7. Goh GX, Tan K, Ang BSP, Wang L-F, Tchoyoson Lim CC. Neuroimaging in zoonotic outbreaks affecting the central nervous system: are we fighting the last war? Am J Neuroradiol. 2020;41:1760–7.

Neuroimaging Update on Traumatic Brain Injury

Apostolos J. Tsiouris and Yvonne W. Lui

Abstract

Traumatic brain injury is a common injury worldwide that affects individuals of all ages. Injuries can range in severity. Timely assessment of injury is important to triage cases that may be severe and imminently life-threatening, and neuroimaging is a critical component to the clinical care of such patients. Injuries may occur in multiple spaces from the extracranial soft tissues to the potential spaces between meningeal layers to the brain parenchyma itself. The neck and intracranial arterial and venous vessels can also be injured with devastating sequelae. CT, CTA, MRI, and MRA can all be useful in the assessment of head injury. In particular, CT is often used as a first-line imaging modality to screen for acute intracranial injury. MRI can be useful in patients who have discordance between symptoms and CT findings as well as in those with more prolonged symptoms or who suffer chronic sequelae of injury. Neuroimaging research is ongoing using MRI to study the underlying pathophysiology of head injury.

Keywords

Head trauma · Brain injury · CT · MRI

Learning Objectives
- Review imaging techniques used to help diagnose and evaluate patients with CNS trauma.
- Compare the utility of CT vs MRI in evaluating TBI patients with a spectrum of brain injuries.
- Show various forms of surgical vs non-surgical intracranial abnormalities resulting from head trauma.

Key Points
- CT is the primary imaging modality utilized to assess patients following CNS trauma in the urgent setting due to availability, speed, and few contraindications.
- Initial CT findings can assist in the appropriate triage of patients that require urgent surgical management and those that would benefit from non-surgical monitoring.
- MRI is useful in patients who suffer from neurologic symptoms out of proportion to initial CT imaging findings and to assist in the detection of brain injuries below the sensitivity of CT.

7.1 Introduction

Traumatic brain injury (TBI) is a leading health concern with approximately 2.8 million reported emergency department visits in 2014 in the United States. Of these, there is an estimated 288,000 TBI-related hospitalizations and 56,800 TBI-related deaths [1]. The majority of these cases involve elderly adults over age 75 years followed by young children [2] with a global incidence estimate of 100–749 cases per 100,000 [3]. These staggering numbers are themselves likely to be

A. J. Tsiouris
Department of Radiology, New York-Presbyterian Hospital—Weill Cornell Medicine, New York, NY, USA
e-mail: apt9001@med.cornell.edu

Y. W. Lui (✉)
Department of Radiology, New York University Langone Health/ Grossman School of Medicine, New York, NY, USA
e-mail: Yvonne.lui@nyulangone.org

© The Author(s) 2024
J. Hodler et al. (eds.), *Diseases of the Brain, Head and Neck, Spine 2024-2027*, IDKD Springer Series, https://doi.org/10.1007/978-3-031-50675-8_7

underestimates as mild severity TBI and head injury in developing areas of the world are generally under-reported and others are not counted among emergency room visits as they may be assessed in outpatient clinics. Regardless, medical imaging is crucial for diagnosis, management, and risk stratification of this important public health problem. This article provides an overview of important imaging findings for various TBI classifications as divided by anatomic location, types of injury, and severity as well as imaging findings of trauma-related intervention. Examples provided also showcase different mechanisms of injury and touch on imaging research in the field of TBI. Overall, this review aims to provide a systematic guide for imaging evaluation and interpretation in TBI-related injuries.

7.2   TBI Clinical Grading

Clinical grading for TBI most commonly uses the Glasgow Coma Scale (GCS), which separates injuries based on three main criteria: eye response (1–4 points), verbal response (1–5 points), and motor response (1–6 points) [4]. Scores are summed and then categorized as mild (13–15), moderate (9–12), and severe (3–8). GCS is shown to be highly correlative with patient morbidity and mortality in the moderate/severe category and helps with initial triage [5]. Despite widespread use across severity categories, GCS is limited in the mild category where a score of 15 does not necessarily indicate an absence of TBI-related symptoms or TBI-related injury. Mild TBI patients may have post-concussive symptoms that are typically self-limited without intervention, although a subgroup can suffer prolonged symptoms.

7.3   Imaging Use and Techniques

7.3.1   Computed Tomography (CT)

The essential initial imaging modality for head trauma is non-contrast computed tomography (CT). For moderate to severe TBI, the American College of Radiology (ACR) deems the non-contrast head CT scan a class 1 recommendation [6]. There are several, commonly used medical decision-making tools including the Canadian CT head rule, New Orleans Criteria, and National Emergency X-Radiography Utilization Study II (NEXUS-II) that help to determine whether a CT scan of the head is indicated in the case of mild TBI [7]. The Pediatric Emergency Care Applied Research Network (PECARN) Head Injury Decision Rule (PR) was published in 2009 by the Pediatric Emergency Care Applied Research Network; this rule is applied in pediatric patients to identify those at low risk for clinically important TBI, so that

CT scan can be safely avoided and therefore reduce exposure to ionizing radiation.

Benefits of CT over other imaging modalities include speed, availability, and high sensitivity for significant injuries requiring immediate intervention or close observation such as intracranial hemorrhage, infarction, herniation, cerebral edema, and skull fracture [8]. Modern CT scans can be performed within just a few seconds and are readily available at essentially all hospital systems on an emergent basis as well as many satellite care centers. The recommended protocol includes using a multidetector CT (MDCT) with axial views, head tilt/gantry angling to reduce ocular lens radiation exposure, 120 kVP, 240 mAs, 22 cm-field of view, with a 2.5- or 5-mm slice thickness. Radiation exposure and dose have been markedly diminished with advances in CT technology. Modern scanners incorporate the use of automatic exposure control systems to optimize acquisition parameters on an individual basis and advanced techniques for image reconstruction to maintain image quality. Typically, CT images are reconstructed and displayed in a multiplanar way using both soft tissue and bone kernels at ~2.5-mm slice thicknesses. Additional 3D reconstructions may also be performed for the calvarial/skull base with axial 0.625 mm sections. Routine use of multiplanar reconstructed (MPR) images has also been supported in the literature to increase CT accuracy in detecting intracranial hemorrhage, especially adjacent to bony surfaces [9]. Comparison with prior relevant imaging is useful to help accurately identify acute findings.

7.3.2   Magnetic Resonance Imaging (MRI)

MRI may be considered for patients with persistent neurologic symptoms but absence of positive findings on nonenhanced CT [10]. Compared with CT, MRI has higher sensitivity for detection of small cortical/parenchymal contusions, axonal injury, and can help age intracranial hemorrhage (acute, subacute, chronic) [6, 11–15]. However, emergent MRI is not as readily available in various hospital systems, takes longer to scan, costs more, requires safety screening prior to scanning, and gives rise to some difficulties in patient monitoring and access during the scan. Recommended routine scanning techniques for nonenhanced brain MRI in cases of head trauma include the following: diffusion-weighted (DWI), T2* gradient recall echo (GRE) or susceptibility-weighted imaging (SWI), T2-weighted fluid-attenuated inversion-recovery (FLAIR), and T2-weighted and T1-weighted sequences. Susceptibility-weighted imaging has been shown to have high sensitivity to hemorrhage, significantly higher than the traditional T2* GRE sequences [16], and DWI can be useful in detecting non-hemorrhagic acute axonal injury [17]. Contrast enhancement is not routinely used; however, contrast may be useful to assess arterial and venous vascular injury as well as other types of meningeal injury [18].

7.3.3 CT or MR Angiography (CTA or MRA)

CTA and MRA are recommended in cases with mechanism of penetrating injury and suspected vascular injury. Such techniques can help detect traumatic pseudoaneurysms, dissection, post-traumatic arteriovenous fistula, venous sinus thrombosis, or other vascular sequela of injury [19–21]. Some hemorrhage patterns on imaging may be signs of serious, underlying injuries such as subarachnoid blood isolated to the basilar cistern, sylvian fissure, or anterior interhemispheric fissures as described later.

7.3.4 Diffusion Tensor Imaging (DTI) and Diffusion Kurtosis Imaging (DKI)

More sophisticated diffusion imaging models including Diffusion Tensor Imaging (DTI) and Diffusion Kurtosis Imaging (DKI) that quantify directional diffusion of water [22] as well as non-Gaussian diffusion [23] can provide information about white matter tracts and other brain tissue microstructure. While diffusion tensor models have been utilized for group-based comparisons in the research arena, there are numerous barriers that have prevented their application in individual patients. For example, DTI has been shown to be very sensitive to axonal microstructural changes; however, the results lack specificity. Changes in mean diffusivity and/or fractional anisotropy may be interpreted as changes in the interrogated white matter microstructural integrity; however, these same types of changes can be visualized in any number of comorbidities or even demographic variation. As a result, accurate and meaningful interpretation of individual DTI examinations is not currently feasible.

7.3.5 Outcome Prediction with Imaging Parameters

Imaging is essential for patients to help with diagnosis, prognosis, and guiding management for various types of traumatic brain injuries. Initial CT or MRI offers rapid evaluation of brain anatomy and helps guide treatment, follow-up imaging monitors recovery or progression of disease, and additional assessment with more advanced techniques better elucidates specify aspects of brain and cerebrovascular physiology and metabolism. CT perfusion, MR perfusion, SPECT, functional MRI (fMRI), PET, and MR spectroscopy (MRS) are only some of the methods where ongoing research is underway to better understand TBI, identify and monitor injury and recovery, and help better predict long-term effects and outcome [12].

7.4 Scalp Lesions

Scalp lacerations, hematomas, or other subcutaneous injuries are common in head trauma patients. Although isolated scalp injury is not often clinically significant, there is 20% association with intracranial injuries even in patients with mild TBI [24]. A visible scalp lesion on cross-sectional imaging directs attention to the site of impact for interpreting radiologists and assists in the detection of minor intracranial bleeds, fractures, or contusions [25]. Location and type of scalp blood (caput succedaneum, subgaleal hematoma, subgaleal hygroma, or cephalohematoma) are important to understand the potential for hemorrhage extension (Table 7.1) [26]. Use of CT soft tissue reconstruction kernel can assess scalp abnormalities with appropriate adjustments in image window and level to differentiate density differences between normal tissue, blood, fluid, and fat. Scalp injuries often also provide a visual clue to mechanism of injury and aid in the search for related intracranial injuries (Fig. 7.1).

Table 7.1 Overview of pediatric scalp fluid collections/hematomas

Lesion type	Caput succedaneum	Subgaleal hematoma	Subgaleal hygroma	Cephalohematoma (extracranial subperiosteal hematoma)
Occurrence	In newborns after vaginal delivery, sometimes associated with delivery assistance such as vacuum extraction	After head trauma (or after birth)	Birth trauma (forceps delivery)	Birth trauma (skull fracture during birth)
Location	Superficial subcutaneous soft tissues of the scalp	Lifts up the galea aponeurotica	Beneath the galea aponeurotica	Subperiosteal (flat skull bones)
Composition	Edema (with microscopic hemorrhages)	Venous blood	Cerebrospinal fluid	Subperiosteal hemorrhage
Clinical presentation	Pitting edema	Diffusely spreading, firm fluctuating mass	–	Well defined, focal, firm mass
Skull fracture		Yes or no	Yes	Yes
Crosses suture lines?	Yes	Yes	Yes	No

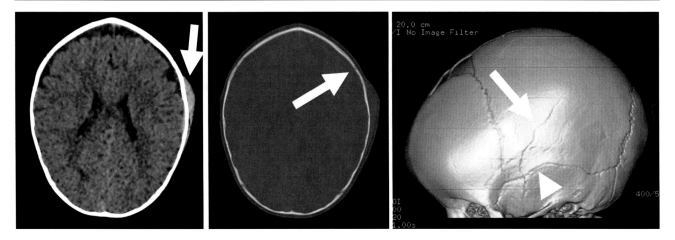

Fig. 7.1 Axial non-contrast head CT demonstrating a small left parietal scalp hematoma (left image, arrow) associated with a subtle underlying non-displaced left parietal bone fracture (center image, arrow) in a young child. 3D volume rendered reconstructions, which increase sensitivity for identifying non-displaced fractures, better depict the linear left parietal bone fracture (right image, arrow) that extends through the left squamosal suture (right image, arrowhead). No intracranial hemorrhage was present

7.5   Skull Fractures

Skull fractures may result from both penetrating and blunt trauma and may be categorized in various ways based on mechanism of injury, topography, complications, and management. Classification can be broken down into the following parameters:

- Shape: linear, comminuted, stellate.
- Depression: depressed, non-depressed, open.
- Anatomic location and extent: skull vault, skull base, craniofacial junction.

The most common fracture shape is linear, often seen in the young pediatric population (<5 years old), typically involving the parietal or basilar skull [27]. Extension of the fracture to suture lines can result in suture diastasis. Fracture complications are dependent on location, extent, and depression. Depressed skull fractures are defined by displacement of the inner and outer tables of the skull on either side of the fracture line. Displacement of the outer table on the one side of the fracture line to or beyond the level of inner table on the other side of the fracture line is particularly concerning for

additional intracranial complications. These occur primarily in the frontoparietal region and are often open, meaning associated with lacerations more superficially and can result in a host of issues including dural tearing, parenchymal contusions, wound infection, and seizure [28]. Comminuted anterior cranial fossa fractures are also associated most highly with CSF leaks [29]. Venous compromise is seen in two thirds of fractures near the dural venous sinus or jugular bulb and can relate to frank laceration of the sinus, mass effect from adjacent extra-axial hematoma, or dural venous sinus thrombosis [19, 30]. Temporal bone and skull base fractures often have more severe complications such as damage to cranial nerves, the craniocervical junction, and middle and inner ear structures [31].

Patients who sustain skull fractures from head trauma are reported to have a 2–5× increased risk of intracranial hemorrhage compared with those without fracture [25, 32]. CT is more sensitive than either skull radiograph or MRI in the detection of fractures. In particular, the combination of excellent depiction of osseous detail, high resolution, and the ability to render maximum intensity projections and surface rendered 3D reconstructions makes CT an optimal tool for the detection of skull fracture [33, 34] (Fig. 7.2).

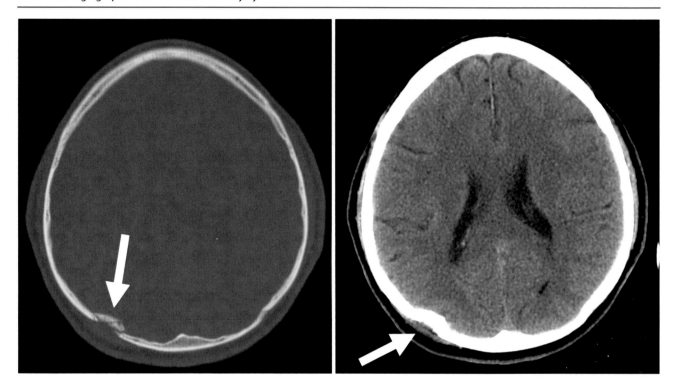

Fig. 7.2 Axial non-contrast head CT demonstrates a focal comminuted depressed posterior right parietal bone fracture (left image, arrow) associated with a small overlying scalp hematoma (right image, arrow) following an assault with a hammer

7.6   Extra-Axial Lesions

Trauma may affect four main extra-axial compartments: epidural, subdural, subarachnoid, and intraventricular spaces.

7.6.1   Epidural Hematoma (EDH)

An epidural hematoma (EDH) is an extracerebral hemorrhagic collection occurring between the superficial dura and inner table of the skull. Because the superficial dura is closely opposed to the inner table, it takes some force to separate them, creating a potential space in which blood may collect. EDHs are commonly associated with fractures that can disrupt and tear the superficial dura, causing damage to meningeal arterial branches embedded in the dura. EDHs classically assume a lenticular shape and typically do not cross suture lines [35, 36] as the dura is invested within the suture. Exceptions to this rule include the vertex EDH that may traverse the sagittal suture as well as pediatric skull fractures with suture diastasis. There is a higher incidence with overlying skull fractures on the same or "coup" side of injury [37–39]. CT is the recommended initial imaging modality as it can show both the extracerebral collection and fractures

with highest sensitivity. The lentiform or biconcave shape can cause mass effect on the adjacent brain parenchyma as hemorrhage accumulates. Clinically, an EDH may be associated with a lucid window, a period of normal neurological function between the time of injury and neurological deterioration. The so-called swirl sign on CT is associated with active bleeding and is characterized by hypodense noncoagulated blood mixed with hyperdense coagulated blood. This radiologic finding is important to communicate to treating providers as patients may undergo rapid decompensation from active arterial bleeding [33, 39].

While classically associated with arterial bleeding, EDHs can arise from either arterial or venous injuries (Table 7.2). Arterial bleeding is most often from the middle meningeal artery, reported in the temporoparietal region in 75% of cases [38]. Bleeding from arterial injury may result in a rapidly expanding hematoma with progressive mass effect, increased intracranial pressure, and potential infarcts which can be surgical emergencies. Treatment often requires urgent decompressive craniotomy in severe cases or embolization of the middle meningeal artery in non-surgical small−/medium-sized EDH cases (Fig. 7.3). Venous origin of EDH is seen in cases of fractures crossing the dural venous sinuses, and bleeding can be seen on either side of the falx cerebri or ten-

Table 7.2 Epidural versus subdural hematoma common characteristics

Epidural hematoma (EDH)	Subdural hematoma (SDH)
"Coup"	"Contrecoup"
Skull fractures seen in ±90% of cases	No correlation with skull fractures
Generally, do not cross suture lines	Can cross suture lines
Not limited by falx or tentorium (may extend from supra- to infratentorial or across midline)	Limited by falx and tentorium (confined to supra- or infratentorial compartment, does not cross midline)
Origin • Arterial (majority, tearing of one or more branches of the meningeal arteries, most commonly the middle meningeal artery) • Venous (minority, laceration of a dural venous sinus, e.g., along the sphenoparietal sinus)	Origin • Venous, laceration of bridging cortical veins
Medical emergency	May be chronic
Mass effect is directly related to the size of the EDH	Mass effect is associated with underlying parenchymal injury not size of SDH
CT is preferred imaging technique because • Rapid accessibility • Shows both the hemorrhage and the skull fracture MR can be useful for • Secondary parenchymal injury (edema, mass effect, herniation)	CT is commonly used to detect and follow SDH size MRI may be useful for • Sensitivity for detecting isodense SDH and staging timing of blood products • Better definition of multicompartment septations that may be present

torium cerebelli [40]. Common locations of venous EDH include the anterior middle cranial fossa, vertex, or occiput resulting from injuries to the sphenoparietal sinus, superior sagittal sinus, and transverse sinus, respectively [38] (Fig. 7.4).

The location of the EDH is crucial to decision-making and management. For instance, posterior fossa EDH can result in early cerebellar compression, effacement of the fourth ventricle, non-communicating hydrocephalus, and/or brainstem compression necessitating emergent decompressive craniectomy and surgical evacuation [41]. Conversely anterior temporal EDH is often indolent, less likely to expand, and thus may be treated well with non-surgical stabilization and monitoring [42].

7.6.2 Subdural Hematoma (SHD)

Subdural hematomas (SDHs) are extracerebral hemorrhagic collections located between the dura and arachnoid membranes. They often arise from tears in bridging cortical veins at the site of crossing the dura. SDH is common in head trauma and seen in up to a third of cases [37]. They are often found on the opposite or contrecoup side of injury and are not generally associated with skull fractures [38]. SDH collections cross sutures but are limited by dural reflections such as the falx or tentorium, giving them the classic concave or crescentic shape [43] (Fig. 7.5).

The imaging appearance of SDHs may range from hyper to hypoattenuating crescentic collections along the inner

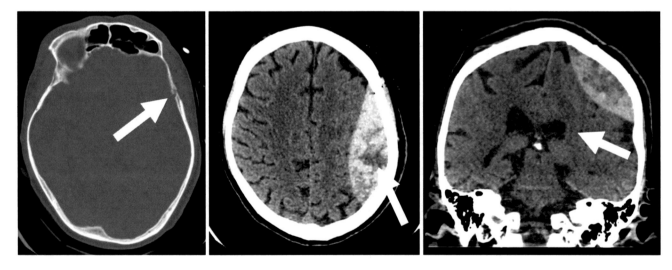

Fig. 7.3 Axial non-contrast head CT demonstrates a jagged non-displaced left temporal bone fracture (left image, arrow) that lacerated the middle meningeal artery. This fracture is associated with a large acute underlying lentiform epidural hematoma with internal "swirl sign" (central image, arrow) compatible with active internal bleeding. The coronal reformation depicts the mass effect on the left parietal lobe, causing compression of the regional sulci and the left ventricular atrium (right image, arrow) as well as mild right-ward subfalcine herniation

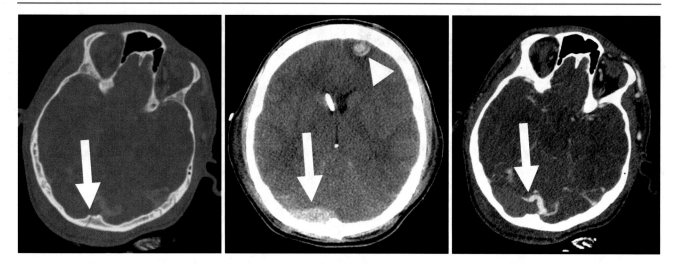

Fig. 7.4 Axial reconstructed bone windows from a CT angiogram of the head demonstrate a non-displaced right occipital bone fracture (left image, arrow) that lacerated the right transverse sinus. This fracture is associated with a moderately sized acute underlying venous epidural hematoma (central image, arrow) that compresses the cerebellum, effaces the fourth ventricle, and causes non-communicating hydroceph- alus that requires emergent ventricular shunting. The angiographic source images show compression and elevation of the co-dominant right transverse sinus (right image, arrow) by the venous epidural hematoma. Additional note is made of a focal contrecoup hemorrhagic brain contusion within the anteromedial left frontal lobe (central image, arrowhead)

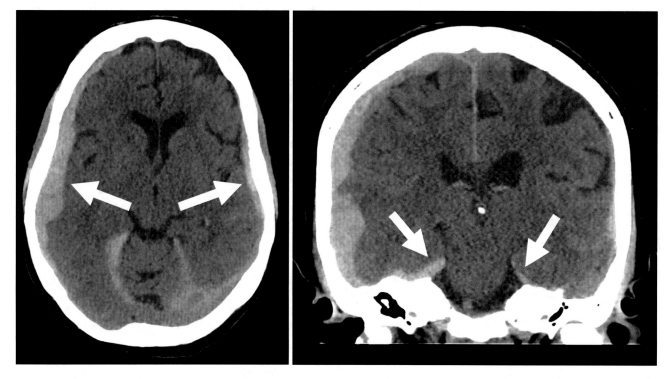

Fig. 7.5 Axial non-contrast head CT demonstrates bilateral crescentic acute SDHs, larger on the right (left image, arrows) causing regional mass effect, sulcal effacement, and mild ventricular compression, with- out frank subfalcine herniation. Coronal reformations show the SDHs extending inferiorly along the cerebellar tentorium (right image, arrows)

table of the calvarium. Although acute bleeds are mostly hyperattenuating, mixed iso- or hypoattenuating blood is not always chronic and may represent hyperacute or unclotted blood, particularly in patients with underlying coagulopa- thies [44]. Looking for layering hematocrit levels can help identify such patients. MRI has better sensitivity in staging the time of bleed especially for subacute/chronic blood prod- ucts as hemoglobin becomes deoxidized, denatured, and enters the extracellular space. A large meta-analysis compar- ing CT and MRI appearances showed hyperattenuating SDH

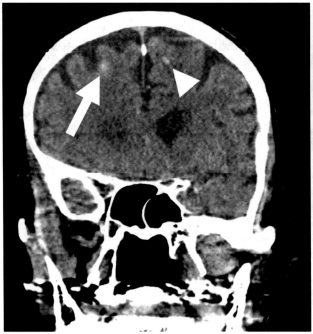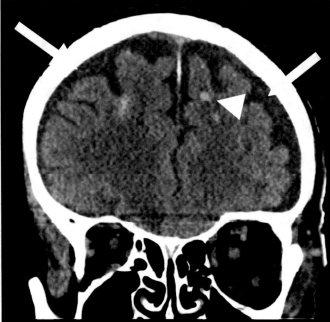

Fig. 7.6 Coronal non-contrast head CT performed on an elderly patient immediately following a fall demonstrates scattered regions of post-traumatic subarachnoid hemorrhage along the right cerebral convexity (left image, arrow) and a small subcortical hemorrhagic axonal injury at the left frontal gray-white interface (left image, arrowhead). The follow-up coronal non-contrast head CT performed the next day again demonstrates stable right frontal subarachnoid hemorrhage and a mild interval increase in the subcortical hemorrhage in the left frontal lobe (right image, arrowhead). In the interim, small bihemispheric subdural hygromas have developed most likely related to occult arachnoid tears (right image, arrows)

after a median of 1–2 days; isoattenuation SDH after 11 days; and hypoattenuating SDH after 14 days [45]. Subacute bleeds have T1 and T2 hyperintense signal on MRI due to presence of extracellular methemoglobin [46]. Chronic SDH may have variable signal and may retain T1 or FLAIR hyperintensity depending on age and internal rebleeding. These chronic collections may also develop enhancing, capillary-rich membranes that help to resorb blood [46]. The vascular membranes are often friable and can lead to development of repeated internal hemorrhage resulting in "acute on chronic" bleeding with mix signal intensity and a complex appearance [47]. Peripheral calcifications may also form in the chronic state.

Subdural hygromas are acute low density extra-axial collections that can mimic chronic subdural hematomas. However, the etiology of hygromas is different since they result from arachnoid damage/tearing causing CSF accumulation in the subdural space. Low density hygromas may occur immediately with trauma but most reports show development days following the initial insult [48, 49] (Fig. 7.6). Hygromas also displace the cortical veins in the subarachnoid space from the inner table of the skull; this finding is particularly important for their diagnosis, as the fluid will be isoattenuating and isointense relative to CSF on CT and MRI, respectively. A combination of subdural hematoma and hygroma (hematohygromas) may also occur, most com-

monly in children, and the two can be difficult to distinguish on imaging.

Management for SDHs depends on size of bleed with common surgical techniques such as burr hole drainage, craniotomy, or port system placement [50]. For smaller and recurrent bleeds, middle meningeal artery embolization may be considered [51]. Differences in imaging features between subdural and epidural hematomas are detailed in Table 7.2.

In pediatric patients, abusive head trauma (AHT) can result in multicompartmental intracranial hemorrhage, classically manifesting as hemorrhages with blood products of varying age, indicating repeated head trauma. Subdural hematomas with internal membranes are particularly characteristic in babies suffering from AHT, usually associated with brain infarctions and retinal hemorrhages. However, non-contrast CT scans are relatively unreliable in determining the age of blood products within subdural hematomas and therefore simply reporting the attenuation of these hematomas rather than attempting to determine their age at initial examinations may be more prudent. Change in the attenuation characteristics of a subdural hemorrhage over time may be more valuable in deciphering the age of the hematoma. AHT should also consider when the clinical history and degree of injury severity are highly discordant. If AHT is suspected, survey imaging of the rest of the body should be pursued to look for prior fractures and other inju-

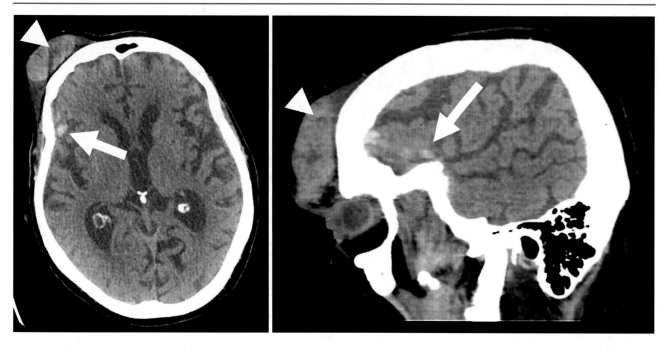

Fig. 7.7 Axial and sagittal images from a non-contrast head CT in an elderly patient with brain atrophy demonstrate a large right frontal scalp hematoma with multifocal underlying "coup" subarachnoid hemorrhage (arrows) in the subjacent right frontal lobe

ries and careful history should be done. Important to note that pediatric patients such as those with coagulopathy or connective tissue disorder can be prone to repeated bleeds and confound diagnosis. When considering AHT, underlying disorders must be excluded carefully.

7.6.3   Traumatic Subarachnoid Hemorrhage (SAH)

Subarachnoid hemorrhage (SAH) after head trauma has a reported incidence of 9–25 cases per 100,000 people annually [52, 53]. This occurs when bleeding is seen between the arachnoid and pia matter usually at the site of injury (coup) (Fig. 7.7) or site opposite of the injury (contrecoup). CT imaging shows nodular or curvilinear foci of hyperattenuation typically along the convexity sulci with decreasing intensity as blood products redistribute over time and are cleared through the arachnoid granulations [54]. On MRI, failure of the normal CSF suppression on T2-weighted FLAIR sequences is useful to detect superficial SAH while SWI can detect the presence of superficial siderosis indicative of prior SAH with hemosiderin staining of the pial surface of the brain. SWI is also sensitive for the detection of central SAH in the basilar cisterns, interpeduncular fossa, or within the ventricles with high sensitivity where T2-weighted FLAIR can be somewhat limited due to pulsation artifact [55]. In general, the presence of SAH without other forms of intracranial hemorrhage has less risk of rapid clinical deterioration and need for surgical intervention [56]; however,

midline SAH (interhemispheric or peri-mesencephalic) has been reported to have worse outcomes and can be associated with diffuse axonal injury [57].

Even in the setting of trauma, isolated SAH in the basilar cisterns should trigger a search for underlying aneurysmal rupture with either CT or MR angiography. Clinically it can be difficult to determine if a ruptured aneurysm led to a fall and subsequent head trauma or if primary head trauma has resulted in subarachnoid hemorrhage. SAH in the interpeduncular or perimesencephalic cisterns may indicate injury to the brainstem [48] or large vessel injury. As blood products are irritating to the vessels, vasospasm can result from traumatic SAH and is more common in severe TBI, reported in about a third of patients [58, 59].

Needless to say, some patients can have a combination of hematomas in different cranial spaces (Fig. 7.8).

7.6.4   Traumatic Intraventricular Hemorrhage (IVH)

Intraventricular hemorrhage (IVH) is reported in about 1–3% in blunt trauma and 10–25% in severe head injury [60, 61]. IVH may result from several mechanisms including injury to subependymal or cortical veins, retrograde reabsorption, or reflux of SAH, or extension of intraparenchymal hemorrhage. Large cohort regression analyses have shown strong correlation between IVH and diffuse axonal injury to the corpus collosum with poor clinical outcomes [57, 62].

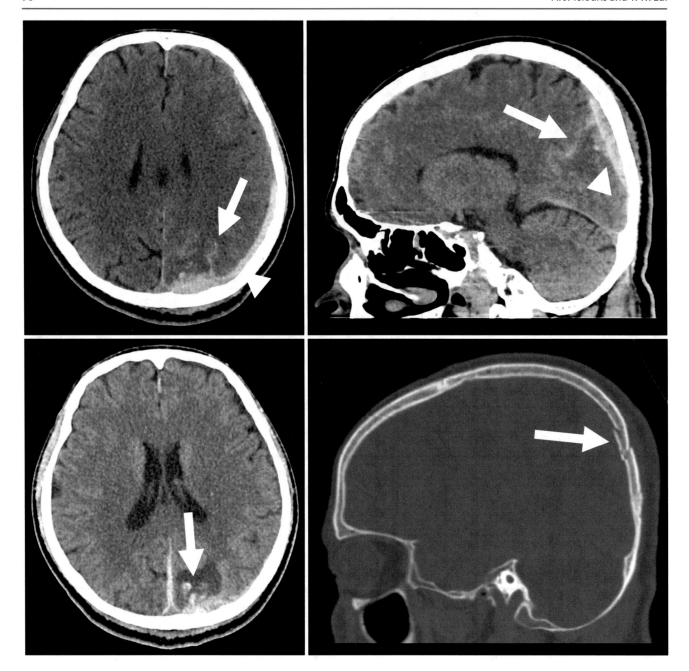

Fig. 7.8 Axial non-contrast head CT demonstrates focal acute SAH within the left parieto-occipital sulcus (top left and right images, arrows) at presentation in a "coup" pattern. This SAH underlies a mildly comminuted depressed left parietal bone fracture (bottom right image, arrow) that indicates the site of the blunt head injury. An associ- ated hemorrhagic contusion with surrounding edema centered within the left cuneus increased in size over time on the 24-h follow-up CT scan (bottom left image, arrow). Lastly, a left hemispheric acute subdu- ral hematoma is present (top left and right images, arrowheads)

On CT, hyperdense layering blood in the ventricles is compatible with IVH. MRI is more sensitive for the identifi- cation of subtle IVH using T2-weighted FLAIR or SWI sequences. In the first 48 h, blood products appear hyperin- tense on the FLAIR sequence then variable in signal as blood becomes more subacute/chronic and SWI shows hypointense area of susceptibility [63, 64]. Both subarachoid and intra- ventricular hemorrhage can result in hydrocephalus (Fig. 7.9).

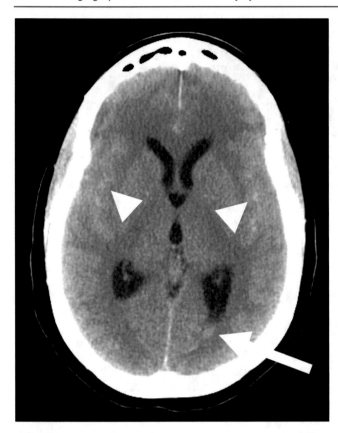

Fig. 7.9 Axial non-contrast head CT performed on a patient extricated from a vehicle following a high-speed motor vehicle collision demonstrates diffuse acute SAH (arrowheads) and a small amount of IVH layering within the occipital horn of the left lateral ventricle (arrow). Also present on this scan is early hydrocephalus related to the SAH

7.7   Intra-Axial Lesions

7.7.1   Hemorrhagic Cerebral Contusions, Coup Versus Contrecoup

Cerebral contusions contribute significantly to morbidity and mortality in the setting of a TBI and constitute about 35% of TBI-related injuries [65]. Brain contusions are focal parenchymal injuries that result from the impact of the brain against the inner table of the skull and can be considered a "bruise" to the brain. The most common locations are at the same (coup) (Fig. 7.10) and opposite (contrecoup) sides of the insult, at areas of irregular bony protrusions mostly involving the anterior and middle cranial fossa [66]. Contusions in the temporal lobe have the worst reported functional outcomes compare to other types of intra- and extra-axial injuries [67].

Essentially all contusions have some component of hemorrhage, but sensitivity in detecting blood varies by imaging technique and protocol. In the hyperacute setting, contusions can appear primarily hypodense on CT indicating edema.

Hyperdense cortical and subcortical hemorrhage may also be present. CT is often used to follow contusions over time that can become more evident as the amount of hemorrhage increases (Fig. 7.11). After the initial 24 h, MRI is more sensitive than CT for the detection of small contusions and defining the extent of hemorrhage and edema, important predictors for clinical outcome. MRI shows a "salt and pepper" appearance of hemorrhagic contusions that may increase in size or "bloom" over the first 48 h following injury [68]. The T2-weighted FLAIR sequence is best for evaluation of contusions mostly involving cerebral edema [38, 66]. SWI or T2* gradient recall echo (GRE) sequences are very sensitive for the detection of hemorrhagic contusions [8], with SWI being far more sensitive than T2* GRE. Contusions are often associated with SAH and must be followed with serial imaging to assess progression of hemorrhage and resulting mass effect/herniation to determine need for surgical intervention [69]. Over time, chronic contusions appear hypodense and atrophic on CT due to the resultant encephalomalacia and gliosis. On MRI, susceptibility artifact within the chronic contusion will persists within the region of encephalomalacia and gliosis due to hemosiderin/ferritin deposition [70] (Fig. 7.12).

Contusions may occur on both the coup and contrecoup sides of blunt traumatic head injury related to the directional force of the trauma. Translational forces from acceleration/deceleration cause the brain to impact the calvarium on the contrecoup side of injury, and these lesions can be larger and more extensive than coup lesions [70].

Table 7.3 provides a review of sequential signal intensity changes that intracranial hemorrhage undergoes on MRI. MRI signal of blood products is largely dependent on three main factors: (1) the fact that hemoglobin is a ferrous (iron-containing) molecule, (2) the number of unpaired electrons associated with the hemoglobin state that dictates its magnetism, and (3) the relative heterogeneity of distribution of hemoglobin (within or outside of red blood cells) which contribute to susceptibility-related local magnetic field distortions.

7.7.2   Diffuse Axonal Injury (DAI)

Diffuse axonal injury (DAI) is a relatively common type of neuronal damage from severe closed head trauma [71, 72]. DAI is clinically defined as head trauma with resulting loss of consciousness 6 h or more that can lead to neurologic degeneration or death. Damage from shear-strain forces in DAI is believed to cause injury to the brain across interfaces where tissue densities differ (e.g., gray and white matter junction) or tissue anchored to adjacent structures (cerebral/cerebellar peduncles or corpus callosum) [72, 73]. The most affected areas of DAI in order of frequency are as follows:

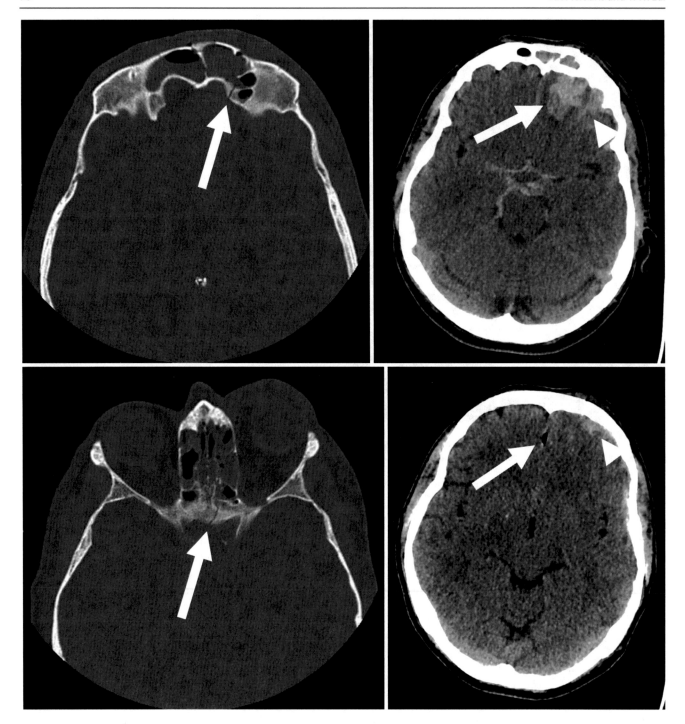

Fig. 7.10 Thin targeted axial bone algorithm images from a maxillofacial CT scan depict a complex comminuted fracture through the left frontal bone and sinus (top left image, arrow). The corresponding non-contrast head CT scan demonstrates a large underlying "coup" hemorrhagic contusion (top right image, arrow) with associated SAH (top right and bottom right images, arrowheads). Contrast is noted within the arteries of the circle of Willis due to the concurrently performed whole body contrast-enhanced trauma CT scan, although a small SAH was also suspected within the suprasellar cistern (top right image). The fracture line extended into the sphenoid bone (bottom left image, arrow) causing a suspected CSF leak in this patient. A focus of interhemispheric air was also present, due to the fracture extending through the air-filled sinuses (bottom right, arrow)

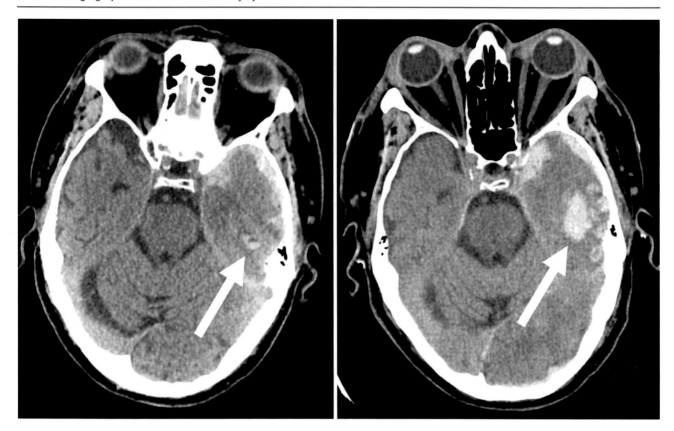

Fig. 7.11 Following a fall from a ladder, a non-contrast CT scan was performed in the emergency department that demonstrates multicompartmental post-traumatic intracranial hemorrhage including a subdural hematoma, SAH, and a small contusion (left image, arrows) within the left lateral temporal lobe. A CT scan performed 12 h later demonstrates a marked interval increase in size of the inferolateral left temporal lobe hemorrhagic contusion (right image, arrow)

gray–white matter junctions, corpus callosum, basal ganglia, brainstem, and mesencephalon. Classification of DAI was first described in 1982 by Adams and colleagues based on location of lesions. DAI grade I (mild) involves microscopic changes in the cerebral cortex, corpus callosum, brainstem, and cerebellum; grade II (moderate) are gross focal lesions in the corpus callosum; and grade III (severe) are focal lesions in the dorsolateral portions of the brainstem involving the superior cerebellar peduncle [74]. Axonal injury in the brainstem is an important indicator for clinical degeneration to coma in DAI patients [73]. Thalamic injury may also occur and are not included in the initial grading system but may result in worse clinical outcomes [75].

Given the clinical importance of DAI and higher associated morbidity and mortality compared to other types of extra-axial injuries or hemorrhagic brain contusions, imaging plays a crucial role in detection and prognosis. As always,

non-contrast head CT is the modality of choice in the acute trauma setting but often underestimates DAI extent especially for non-hemorrhagic lesions [72]. Only around 10% of patients with DAI show hemorrhagic lesions initially (Fig. 7.13), which then can become more apparent in weeks following injury as these areas begin to atrophy and undergo gliosis with ex-vacuo ventricular dilatation [76]. Thus, when patients have clinical findings discrepant with initial CT imaging, MRI is often used to improve sensitivity in evaluation. In the acute setting, DWI sequences can show non-hemorrhagic lesions in areas of cytotoxic or vasogenic edema [17]. Greater degrees of signal abnormality in the corpus callosum and brainstem (grade II and III lesions) have been shown to correlate with length of comatose state [77]. For hemorrhagic lesions, susceptibility-weighted sequences can detect microhemorrhages with some reports showing SWI to be six times as sensitive as T2* GRE imaging [78]

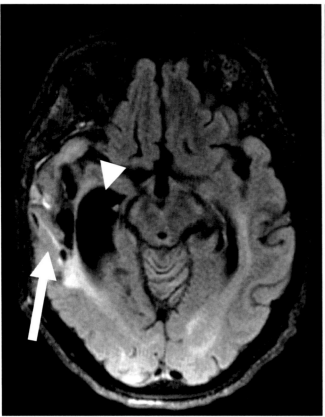 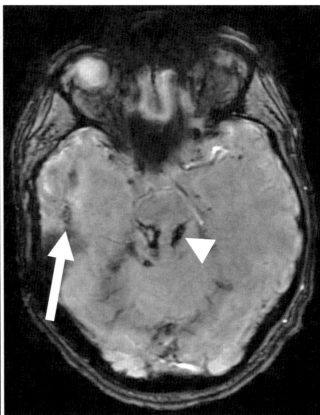

Fig. 7.12 T2-weighted FLAIR (left image) and SWI (right image) MR sequences demonstrate extensive chronic hemorrhagic encephalomalacia within the lateral right temporal lobe (arrows) in a patient with a severe TBI following a high-speed motor vehicle collision. There is associated ex-vacuo dilatation of the temporal horn of the right lateral ventricle (left image, arrowhead). Additionally, there is evidence of chronic hemorrhagic axonal injury involving the superior cerebellar peduncles (right image, arrowheads)

Table 7.3 Sequential signal intensity changes of intracranial hemorrhage on MRI (1.5 T)

	Hyperacute hemorrhage	Acute hemorrhage	Early subacute hemorrhage	Late subacute hemorrhage	Chronic hemorrhage
What happens	Blood leaves the vascular system (extravasation)	Deoxygenation with formation of deoxy-Hb	Clot retraction and deoxy-Hb is oxidized to met-Hb	Cell lysis (membrane disruption)	Macrophages digest the clot
Time frame	<12 h	Hours–days (weeks in center of hematoma)	A few days	4–7 days–1 month	Weeks–years
Red blood cells	Intact erythrocytes	Intact, but hypoxic erythrocytes	Still intact, severely hypoxic	Lysis (solution of lysed cells)	Gone; encephalomalacia with proteinaceous fluid
State of Hb	Intracellular oxy-Hb (HbO$_2$)	Intracellular deoxy-Hb (Hb)	Intracellular met-Hb (HbOH) (occurs initially at periphery of clot)	Extracellular met-Hb (HbOH)	Hemosiderin (insoluble) and ferritin (water soluble)
Oxidation state	Ferrous (Fe^{2+}) no unpaired e–	Ferrous (Fe^{2+}) 4 unpaired e–	Ferric (Fe^{3+}) 5 unpaired e–	Ferric (Fe^{3+}) 5 unpaired e–	Ferric (Fe^{3+}) 2000 × 5 unpaired e–
Magnetic properties	Diamagnetic ($c < 0$)	Paramagnetic ($c > 0$)	Paramagnetic ($c > 0$)	Paramagnetic ($c > 0$)	FeOOH is superparamagnetic
SI on T1WI	≈ or ↓	≈ (or ↓) (no PEDD interaction)	↑↑ (PEDD interaction)	↑↑ (PEDD interaction)	≈ (or ↓) (no PEDD interaction)
SI on T2WI	↑ (essentially imaging of high-water content of blood, plasma)	↓ T2 PRE (susceptibility effect from concentration of Hb inside RBCs)	↓↓ T2 PRE (susceptibility effect from concentration of Hb inside RBCs)	↑↑ No T2 PRE (more homogenous distribution across intracellular and extracellular compartments after cell lysis reduces local susceptibility effects)	↓↓ T2 PRE (susceptibility effect)

Legend: *Hb* hemoglobin, *e* electron, *FeOOH* ferric oxyhydroxide, ↑ increased SI relative to normal gray matter, ↓ decreased SI relative to normal gray matter, *PRE* proton relaxation enhancement, *PEDD* proton-electron dipolar-dipolar

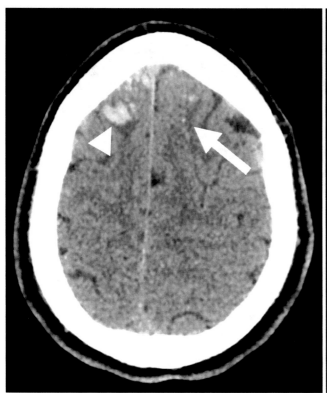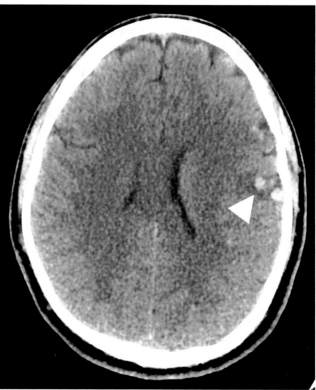

Fig. 7.13 Axial non-contrast head CT images performed on a comatose patient with a severe TBI demonstrate bilateral frontal lobe acute hemorrhagic contusions in the frontal lobes (top left and right images, arrowheads) as well as multifocal punctate acute microhemorrhages in a linear pattern in the left superior frontal gyrus compatible with traumatic hemorrhagic axonal shear injuries (top left image, arrow). T2-weighted FLAIR demonstrates multifocal regions of white matter edema within the left superior frontal gyrus (middle left image, arrow) associated with numerous foci of microhemorrhage on SWI within the bilateral superior frontal gyri (lower left image, arrows) confirming the hemorrhagic axonal shear injuries. The T2-weighted FLAIR sequence also depicts a focal region of cortical/subcortical edema (middle right image, arrow) corresponding to cortical hemorrhage on the SWI (lower right image, arrow) within the posterolateral left frontal lobe confirming a hemorrhagic contusion

(Fig. 7.14). Bland T2 hyperintense white matter lesions may be present in patients with DAI but are nonspecific findings and can also be seen in nontraumatic causes such as ischemia, demyelination, migraines, vasculopathies, etc. A linear pattern along the vectors of the force applied to the brain and an association of these T2 hyperintensities with regions of diffusion restriction and microhemorrhage are important to distinguish DAI from other nonspecific causes [79]. More focal regions of traumatic axonal injury (TAI) which may be seen on MRI are also now understood to occur in less severe clinical cases.

Diffusion tensor imaging (DTI) has emerged as an MRI technique that can study white matter and potential white matter injury. DTI uses orthogonal diffusion vectors and can measure directional diffusion. In group studies, DTI has been shown to demonstrate anisotropy changes in white matter in patients with TBI compared with controls even in the absence of T2 FLAIR and susceptibility abnormalities [80, 81]. Changes in fractional anisotropy after TBI can be confusing (elevated vs depressed compared with normal), and this inconsistency is now believed to relate to timing after injury. Clinical use of DTI as a TAI biomarker remains challenging due to heterogeneity in data acquisition and analysis methods, variance across the normal population, and heterogeneity of head injuries. Ongoing research is still underway to better understand and characterize white matter injury using multicompartment diffusion modeling and to try to identify potential clinical uses.

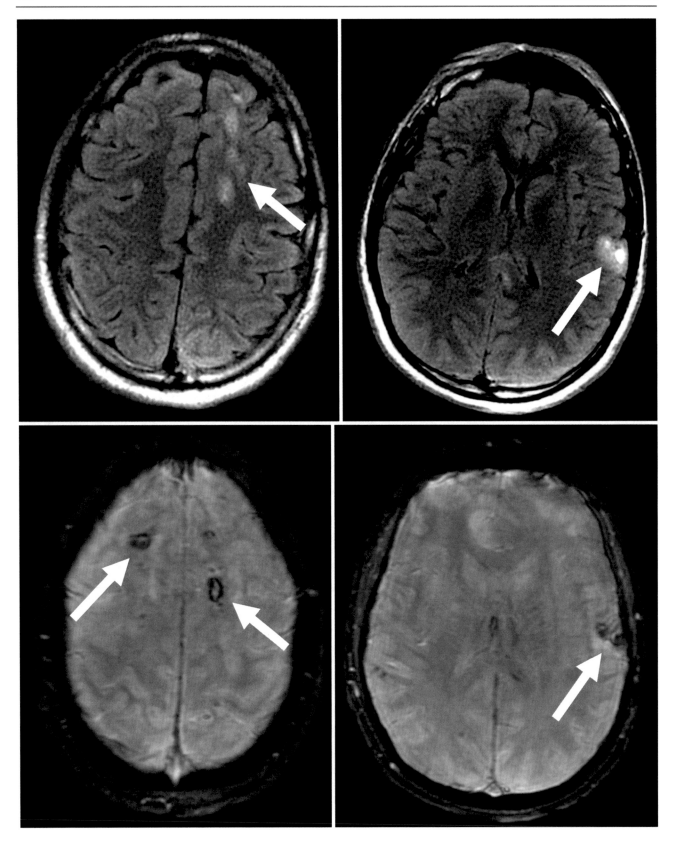

Fig. 7.13 (continued)

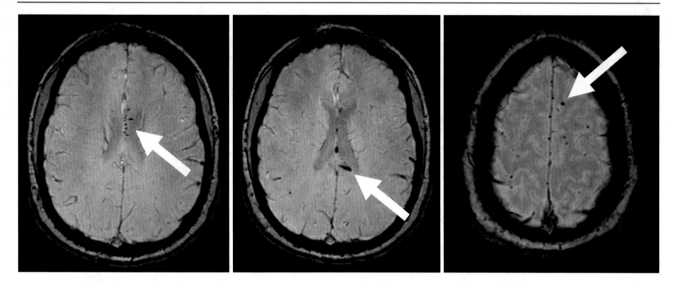

Fig. 7.14 SWI demonstrates numerous punctate and linear foci of susceptibility compatible with traumatic hemorrhagic axonal shear injuries within the subcortical white matter of the left frontal lobe and the corpus callosum (arrows) in a young male patient that suffered a moderate TBI following a motorcycle accident

7.8 Vascular Injury

Vascular injuries may occur with head trauma including arterial dissection, pseudoaneurysm, active extravasation, vascular occlusion, carotid cavernous fistula, dural arteriovenous fistula, and venous thrombosis. Patients with severe DAI and cerebral edema may also develop diffuse vascular injury, which is shown when dark areas of SWI susceptibility artifact surround engorged veins indicating areas of venous stasis [82]. Several guidelines exist for imaging use when vascular injury is suspected including the Denver and Western Trauma Association criteria. Consensus is that any head trauma with a skull base fracture or penetration neck injury extending through the carotid canal, particularly zone III (through superior angle of mandible) should be further evaluated with angiography [83].

7.8.1 Carotid Artery-Cavernous Sinus Fistula (CCF)

Carotid artery-cavernous sinus fistula (CCF) can have different etiologies but occur in the setting of trauma when the cavernous segment of the internal carotid artery is injured result in a direct communication between the arterial system and the venous system of the cavernous sinus. This fistulous connection may lead to dilation of the cavernous sinus and secondary enlargement of the superior ophthalmic vein (SOV) and inferior petrosal sinus [8]. Characteristic imaging shows enlarged cavernous sinus or ipsilateral SOV with multiple flow voids on MRI and clinical symptoms include injected conjunctiva, pulsatile exophthalmos, and periorbital edema (Fig. 7.15).

7.8.2 Traumatic Aneurysms

Post-traumatic intracranial aneurysms are rare, accounting for <1% of all aneurysms and occur most commonly in children [84]. Common locations include the cavernous and infraclinoid internal carotid artery as well as the anterior cerebral artery. As with all intracerebral aneurysms, standard assessments include CTA/MRA and catheter digital subtraction angiography.

7.8.3 Traumatic Vascular Dissection

Damage to the intimal layer of an artery may result in the creation of a false lumen with blood diverting into the media through the dissection flap. Sometimes even minor neck injury can result in cervical vascular dissections with resultant potential vascular compromise of the brain. Intracranial dissection is less common, and severe cases can be associated with adjacent fractures causing direct damage to the vessels or result from rotational force in blunt head trauma [85]. The incidence of internal carotid and vertebral artery dissections in the setting of head trauma is 0.86% and 0.53%, respectively [86].

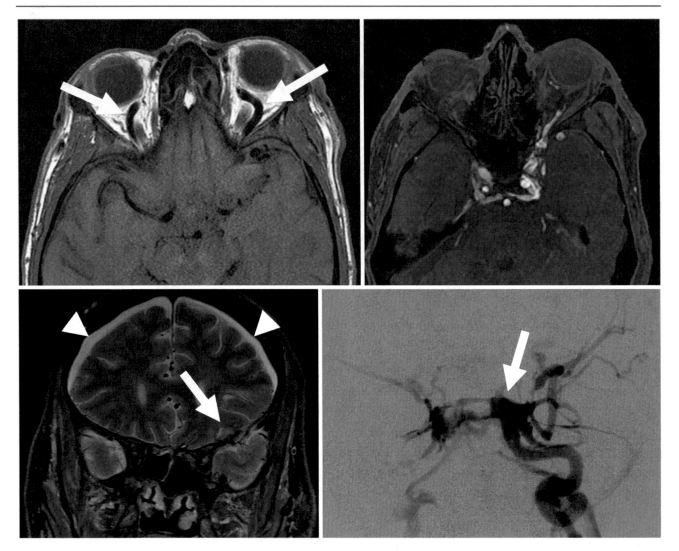

Fig. 7.15 A young male patient developed bilateral ocular proptosis and chemosis while hospitalized for a recent severe TBI with non-displaced skull base fracture. The axial T1-weighted MR image demonstrates enlargement of the bilateral superior ophthalmic veins, left more than right (top left image, arrows). The coronal T2-weighted image demonstrates small bilateral post-traumatic subdural hygromas (bottom left image, arrowheads) and a small inferior left frontal hemorrhagic contusion (bottom left image, arrow). The time-of-flight gradient echo MRA demonstrates arterialized flow-related enhancement within the bilateral cavernous sinuses and left superior ophthalmic vein (top right image, arrows). The left ICA arterial phase digital subtraction catheter angiogram (anteroposterior projection) confirmed the presence of a direct carotid cavernous fistula with pronounced early arterial phase opacification of the cavernous sinuses and ophthalmic veins (bottom right image, arrows)

CTA and MRA are the most commonly utilized imaging modalities and are highly accurate in the assessment of the integrity of the cervical arteries and to assess for luminal narrowing. Anatomic black-blood MRI sequences may also show a high intensity "crescent sign" on T1-weighted and T2-weighted sequences indicating an intramural hematoma at the site of the dissection with a concomitant flow void or abnormal contour on MRA [87] (Fig. 7.16). Ultrasound is also being increasingly used for detection, particularly with B mode and color flow doppler. Conventional catheter angiography remains a useful tool for diagnosing cervical and intracranial arterial dissections and may show features such as the "string sign" or "flame shaped tapering," however in current practice is reserved primarily for endovascular therapy.

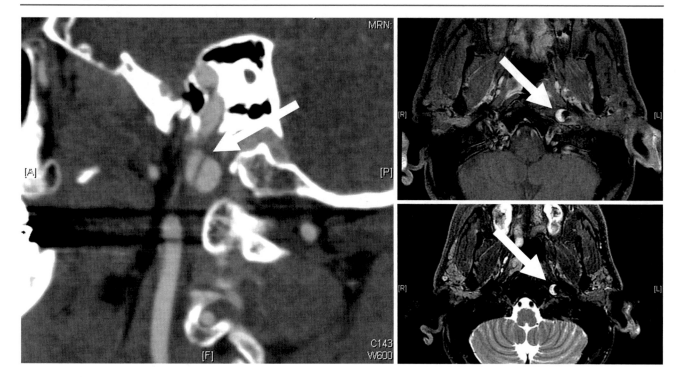

Fig. 7.16 CTA was performed in a young patient complaining of left neck pain following a concussion while playing ice hockey. The CTA demonstrates a linear intimal flap and pseudoaneurysm of the distal left internal carotid artery located directly below the skull base compatible with a traumatic dissection and pseudoaneurysm (left image, arrows). Crescentic T1 and T2 hyperintensity are also present on the anatomic T1-weighted and T2-weighted sequences performed through the upper neck that represented the subintimal hematoma and confirmed a traumatic ICA dissection (right images, arrows)

7.9 Secondary Complications

7.9.1 Definition

Secondary intracranial complications are worth discussing and can be clinically critically important. These are sequelae that result as a series of pathophysiologic events triggered by the initial injury that then may lead to further tissue injury and neuron loss.

7.9.2 Intracranial Hypertension

Intracranial hypertension may result after head trauma due to swelling, edema, or hemorrhage and can continue to increase in the initial days after injury, leading to progressive and sometimes precipitous decline. Suspicious imaging findings include diffuse sulcal effacements, compression of the ventricles, enlarging hematomas, and/or herniation. These findings have been found to have a linear relationship with increased intracranial pressure and can help guide manage-

ment including placement of ICP monitors, need for neuro ICU care with close ICP monitoring, surgical intervention such as CSF drainage, hematoma evacuation, or decompressive craniotomy [98].

7.9.2.1 Brain Herniation

Profound intracranial hypertension may lead to multiple secondary injuries of which brain herniation is the most dangerous. The mass effect from increased pressure can result in obliteration of the basal cisterns, subarachnoid spaces, and non-communicating hydrocephalus if ventricular outflow is obstructed. Compression of important vascular structures can lead to brain infarction thus leading to a cascade of neurologic damage. Herniation patterns are described in Table 7.4.

7.9.2.2 Secondary Brainstem Hemorrhage (Duret Hemorrhage)

Rapid downward cerebral herniation can lead to a devastating effect, hemorrhage within a compressed brainstem. CT findings show hyperdense blood in the brainstem typically in

Table 7.4 Cerebral herniation types

Type of herniation	Subfalcine (cingulate)	Tonsillar	Descending transtentorial	Ascending transtentorial	Uncal	External
Definition	Medial cingulate gyrus displacement under inferior free margin of the falx	Downward displacement of cerebellar tonsil(s) through foramen magnum	Downward shift of diencephalon, mesencephalon, and upper brainstem	Superior displacement of the vermis through the tentorial incisura	Herniation of medial temporal lobe through tentorial notch	Brain tissue extrudes externally through a skull defect
Cause	Supratentorial mass (e.g., EDH, SDH, mass lesion, ...)	Posterior fossa mass lesion or supratentorial mass effect	Supratentorial mass effect	Posterior fossa mass lesion	Temporal mass lesion, e.g., focal hematoma	Increased ICP in association with a traumatic or surgical skull defect Occasionally can occur with postoperative pressure gradient and shifts without frank elevation of ICP
Imaging	• Unilateral intracranial mass or lesion • Falx bowing • Compressed ipsilateral lateral ventricle • Enlarged contralateral ventricle (obstructed foramen of Monro)	• Inferior displacement of cerebellar tonsils • Obliterated cisterna magna	• Obliterated peri-mesencephalic cisterns with plugging of tentorial incisura • Downward shift of pineal calcification • Foreshortened and compressed brainstem	• Obliterated fourth ventricle • Effaced superior cerebellar and quadrigeminal cisterns	• Obliterated suprasellar cistern • Mesencephalon shifts to opposite side • Widening of ipsilateral CPA cistern • Hydrocephalus (due to aqueductal obstruction)	• Extracranial displacement of brain tissue • Bone defect
Potential vascular structures compromised	ACA (pericallosal and callosomarginal arteries)	PICA	PCA	SCA	Contralateral PCA	Venous infarction (propensity to hemorrhage)
Other complications	Intracranial hypertension may cause descending transtentorial h	Hydrocephalus and syringomyelia	Duret (brainstem) hemorrhage	Hydrocephalus	Progression to descending transtentorial herniation	Pressure necrosis with swelling of the adjacent brain at the margins of the defect

the lower midbrain/ventral pons. A recent large meta-analysis implicated damage to anteromedial basilar artery perforators after sudden descending herniation [88] as the main cause. Outcome in the setting of Duret hemorrhage is poor and often fatal.

7.9.3   Ischemia and Infarction

Post-traumatic ischemia is another secondary effect of trauma that leads to poorer clinical outcomes. MRI is most sensitive to detect secondary ischemic injury as areas of increased signal intensity on T2-weighted images with corresponding restricted diffusion [89]. The most common post-

traumatic ischemic injury is inflicted on the ipsilateral posterior cerebral artery territory due to supratentorial mass effect. Causes can be extra-axial or intracranial hemorrhage resulting in mass effect and downward transtentorial herniation. Buildup of supratentorial pressure and mass effect may ultimately lead to impingement of the posterior cerebral artery between the free edge of the tentorium and the herniating brain. Anterior cerebral artery impingement can occur along the free edge of the falx in the setting of subfalcine herniation. Frank compression of the middle cerebral artery is less common [89, 90]. More distal vessel compromise can also occur relating to vasospasm in the setting of acute subarachnoid hemorrhage.

7.9.4   Infections

Penetrating head trauma (Figs. 7.17 and 7.18) involving contaminated foreign objects or the introduction of non-sterile portions of the patient's own anatomy (paranasal sinuses, skin, etc.), which then penetrate the intracranial compartment can introduce bacteria and other infectious agents. The spectrum of post-traumatic infection ranges from local wound/scalp infection and cellulitis to more hazardous intracranial infections such as meningitis, ventriculitis, cerebritis,

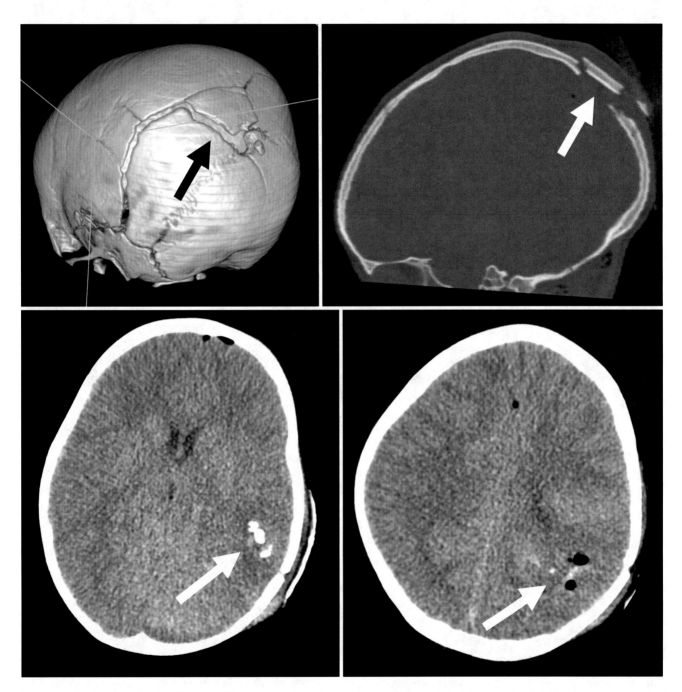

Fig. 7.17 Gunshot wound to the left parietal lobe by a stray bullet in a young child, initial non-contrast CT scan. The 3D volume rendered reconstructed CT scan through the skull and the sagittal CT scan reconstructed images demonstrate a complex elevated comminuted fracture through the bilateral parietal bones (top left and right images, arrows). Axial non-contrast CT scan images demonstrate the bullet fragments lodged within the left parietal lobe associated with multiple foci of intracranial air and microhemorrhage (bottom left and right images, arrows). The non-contrast CT scan also shows diffuse sulcal effacement and ventricular compression compatible with diffuse cerebral edema and raised ICP

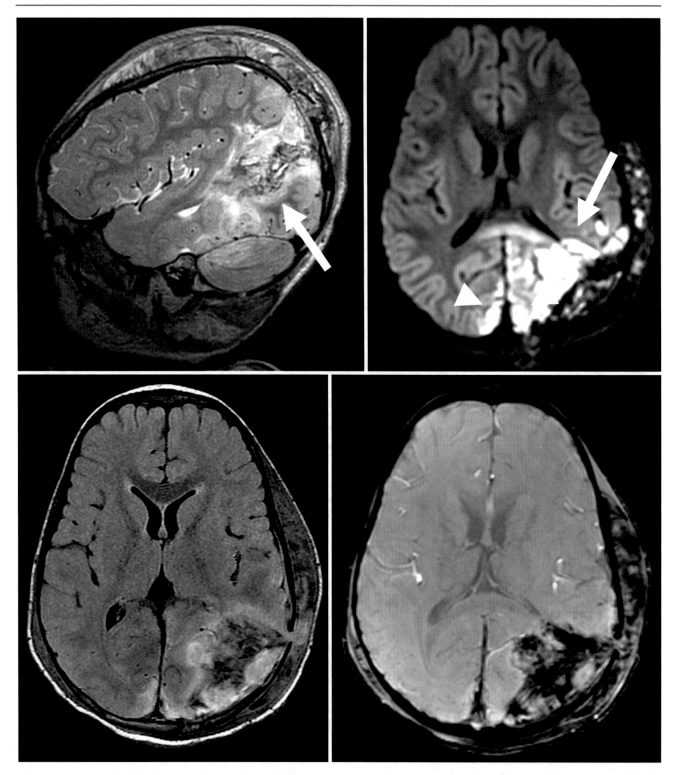

Fig. 7.18 Gunshot wound to the left parietal lobe by a stray bullet in a young child, follow-up MRI scan. Extensive edema and hemorrhage are present within the left parietal lobe along the bullet track (top left image, arrow). The diffusion-weighted images demonstrate a large left parietal contusion/infarction (top right image, arrow). Note the bilateral paramedial occipital lobe infarction from herniation and compression of the posterior cerebral arteries (top right image, arrowheads). T2-weighted FLAIR (bottom left image) and SWI (bottom right image) show the related edema and hemorrhage in the left parietal lobe

and abscess [91]. Imaging findings may show abnormal enhancement of the leptomeninges, ventricles, or a rim enhancing collection, respectively, on contrast-enhanced studies, with MRI having greater sensitivity. Classically, areas of pyogenic infection will carry signature restricted diffusion.

7.10 Post-traumatic Sequelae

7.10.1 Post-traumatic Encephalomalacia

In the later phases after serious head trauma, many chronic changes can occur to the brain. Post-traumatic encephalomalacia is the long-term result of brain tissue loss and death. After the initial insult, the damaged brain tissue undergoes gliosis or scarring often with surrounding cystic cavitation commonly called encephalomalacia [92]. The most common areas of post-traumatic encephalomalacia are the anterior and basal portions of the temporal lobes as these are often injured from contusions from the impact against the skull base [93]. CT imaging reveals atrophic hypodense regions, and MRI demonstrates gliotic T2 hyperintense and/or cystic regions that correlate to the post-traumatic contusions and/or infarctions. Long-term clinical symptoms from encephalomalacia depend on the extent and location of the injury, as well as individual factors such as age and plasticity of the brain at the time of injury. Deficits may vary but can include chronic focal neurological deficits, behavioral changes, and seizures, and may result in life-long disability [93].

7.10.2 Traumatic CSF Leak

Cerebral spinal fluid (CSF) leak is another complication seen in up to 2% after head trauma, with 12–30% reported in cases involving skull base fractures [94]. Leaks may also occur at the cribriform plate and along the walls of the frontal sinuses often associated with fractures that involve communications between the paranasal sinuses and intracranial compartment [95]. CSF leaks can be difficult to detect but signs of pneumocephalus can help point to areas of potential leak. Persistent sinus opacification adjacent to a fracture can be another important clue. If CSF leak is suspected into the paranasal sinuses, nasopharynx, or nasal passages, sampling of nasal fluid and testing for beta-2 transferrin can be done for confirmation. Chronic CSF leaks may present with intracranial hypotension and its concomitant imaging findings or recurrent meningitis. Both CT and MR, contrast-enhanced cisternography,and/or myelography can be useful to try to localize leaks.

7.10.3 Growing Skull Fracture

Growing fractures are rare though may occur in pediatric patients [96]. Incidence is reported as about <0.05–1.6% of cases. Findings include a fracture line which continues to widen due to increased extra-axial brain herniation from the skull defect. These cases may be associated with meningoceles and/or encephalomalacia as the herniated brain parenchyma begins to infarct [97].

7.10.4 Diabetes Insipidus (DI)

Trauma to the pituitary infundibulum can result in central diabetes insipidus (DI). Evaluation of the pituitary gland is typically done with dedicated MRI. Healthy patients typically have T1 hyperintensity in the posterior pituitary gland. Lack of this bright spot may be seen in DI though the finding is nonspecific [98]. Findings of an ectopic posterior pituitary can be seen congenitally; however, in the setting of a history of significant head trauma and acute onset DI, can indicate a proximal stump from a transected infundibulum or a retracted stalk.

7.11 Concluding Remarks

Cross-sectional imaging for patients who sustain craniocerebral trauma is an essential tool for prognosis and management. Both CT and MRI have revolutionized our ability to detect the sequelae of acute head trauma inside the cranial vault and determine the potential effects on the brain. Unenhanced CT is a critical tool for initial diagnosis of severity and extent of injury as well as to appropriately triage patients that need close monitoring and/or immediate neurosurgical intervention. CT is the primary imaging modality because of its speed, availability, lack of contraindications, and high sensitivity for hemorrhage and fractures. MRI is useful in many circumstances and provides unparalleled tissue contrast without ionizing radiation. MRI is used in situations such as assessing complications, working up patients with clinical and CT discordance, and as a more sensitive tool to detect intracranial injury. Overall, given the high incidence of TBI-related injuries globally especially in elderly and young populations, imaging continues to be crucial for diagnosis and understanding patterns of injury to provide optimal management for these patients.

Take-Home Messages
- Traumatic brain injury is common and can affect individuals of all ages.
- Neuroimaging is critical for assessment and triage of patients who have sustained head trauma.
- CT and MRI are complementary: CT is widely available in emergency settings and MRI is sensitive to more subtle injuries.

References

1. Peterson AB, Zhou H, Thomas KE. Disparities in traumatic brain injury-related deaths-United States, 2020. J Saf Res. 2022;83:419–26.
2. Capizzi A, Woo J, Verduzco-Gutierrez M. Traumatic brain injury: an overview of epidemiology, pathophysiology, and medical management. Med Clin North Am. 2020;104:213–38.
3. Haarbauer-Krupa J, Pugh MJ, Prager EM, et al. Epidemiology of chronic effects of traumatic brain injury. J Neurotrauma. 2021;38:3235–47.
4. Teasdale G, Maas A, Lecky F, et al. The Glasgow coma scale at 40 years: standing the test of time. Lancet Neurol. 2014;13:844–54.
5. Brown JB, Forsythe RM, Stassen NA, et al. Evidence-based improvement of the National Trauma triage protocol: the Glasgow coma scale versus Glasgow coma scale motor subscale. J Trauma Acute Care Surg. 2014;77:95–102.
6. Shih RY, Burns J, Ajam AA, et al. ACR Appropriateness Criteria® head trauma: 2021 update. J Am Coll Radiol. 2021;18:S13–36.
7. Mower WR, Gupta M, Rodriguez R, et al. Validation of the sensitivity of the National Emergency X-Radiography Utilization Study (NEXUS) head computed tomographic (CT) decision instrument for selective imaging of blunt head injury patients: an observational study. PLoS Med. 2017;14:e1002313.
8. Wintermark M, Sanelli PC, Anzai Y, et al. Imaging evidence and recommendations for traumatic brain injury: conventional neuroimaging techniques. J Am Coll Radiol. 2015;12:e1–14.
9. Wei SC, Ulmer S, Lev MH, et al. Value of coronal reformations in the CT evaluation of acute head trauma. AJNR Am J Neuroradiol. 2010;31:334–9.
10. Ayhan KA, Celik SE, Dalbayrak S, Yilmaz M, Akansel G, Tireli G. Magnetic resonance imaging finding in severe head injury patients with normal computerized tomography. Turk Neurosurg. 2008;18(1):1–9.
11. Gentry LR, Godersky JC, Thompson B, et al. Prospective comparative study of intermediate-field MR and CT in the evaluation of closed head trauma. AJR Am J Roentgenol. 1988;150:673–82.
12. Han JS, Kaufman B, Alfidi RJ, et al. Head trauma evaluated by magnetic resonance and computed tomography: a comparison. Radiology. 1984;150:71–7.
13. Paterakis K, Karantanas AH, Komnos A, et al. Outcome of patients with diffuse axonal injury: the significance and prognostic value of MRI in the acute phase. J Trauma. 2000;49:1071–5.
14. Kelly AB, Zimmerman RD, Snow RB, et al. Head trauma: comparison of MR and CT—experience in 100 patients. AJNR Am J Neuroradiol. 1988;9:699–708.
15. Chiara Ricciardi M, Bokkers RPH, Butman JA, et al. Trauma-specific brain abnormalities in suspected mild traumatic brain injury patients identified in the first 48 hours after injury: a blinded magnetic resonance imaging comparative study includ-

ing suspected acute minor stroke patients. J Neurotrauma. 2017;34:23–30.
16. Huang YL, Kuo YS, Tseng YC, et al. Susceptibility-weighted MRI in mild traumatic brain injury. Neurology. 2015;84:580–5.
17. Hergan K, Schaefer PW, Sorensen AG, et al. Diffusion-weighted MRI in diffuse axonal injury of the brain. Eur Radiol. 2002;12:2536–41.
18. Kim SC, Park SW, Ryoo I, et al. Contrast-enhanced FLAIR (fluid-attenuated inversion recovery) for evaluating mild traumatic brain injury. PLoS One. 2014;9:e102229.
19. Slasky SE, Rivaud Y, Suberlak M, et al. Venous sinus thrombosis in blunt trauma: incidence and risk factors. J Comput Assist Tomogr. 2017;41:891–7.
20. Netteland DF, Sandset EC, Mejlænder-Evjensvold M, et al. Cerebral venous sinus thrombosis in traumatic brain injury: a systematic review of its complications, effect on mortality, diagnostic and therapeutic management, and follow-up. Front Neurol. 2023;13:1079579.
21. Rischall MA, Boegel KH, Palmer CS, et al. MDCT venographic patterns of dural venous sinus compromise after acute skull fracture. AJR Am J Roentgenol. 2016;207:852–8.
22. Xiong KL, Zhu YS, Zhang WG. Diffusion tensor imaging and magnetic resonance spectroscopy in traumatic brain injury: a review of recent literature. Brain Imaging Behav. 2014;8:487–96.
23. Jensen JH, Helpern JA. MRI quantification of non-gaussian water diffusion by kurtosis analysis. NMR Biomed. 2010;23:698–710.
24. Hamrah H, Mehrvarz S, Mirghassemi AM. The frequency of brain CT-scan findings in patients with scalp lacerations following mild traumatic brain injury; A cross-sectional study. Bull Emerg Trauma. 2018;6:54–8.
25. Malli N, Ehammer T, Yen K, et al. Detection and characterization of traumatic scalp injuries for forensic evaluation using computed tomography. Int J Legal Med. 2013;127:195–200.
26. Ojumah N, Ramdhan RC, Wilson C, et al. Neurological neonatal birth injuries: a literature review. Cureus. 2017;9.
27. Wang H, Zhou Y, Liu J, et al. Traumatic skull fractures in children and adolescents: a retrospective observational study. Injury. 2018;49:219–25.
28. Satardey R, Balasubramaniam S, Pandya J, et al. Analysis of factors influencing outcome of depressed fracture of skull. Asian J Neurosurg. 2018;13:341–7.
29. Archer JB, Sun H, Bonney PA, et al. Extensive traumatic anterior skull base fractures with cerebrospinal fluid leak: classification and repair techniques using combined vascularized tissue flaps. J Neurosurg. 2016;124:647–56.
30. Rivkin MA, Saraiya PV, Woodrow SI. Sinovenous thrombosis associated with skull fracture in the setting of blunt head trauma. Acta Neurochir. 2014;156:999–1007.
31. Dreizin D, Sakai O, Champ K, et al. CT of skull base fractures: classification systems, complications, and management. Radiographics. 2021;41:762–82.
32. Faried A, Halim D, Widjaya IA, et al. Correlation between the skull base fracture and the incidence of intracranial hemorrhage in patients with traumatic brain injury. Chin J Traumatol. 2019;22:286–9.
33. Nakahara K, Shimizu S, Utsuki S, et al. Linear fractures occult on skull radiographs: a pitfall at radiological screening for mild head injury. J Trauma. 2011;70:180–2.
34. Ringl H, Schernthaner R, Philipp MO, et al. Three-dimensional fracture visualisation of multidetector CT of the skull base in trauma patients: comparison of three reconstruction algorithms. Eur Radiol. 2009;19:2416–24.
35. Gupta VK, Seth A. "Swirl Sign" in extradural hematoma. World Neurosurg. 2019;121:95–6.
36. Rincon S, Gupta R, Ptak T. Imaging of head trauma. Handb Clin Neurol. 2016;135:447–77.

37. Tallon JM, Ackroyd-Stolarz S, Karim SA, et al. The epidemiology of surgically treated acute subdural and epidural hematomas in patients with head injuries: a population-based study. Can J Surg. 2008;51:339–45.

38. Parizel PM, Van Goethem JW, Özsarlak Ö, et al. New developments in the neuroradiological diagnosis of craniocerebral trauma. Eur Radiol. 2005;15:569–81.

39. Amoo M, Henry J, Alabi PO, et al. The "swirl sign" as a marker for haematoma expansion and outcome in intra-cranial haemorrhage: a meta-analysis. J Clin Neurosci. 2021;87:103–11.

40. Parker SL, Kabani AA, Conner CR, et al. Management of venous sinus-related epidural hematomas. World Neurosurg. 2020;138:e241–50.

41. Su TM, Lee TH, Lee TC, et al. Acute clinical deterioration of posterior fossa epidural hematoma: clinical features, risk factors and outcome. Chang Gung Med J. 2012;35:271–80.

42. Gean AD, Fischbein NJ, Purcell DD, et al. Benign anterior temporal epidural hematoma: indolent lesion with a characteristic CT imaging appearance after blunt head trauma. Radiology. 2010;257:212–8.

43. Carroll JJ, Lavine SD, Meyers PM. Imaging of subdural hematomas. Neurosurg Clin N Am. 2017;28:179–203.

44. Lim M, Kheok SW, Lim KC, et al. Subdural haematoma mimics. Clin Radiol. 2019;74:663–75.

45. Sieswerda-Hoogendoorn T, Postema FAM, Verbaan D, et al. Age determination of subdural hematomas with CT and MRI: a systematic review. Eur J Radiol. 2014;83:1257–68.

46. Senturk S, Guzel A, Bilici A, et al. CT and MR imaging of chronic subdural hematomas: a comparative study. Swiss Med Wkly. 2010;140:335–40.

47. Honda Y, Sorimachi T, Momose H, et al. Chronic subdural haematoma associated with disturbance of consciousness: significance of acute-on-chronic subdural haematoma. Neurol Res. 2015;37:985–92.

48. Zanini MA, De Lima Resende LA, De Souza Faleiros AT, et al. Traumatic subdural hygromas: proposed pathogenesis based classification. J Trauma. 2008;64:705–13.

49. Yu J, Tang J, Chen M, et al. Traumatic subdural hygroma and chronic subdural hematoma: a systematic review and meta-analysis. J Clin Neurosci. 2023;107:23–33.

50. Brennan PM. Treatment decision making in acute subdural haematoma. Lancet Neurol. 2022;21:581–2.

51. Ironside N, Nguyen C, Do Q, et al. Middle meningeal artery embolization for chronic subdural hematoma: a systematic review and meta-analysis. J Neurointerv Surg. 2021;13:951–7.

52. Edjlali M, Rodriguez-RéGent C, Hodel J, et al. Subarachnoid hemorrhage in ten questions. Diagn Interv Imaging. 2015;96:657–66.

53. León-Carrión J, Domínguez-Morales MDR, Barroso y Martín JM, et al. Epidemiology of traumatic brain injury and subarachnoid hemorrhage. Pituitary. 2005;8:197–202.

54. Fainardi E, Chieregato A, Antonelli V, et al. Time course of CT evolution in traumatic subarachnoid haemorrhage: a study of 141 patients. Acta Neurochir. 2004;146:257–63.

55. Verma RK, Kottke R, Andereggen L, et al. Detecting subarachnoid hemorrhage: comparison of combined FLAIR/SWI versus CT. Eur J Radiol. 2013;82:1539–45.

56. Griswold DP, Fernandez L, Rubiano AM. Traumatic subarachnoid hemorrhage: a scoping review. J Neurotrauma. 2022;39:35–48.

57. Mata-Mbemba D, Mugikura S, Nakagawa A, et al. Traumatic midline subarachnoid hemorrhage on initial computed tomography as a marker of severe diffuse axonal injury. J Neurosurg. 2018;129:1317–24.

58. Busl KM. Subarachnoid Hemorrhage. Continuum (Minneap Minn). 2021;27:1201–45.

59. Perrein A, Petry L, Reis A, et al. Cerebral vasospasm after traumatic brain injury: an update. Minerva Anestegiol. 2015;81:1219–28.

60. Abraszko RA, Zurynski YA, Dorsch NW. The significance of traumatic intraventricular haemorrhage in severe head injury. Br J Neurosurg. 1995;9:769–74.

61. Li CY, Chuang CC, Chen CC, et al. The role of intraventricular hemorrhage in traumatic brain injury: a novel scoring system. J Clin Med. 2022;11:2127.

62. Matsukawa H, Shinoda M, Fujii M, et al. Intraventricular hemorrhage on computed tomography and corpus callosum injury on magnetic resonance imaging in patients with isolated blunt traumatic brain injury. J Neurosurg. 2012;117:334–9.

63. Wu Z, Li S, Lei J, et al. Evaluation of traumatic subarachnoid hemorrhage using susceptibility-weighted imaging. AJNR Am J Neuroradiol. 2010;31:1302–10.

64. Sohn C-H, Baik S-K, Lee H-J, et al. MR imaging of hyperacute subarachnoid and intraventricular hemorrhage at 3T: a preliminary report of gradient echo T2*-weighted sequences. AJNR Am J Neuroradiology. 2005;26:662–5.

65. Shafiei M, Sabouri M, Veshnavei HA, et al. Predictors of radiological contusion progression in traumatic brain injury. Int J Burns Trauma. 2023;13:58–64.

66. Toyama Y, Koboyashi T, Nishiyama Y, et al. CT for acute stage of closed head injury. Radiat Med. 2005;23:309–16.

67. Yue JK, Winkler EA, Puffer RC, et al. Temporal lobe contusions on computed tomography are associated with impaired 6-month functional recovery after mild traumatic brain injury: a TRACK-TBI study. Neurol Res. 2018;40:972–81.

68. Alahmadi H, Vachhrajani S, Cusimano MD. The natural history of brain contusion: an analysis of radiological and clinical progression. J Neurosurg. 2010;112:1139–45.

69. Kurland D, Hong C, Aarabi B, et al. Hemorrhagic progression of a contusion after traumatic brain injury: a review. J Neurotrauma. 2012;29:19–31.

70. Sriyook A, Gupta R. Imaging of head trauma: pearls and pitfalls. Radiol Clin N Am. 2023;61:535–49.

71. Hammoud DA, Wasserman BA. Diffuse axonal injuries: pathophysiology and imaging. Neuroimaging Clin N Am. 2002;12:205–16.

72. Su E, Bell M. Diffuse axonal injury. Translational research in traumatic brain injury boca. Raton, FL: CRC Press/Taylor and Francis Group; 2016. [Epub ahead of print]

73. Li XY, Feng DF. Diffuse axonal injury: novel insights into detection and treatment. J Clin Neurosci. 2009;16:614–9.

74. Adams JH, Graham DI, Murray LS, et al. Diffuse axonal injury due to nonmissile head injury in humans: an analysis of 45 cases. Ann Neurol. 1982;12:557–63.

75. Abu Hamdeh S, Marklund N, Lannsjö M, et al. Extended anatomical grading in diffuse axonal injury using MRI: hemorrhagic lesions in the substantia nigra and mesencephalic tegmentum indicate poor long-term outcome. J Neurotrauma. 2017;34:341–52.

76. Provenzale JM. Imaging of traumatic brain injury: a review of the recent medical literature. AJR Am J Roentgenol. 2010;194:16–9.

77. Zheng WB, Liu GR, Li LP, et al. Prediction of recovery from a post-traumatic coma state by diffusion-weighted imaging (DWI) in patients with diffuse axonal injury. Neuroradiology. 2007;49:271–9.

78. Tong KA, Ashwal S, Obenaus A, et al. Susceptibility-weighted MR imaging: a review of clinical applications in children. AJNR Am J Neuroradiol. 2008;29:9–17.

79. Shetty T, Nguyen JT, Cogsil T, et al. Clinical findings in a multicenter MRI study of mild TBI. Front Neurol. 2018;9:836.

80. Chan JHM, Tsui EYK, Peh WCG, et al. Diffuse axonal injury: detection of changes in anisotropy of water diffusion by diffusion-weighted imaging. Neuroradiology. 2003;45:34–8.

81. Hulkower MB, Poliak DB, Rosenbaum SB, et al. A decade of DTI in traumatic brain injury: 10 years and 100 articles later. AJNR Am J Neuroradiol. 2013;34:2064–74.

82. Iwamura A, Taoka T, Fukusumi A, et al. Diffuse vascular injury: convergent-type hemorrhage in the supratentorial white matter on susceptibility-weighted image in cases of severe traumatic brain damage. Neuroradiology. 2012;54:335–43.

83. Sperry JL, Moore EE, Coimbra R, et al. Western trauma association critical decisions in trauma: penetrating neck trauma. J Trauma Acute Care Surg. 2013;75:936–40.

84. Bhaisora KS, Behari S, Godbole C, et al. Traumatic aneurysms of the intracranial and cervical vessels: a review. Neurol India. 2016;64(Suppl):S14–23.

85. Simon LV, Nassar AK. Vertebral artery injury; 2023.

86. Schievink WI. Spontaneous dissection of the carotid and vertebral arteries. N Engl J Med. 2001;344:898–906.

87. Hakimi R, Sivakumar S. Imaging of carotid dissection. Curr Pain Headache Rep. 2019;23

88. Beucler N, Cungi PJ, Dagain A. Duret brainstem hemorrhage after transtentorial descending brain herniation: a systematic review and meta-analysis. World Neurosurg. 2023;173:251–262.e4.

89. Server A, Dullerud R, Haakonsen M, et al. Post-traumatic cerebral infarction. Neuroimaging findings, etiology and outcome. Acta Radiol. 2001;42:254–60.

90. Wang WH, Hu LS, Lin H, et al. Risk factors for post-traumatic massive cerebral infarction secondary to space-occupying epidural hematoma. J Neurotrauma. 2014;31:1444–50.

91. Vakil MT, Singh AK. A review of penetrating brain trauma: epidemiology, pathophysiology, imaging assessment, complications, and treatment. Emerg Radiol. 2017;24:301–9.

92. Castellani RJ, Smith M, Bailey K, et al. Neuropathology in consecutive forensic consultation cases with a history of remote traumatic brain injury. J Alzheimers Dis. 2019;72:683–91.

93. Kazim SF, Shamim MS, Tahir MZ, et al. Management of penetrating brain injury. J Emerg Trauma Shock. 2011;4:395–402.

94. Phang SY, Whitehouse K, Lee L, et al. Management of CSF leak in base of skull fractures in adults. Br J Neurosurg. 2016;30:596–604.

95. Hofmann E, Behr R, Schwager K. Imaging of cerebrospinal fluid leaks. Klin Neuroradiol. 2009;19:111–21.

96. Drapkin AJ. Growing skull fracture: a posttraumatic neosuture. Childs Nerv Syst. 2006;22:394–7.

97. Ersahin Y, Gulmen V, Palali I, et al. Growing skull fractures (craniocerebral erosion). Neurosurg Rev. 2000;23:139–44.

98. Makulski DD, Taber KH, Chiou-Tan FY. Neuroimaging in posttraumatic hypopituitarism. J Comput Assist Tomogr. 2008;32:324–8.

Differential Diagnosis of Intracranial Masses

8

Fabrice Bonneville, H. Rolf Jäger, and James G. Smirniotopoulos

Abstract

The differential diagnosis of cerebral mass lesions includes neoplastic, inflammatory, infective, and vascular lesions, as well as incidental developmental anomalies. A differential diagnostic approach should be based on the patient's mode of presentations and prior clinical history, as well as on a systematic analysis of imaging patterns. This includes anatomical features, such as intra- vs. extra-axial, predominant gray matter or white matter involvement, supra-versus infratentorial, single vs. multiple, as well as signal characteristics on standard MR sequences, enhancement patterns, and findings on diffusion-weighted imaging, and hemorrhage-sensitive and perfusion sequences. Here we will discuss primary and secondary cerebral neoplasms in broad terms and illustrate the most important tumor mimics.

Keywords

Intracranial masses · Differential diagnosis · Glioma
Astrocytoma · Lymphoma · Tumefactive demyelination
Meningioma · Metastasis · Schwannoma · Ganglioglioma
Edema · Contrast enhancement · MRI · CT

Learning Objects
- Distinguish intra-axial from extra-axial and intra-ventricular masses.
- Describe secondary effects: "volume effect" and perilesional vasogenic edema.
- Distinguish metastatic disease at gray–white junction from deeper infiltrating gliomas.
- Become aware of the most important non-neoplastic tumor mimics.

8.1 Introduction

Interpretation of imaging of cerebral mass lesion requires knowledge about the patient's clinical presentation and prior medical history as well as a systematic approach and awareness of tumor mimics. Pattern analysis is preferable to pattern recognition: progression of clinical course (acute-rapid, subacute-smoldering, chronic-prolonged); location of lesion (intra- vs. extra-axial); secondary effects (volume, edema, herniation); enhancement (solid, ring-like or leading edge, non-enhancing); blood-products;, MR perfusion, MR spectroscopy (MRS); diffusion-weighted Imaging (DWI and ADC values); response to treatment.

8.2 Time Course of Disease

Cerebrovascular events usually present acutely; they may include epidural, subdural, subarachnoid, or intraparenchymal hemorrhage (deep or lobar) or ischemic (aphasia, motor deficit, etc.) and have typical, mostly unequivocal imaging features. However, late subacute ischemic or hemorrhagic lesions may lack these typical features and may mimic mass lesions.

F. Bonneville (✉)
Department of Neuroradiology, University Hospital of Toulouse, Toulouse, France
e-mail: Bonneville.f@chu-toulouse.fr

H. R. Jäger
UCL Queen Square Institute of Neurology, The National Hospital for Neurology and Neurosurgery and University College Hospital (UCH), London, UK
e-mail: r.jager@ucl.ac.uk

J. G. Smirniotopoulos
Department of Radiology, Sigma Healthcare Consulting, Silver Spring, MD, USA

© The Author(s) 2024
J. Hodler et al. (eds.), *Diseases of the Brain, Head and Neck, Spine 2024-2027*, IDKD Springer Series,
https://doi.org/10.1007/978-3-031-50675-8_8

The clinical presentation of brain tumors is variable ranging from absent (incidental discovery), minor symptoms, focal deficits, to rapid onset neurological decline. Epilepsy is a common presentation of brain tumors, as are symptoms of increased mass (nausea and vomiting) and cognitive decline. Occasionally, an intertumoral hemorrhage can lead to an acute presentation.

Pseudotumors, which include vascular, inflammatory, and infective lesions, have also a variable time course, and some lesions (such as enlarge perivascular spaces) are discovered incidentally.

> **Key Point**
> • Every image should be interpreted in the clinical context for each patient. When things are inconsistent, expand your differential diagnosis.

8.3   Intra-axial Vs. Extra-axial

Intra-axial lesions involve the parenchyma of the brain (including brainstem and cerebellum). They may follow an anatomic distribution (e.g., vascular territory for ischemia/infarction) or non-anatomic distribution (abscess). Diffuse gliomas will expand the infiltrated gray matter, white matter and tracts, causing effacement of ventricles and sulci, midline shift, or hydrocephalus (Fig. 8.1). Extra-axial lesions will displace the brain away from the skull—often enlarging the subarachnoid cisternal spaces at the edges adjacent to the mass (Fig. 8.2).

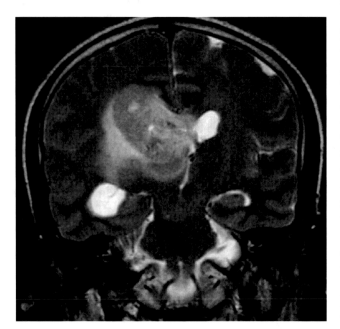

Fig. 8.1 Intra-axial tumor (glioblastoma). Coronal T2-weighted image shows hyperintense right frontal mass lesion with surrounding peritumoral oedema, mass effect on the ventricle and midline shift

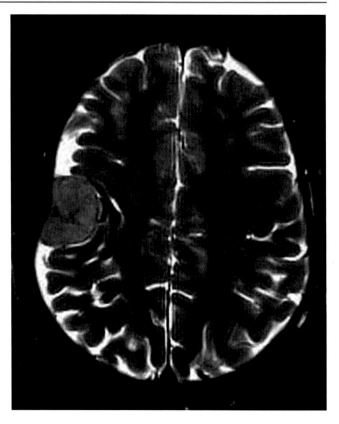

Fig. 8.2 Extra-axial mass (meningioma). Axial T2-weighted MR shows a right-side gray-matter signal intensity hemispheric-shape mass with enlargement of the subarachnoid space at it's margins. There is underlying hyperostosis

8.4   Pattern Analysis

Radiology (also pathology and dermatology) are often taught using "pattern recognition." This works well once you have accumulated—through experience—a built-in library of "patterns" that you may match with an unknown case. Another approach is break down of the imaging features, analyze them separately, and then synthesize a differential diagnosis. Patterns of contrast enhancement may suggest more specific diagnoses: gyral gray-matter enhancement occurs with reperfusion after ischemia, post-ictal or seizures, and meningoencephalitis; ring enhancement implies "central necrosis"—but may be seen with an organized abscess as well as neoplasms [1].

8.5   Neoplastic Vs. Non-neoplastic Disease

Neoplastic diseases are usually "tumefactive"—they take up space ("positive volume effect") and displace adjacent structures causing secondary damage and herniation. Both primary and secondary (metastatic) lesions may have added volume from accumulation of interstitial fluid—

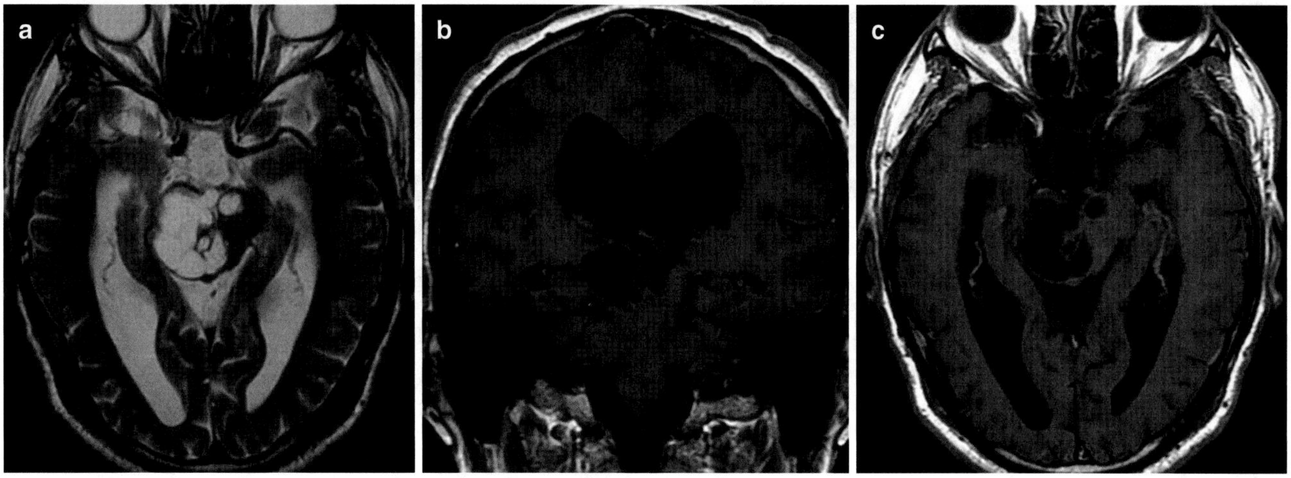

Fig. 8.3 Dilated perivascular Virchow-Robin spaces in a 36-year-old man with intracranial hypertension. (**a**) Axial T2 image shows a multiloculated hyperintense mass lesion in the mesencephalon responsible of hydrocephalus, with hyperintense signal intensity identical to CSF. (**b**) Coronal T1-weighted and (**c**) axial post-gadolinium T1-weighted images reveal no enhancement and also demonstrate that signal intensity of the lesion follows CSF. This pattern, in this location is typical for a cluster of dilated perivascular spaces. If usually asymptomatic, they have been reported to be a source of non-communicating hydrocephalus when located in the midbrain

brain edema—most often due to abnormal increased permeability from breakdown of the blood–brain barrier (BBB): vasogenic edema. When large enough, tumefactive dilated perivascular spaces, though non-neoplastic, may also have mass effect (Fig. 8.3). In contrast, inflammatory demyelination often has minimal or neutral "volume neutral." Chronic destructive processes (demyelination, healed viral infections, old infarcts) have "negative volume effect."

Tumefactive demyelinating lesions (TDLs) are a frequent differential dilemma. If correctly identified, they should not be biopsied. Instead, a trial of immune-modulating therapy should be given. Features suggesting a TDL (instead of a neoplasm) include: lesion centered in white matter (including corpus callosum); central-vein sign; "garland-like" or incomplete rim enhancement ("open-ring" or "horseshoe"); less than expected volume effect; rCBV lower than neoplasm; ADC values higher than neoplasm (GBM or lymphoma)Cho/Naa ratio lower than neoplasm; and, non-contrast CT showing low attenuation (compared to solid portions of GBM and hyper-attenuation of lymphoma [2–4] (Fig. 8.4).

> **Key Point**
> • Chronic destructive lesions cause a loss of brain volume or "negative volume effect," with compensatory enlargement of ventricles and sulci. Adding cells (blood, pus, neoplasm) usually cause proportionate "positive volume effect" with compression of ventricles and effacement of sulci.

> **Key Point**
> • Tumefactive demyelination may be distinguished from a neoplasm by paucity of mass effect; minimal/no perilesional edema; "open ring" enhancement; increased ADC; and low perfusion values.

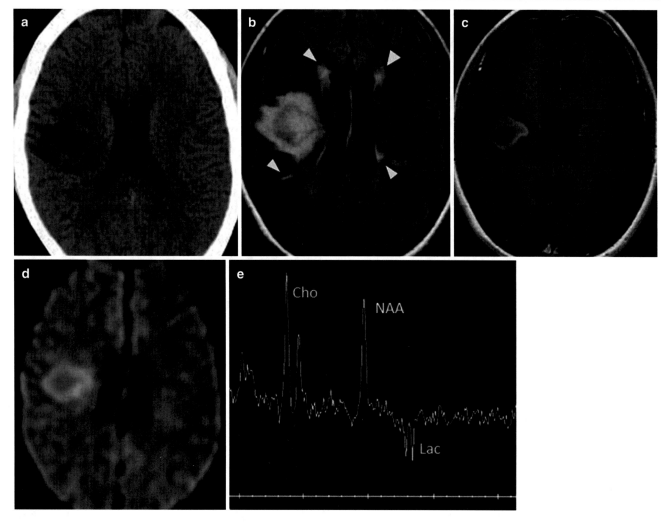

Fig. 8.4 Pseudotumoral multiple sclerosis in a 24-year-old woman with left hemiparesis. (**a**) Non-contrast head CT shows large mass lesion in the right frontal lobe. (**b**) Axial FLAIR demonstrates surrounding vasogenic oedema and depicts additional periventricular and subcortical white matter hyperintensities (arrowheads), fulfilling the McDonald's criteria for dissemination in space. (**c**) Axial post-gadolinium T1-weighted image reveals rim enhancement of the large lesion, but not of the small ones. Of note, there is no mass effect on the adjacent sulci and ipsilateral ventricle. This feature is suggestive of demyelinating lesion and would be unlikely in case of a tumor this size. (**d**) Axial diffusion-weighted image shows peripheral hyperintensity, which is commonly observed in acute demyelinating lesion. (**e**) Long TE MR spectroscopy demonstrates typical findings of acute demyelinating lesion with the presence of the inverted doublet of lactate, together with elevated choline and decreased NAA with a ratio Cho/NAA between 1 and 2

8.6 Single Vs. Many Lesions

The vast majority of intracranial lesions may present as a single/solitary mass: primary neoplasm; hematoma; abscess; infarction. Multiple lesions primarily occur as part of a systemic disease: inflammatory; toxic; metabolic; genetic; or hematogenous dissemination (Fig. 8.5). Hematogenous dissemination of infection and metastatic neoplasms can present with solid nodular as well as ring-enhancing lesions. Approximately 40–60% of patients with hematogenous metastasis will present initially with a single or solitary metastasis [5]. Inflammatory and autoimmune diseases (without infection) typically show multiple lesions: multiple sclerosis—MS, Acute Disseminated Encephalomyelitis—ADEM (Fig. 8.6).

Key Point
- Multiple lesions have many possible causes—some neoplastic, others toxic, metabolic, inflammatory, or genetic.

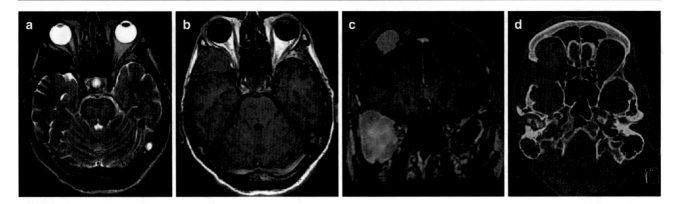

Fig. 8.5 A 69-year-old female patient with multiple myeloma and diplopia. (**a**) Axial T2-weighted image, (**b**) axial unenhanced T1W image, (**c**) coronal T1W image post-contrast, and (**d**) CT with bone window settings. T2 hypointense and T1 gray matter isointense mass centered on the right sphenoid is protruding into the right orbit, displacing the right lateral rectus muscle anteriorly. The coronal post-contrast images demonstrate enhancement of this mass and additional enhancing lesions in the right frontal bone. CT shows bone destruction. The appearance is consistent with multiple myeloma deposits

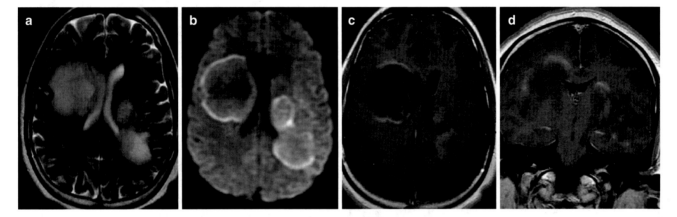

Fig. 8.6 Pseudotumoral acute disseminated encephalomyelitis (ADEM) in a 29-year-old woman with rapidly progressive left hemiparesis and confusion. (**a**) Axial T2-weighted image shows multiple large lesions in the deep brain, sparing the corpus callosum, with minimal mass effect on the ventricles. (**b**) Diffusion-weighted image demonstrates hyperintense rim around each lesion. (**c**) Axial and (**d**) coronal post-gadolinium T1-weighted images illustrate open-ring enhancement of the lesions, a feature suggestive of acute demyelination. ADEM is the favored diagnosis because all the lesions appear the same way and especially because all of them are enhancing

8.7   Metastatic Disease

Hematogenous dissemination of tumor cells is the most common mechanism for brain metastasis; other routes include dissemination via the CSF. The brain requires about 20% of our cardiac output. It is a vast "filtration bed" where platelet thrombi, clots, and tumor emboli may lodge. The majority of these "particulates" will lodge in two places: in the subcortical gray–white matter junction; and, in the penetrating vessels that supply the deep gray matter [6]. Within the brain parenchyma, metastases are remarkably well localized, round solid or ring enhancing, often with a rim of reactive gliosis, and surrounded by perilesional vasogenic edema. Survival of patients presenting with parenchymal brain metastasis has been short in the past, but the advent of new treatments (immunotherapy and stereotactic radiosurgery) has led to a much better prognosis.

> **Key Point**
> - Metastatic lesions are usually peripheral cortical or subcortical, round, and well-demarcated with enhancement and perilesional vasogenic edema. At initial presentation with metastatic disease, 40–60% of patients will have a single or solitary (only brain) metastatic lesion.

8.8   Primary Neoplasms

8.8.1   Extra-axial Neoplasms

Extra-axial neoplasms arise from the supporting tissues of the meninges (meningioma) and the nerves passing from central to peripheral (schwannoma). These are the two most common extra-axial and most common non-glial tumors. They occur anywhere around the cerebral convexities, along the falx and tentorium, and on the skull base. Meningiomas arise from the arachnoid and usually have a broad base of attachment to the adjacent dura—giving them a hemispheric or "globose" shape (Fig. 8.7). A second morphology is the "en plaque" meningioma—a thickening growing along the inner table of the skull like a flat bread (pita bread). Meningiomas usually maintain a homogenous CT high attenuation, and MR gray-matter-like signal intensity, and enhancement as they grow larger. They are commonly associated with adjacent hyperostosis and an enhancing "dural tail" [7]. Intra-axial vasogenic edema occurs in about 50% of meningiomas and is only loosely correlated with histology [8]. It is more often seen when the tumor does not have a clear visible CSF-cleft, has high signal intensity on T2 and a pial blood supply (rather than dural-only) (Fig. 8.8) [9]. On perfusion imaging, they usually have increased rCBV and rCBF—while showing prolonged MTT.

Schwannomas arise from the peripheral portions of the cranial nerves [3–12]—so they are ventral to the brainstem,

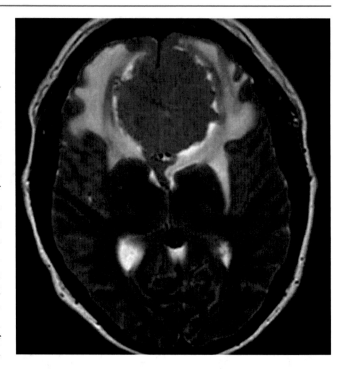

Fig. 8.8 Meningioma. Axial T2-weighted MR shows a bi-frontal soft-tissue mass centered on the falx, with non-specific gray-matter signal intensity. There is bi-frontal intra-axial vasogenic edema that skirts the gray matter of the lenticular nuclei. Meningiomas easily infiltrate through the dura (not a sign of malignancy)—while other lesions (metastasis) usually do not

most commonly in the posterior fossa. The most common site of origin is the inferior division of the vestibular nerve, at the apex of the internal auditory canal (IAC)—VS (vestibular Schwannoma). The tumors will compress the adjacent cochlear nerve—causing high-frequency hearing loss; but, vestibular dysfunction may be retained. They grow out of the IAC into the cerebellopontine angle (CPA) cistern—where they present the bulk of the mass (Fig. 8.9). Like meningiomas VS will show avid enhancement. However, unlike meningioma, large schwannomas become heterogenous from benign cystic/necrotic degeneration. There are no imaging signs that reliably predict tumor growth, but larger tumors at presentation tend to grow faster [11].

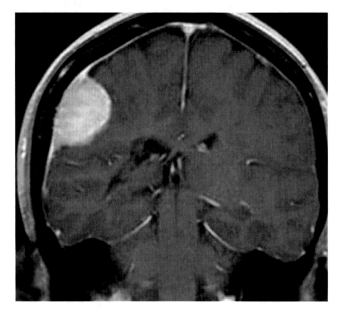

Fig. 8.7 Meningioma. Coronal T1-weighted MR after gadolinium. This globose meningioma shows a sharply-demarcated, hemispheric, extra-axial lesion with overlying calvarial thickening (hyperostosis). The nearby adjacent dura is slightly thickened with avid enhancement—the "dural tail." This represents a reactive process, not neoplastic infiltration

Key Point

Meningiomas usually remain homogeneous, even when large. Vestibular schwannomas are distinguished by location at a nerve (e.g., arising within the internal auditory canal); and, they often become heterogeneous as they grow and enlarge. Almost all extra-axial and non-glial neoplasms show contrast enhancement.

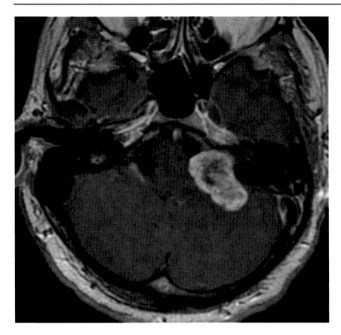

Fig. 8.9 Vestibular schwannoma. Axial T1-weighted MR after gadolinium shows a heterogeneously enhancing left-sided mass in the cerebellopontine angle cistern with a component inside an enlarged internal auditory canal

8.8.2 Intra-axial Neoplasms

The overwhelming majority of primary intra-axial neoplasms arise from the glia—or glial cell precursors, and the 2021 WHO classification of brain tumors is heavily based on molecular features, in particular the presence of IDH and 1p/19q mutations [13]. Glial CNS neoplasms are discussed elsewhere in details in the course.

Here, we would merely like to highlight a few imaging features that are important for the differential diagnosis: A T2/FLAIR mismatch is a sensitive sign for an IDH mutant astrocytoma (but it is present only in about 50% of these tumors, so that absence of this sign does not exclude an astrocytoma) [14] (Fig. 8.10). Oligodendrogliomas (IDH mutant 1p19q deleted) show frequently intratumoral calcification and are commonly located in the frontal lobes with involvement of the cortex and subcortical white matter

(Fig. 8.11). The classical picture of GBMs is that of an irregularly enhancing tumor often with a necrotic center, surrounding white matter infiltration/edema. However, with the increased molecular diagnosis of GBMs (IDH wild-type), it has become apparent that GBMs can also present as non-enhancing infiltrative tumors. A further entity of note are gliomas with H3 K27 mutations, which involve usually midline structures [15] (Fig. 8.12).

Lymphoma is another common CNS neoplasm, which is important to distinguish from glial neoplasm. The majority (80–85%) of primary CNS lymphomas are diffuse large B-cell Lymphomas, Epstein–Barr virus negative (EBV-). These can be solitary or multiple (30–50%) and are usually hypointense to gray matter on T2W imaging, have a low ADC, and enhance homogeneously [16] (Fig. 8.13). On MR perfusion imaging, lymphomas show typically a mildly elevated rCBV (much less than, e.g., GBMs) and a marked T1 leakage effect. EVB + B-cell lymphomas account for approximately 10% of lymphomas and are associated with immune deficiency (e.g., post-transplant, autoimmune conditions, HIV), show irregular ring enhancement, have variable ADC values, and may contain hemorrhagic components. Other forms of lymphoma include secondary CNS lymphoma (usually with ependymal and meningeal involvement), intravascular B-cell lymphoma, dural lymphoma, and lymphomatosis cerebri.

Intraventricular neoplasms include colloid cysts (at the foramen of Monro/third ventricle), meningiomas (typically in the trigone of the third ventricle), choroid tumors and ependymomas (lateral ventricle in children, fourth ventricle in adults), central neurocytoma (lateral ventricle, involvement of the septum pellucidum), and metastases (choroidal/ependymal). Neurocytomas that occur in younger adults show frequently restricted diffusion and contain calcifications (Fig. 8.14).

Tumor mimics are important in the differential diagnosis and we include here a pictorial panel with detailed descriptions of such lesions of vascular origin (Figs. 8.15, 8.16, and 8.17), inflammatory origin (Figs. 8.18 and 8.19), or infectious origin (Figs. 8.20 and 8.21).

Fig. 8.10 Low-grade astrocytoma (grade 2) in a 47-year-old male patient present new onset epilepsy. (**a**) Axial T2W, (**b**) FLAIR, (**c**) T1 post-contrast, and (**d**) rCBV map of DSC perfusion imaging. A left temporal and insular mass lesions appear homogeneously hyperintense on T2 w images. The FLAIR image shows a hyperintense rim with a hypointense center (T2/FLAIR mismatch), which is typical for an IDH mutant astrocytoma. Post-contrast T1 W image shows no enhancement, and the rCBV does not contain any areas of increased rCBV

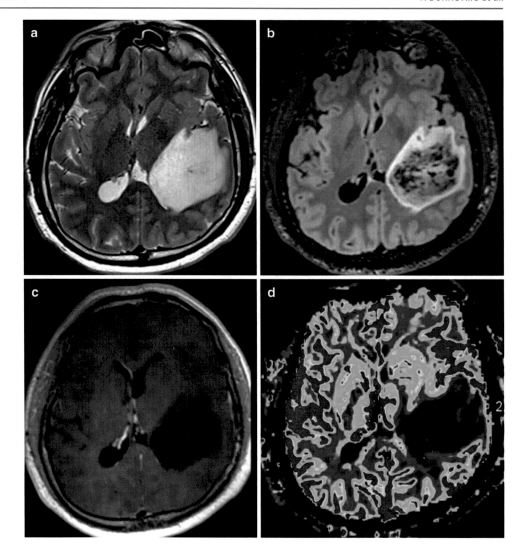

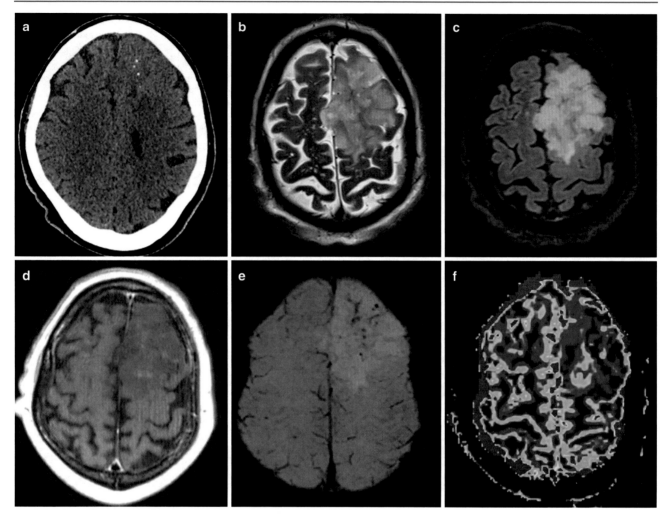

Fig. 8.11 Oligodendroglioma in a 57-year-old male patient presenting with epilepsy. (**a**) Axial CT, (**b**) axial T2-weighted image, (**c**) FLAIR, (**d**) post-contrast T1-weighted, (**e**) SWI image, and (**f**) rCBV map of DSC perfusion. A heterogenous T2/FLAIR hyperintense left frontal mass involving cortex and subcortical white matter contains punctate calcification (**a**) which causes signal drop out on the SWI sequence (**e**). There is faint enhancement (**d**) and mildly raised rCBV (**f**). This is an oligodendroglioma. Mild enhancement and mildly elevated rCBV values can also be seen in low-grade (WHO grade 2) oligodendrogliomas due to the typical intratumoral "chicken wire" vessels

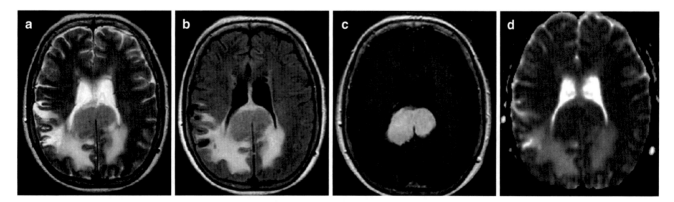

Fig. 8.12 Biopsy-proven lymphoma in a 64-year-old female patient with progressive cognitive decline and headaches. (**a**) Axial T2-weighted, (**b**) FLAIR, (**c**) T1 post-contrast, and (**d**) ADC map demonstrate a mass lesion in the splenium with surrounding oedema. The mass is of intermediate intensity on T2W and FLAIR images (**a** and **b**), enhances homogenously (**c**), and has a relatively low ADC. These features in this location suggest a primary CNS lymphoma

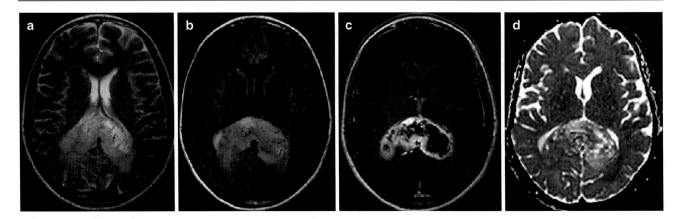

Fig. 8.13 Glioblastoma in a 59 year-old male patient with cognitive decline. (**a**) Axial T2-weighted, (**b**) FLAIR, (**c**) T1 post-contrast, and (**d**) ADC map. There is a mass lesion in the splenium which is predominantly hyperintense on T2 and FLAIR images (**a** and **b**). These images also contain some vascular flow voids. Following IV gadolinium, the mass enhances heterogeneously with a characteristic necrotic center (**c**). The ADC map is heterogeneous but contains predominantly areas of increased ADC values. Biopsy confirmed a glioblastoma

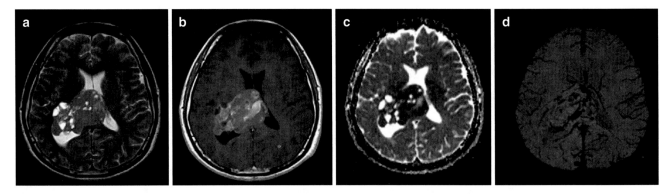

Fig. 8.14 Central neurocytoma in a 42-year-old man with intracranial hypertension, headaches, and blurry vision. (**a**) Axial T2-weighted image, (**b**) axial T1 pre-contrast, (**c**) ADC map, and (**d**) SWI image demonstrate an intraventricular heterogeneous mass lesion, involving the septum pellucidum and extending in the right ventricle. Heterogeneity with areas of spontaneous T1 hyperintensity, low ADC, and hypointensity on SWI is suggestive of the diagnosis

Fig. 8.15 Subacute stroke in a 57-year-old man with subacute vertigo and headaches since 7 days. (**a**) Axial FLAIR shows abnormal heterogeneous cortico-subcortical hyperintensity in the left cerebellar hemisphere, better delineated on (**b**) axial diffusion-weighted Image. (**c**) Axial post-contrast T1-weighted image reveals peripheral enhancement, erroneously suggesting a tumor. (**d**) Coronal T2-weighted image demonstrates sharp borders of this cortico-subcortical lesion, not crossing the midline, strictly limited to the PICA territory, which is in favor of an ischemic stroke

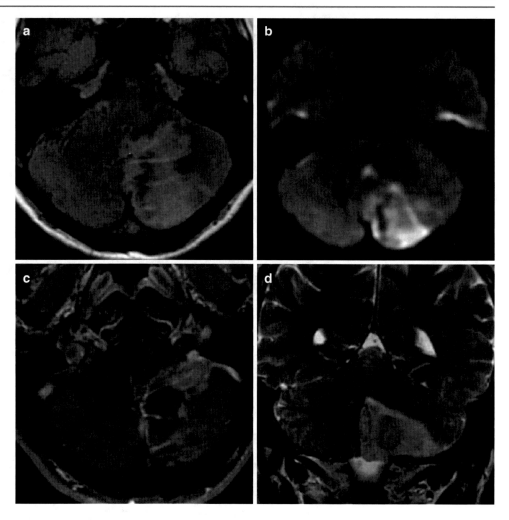

Fig. 8.16 Giant thrombosed aneurysm in a 72-year-old woman with cognitive impairment and headaches. Axial T1-weighted images (**a**) before and (**b**) after gadolinium injection reveal a huge non-enhancing mass lesion in the left frontal lobe with mass effect on the ipsilateral ventricle and minimal midline shift. Spontaneous hyperintensity at the periphery of the lesion is suggestive of thrombus. (**c**) Axial FLAIR demonstrates heterogeneous hypointensity of the mass lesion, which is in favor of a thrombosed aneurysm, as confirmed by (**d**) anteroposterior view of left internal carotid artery digital subtracted angiogram

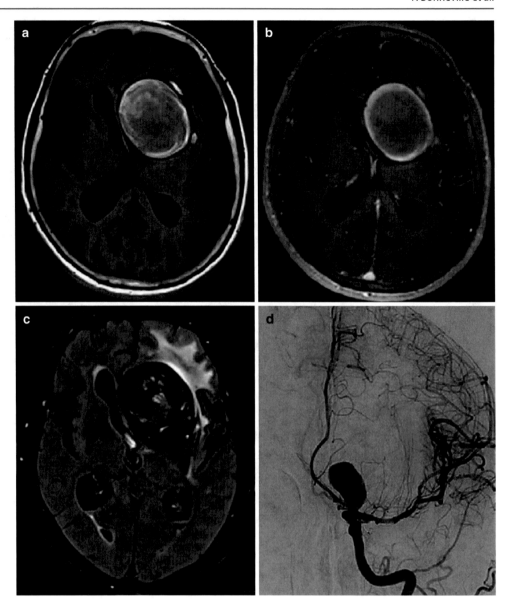

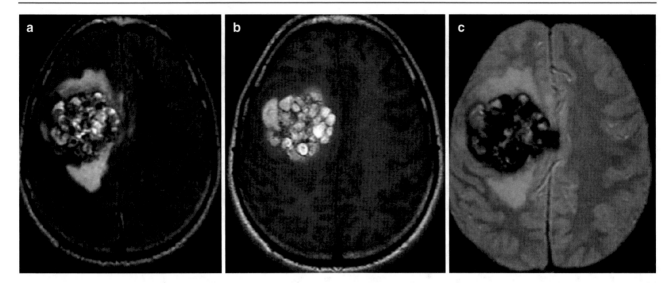

Fig. 8.17 Giant cavernoma in a 29-year-old man with seizures. (**a**) Axial FLAIR reveals a giant right frontal heterogeneous mass lesion in the right frontal lobe, surrounded by vasogenic edema. (**b**) Axial T1-weighted image demonstrates spontaneous hyperintensity of this multilobulated mass, formed by a cluster of multiple dilated "caverns," filled with blood, as confirmed by the marked hypointensity observed on (**c**) axial gradient echo T2* image

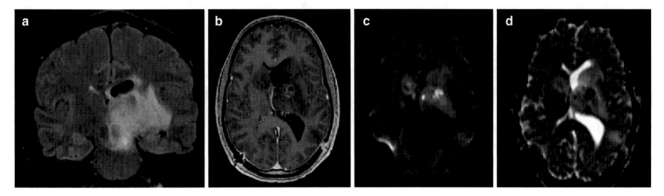

Fig. 8.18 Behcet's disease in a 31-year-old man with right hemiparesia and confusion. (**a**) Coronal FLAIR, (**b**) axial enhanced T1-weighted image, (**c**) DWI image, and (**d**) ACD demonstrate a partially enhancing lesion centered on the left basal ganglia extending across the midline and inferiorly into the midbrain. There is patchy enhancement and partially restricted diffusion. This is an inflammatory mass in the context of Behcet's disease

Fig. 8.19 Sarcoidosis in a 42-year-old woman with left hemiparesis. (**a**) Coronal post-contrast T1-weighted image reveals a dura-based mass lesion mimicking a meningioma. The lack of adjacent bony reaction and of typical dural-tail sign is suspicious. (**b**) Coronal T2 demonstrates mark hypointensity, a feature that may suggest chronic inflammation, as observed in systemic diseases, and in particular in sarcoidosis

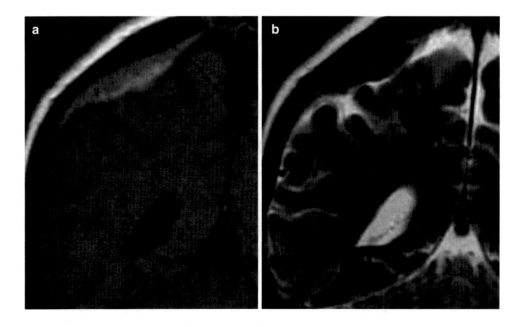

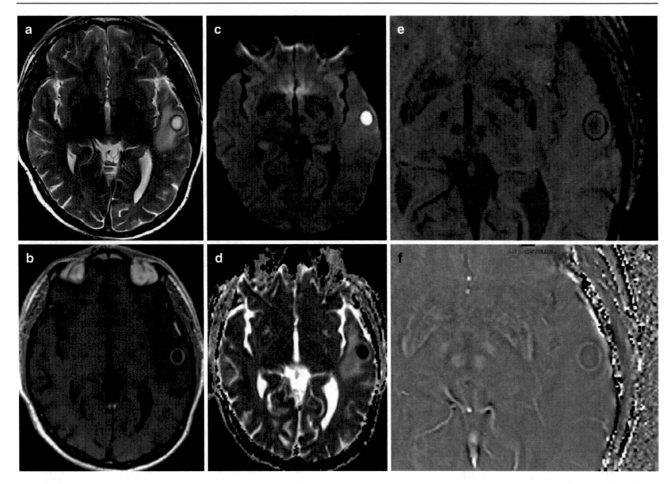

Fig. 8.20 Bacterial abscess in a 48-year-old woman with seizures. (**a**) Axial T2-weighted image, (**b**) Axial post-contrast T1-weighted, (**c**) DWI and (**d**) ADC map, (**e**) SWI image with minimal intensity projection, and (**f**) phase images of SWI sequence. There is a ring-enhancing lesion in the left temporal lobe with surrounding oedema (**a** and **b**) showing central restricted diffusion (**c** and **d**) and a double rim sign on SWI images (**e** and **f**). These features a typical for a bacterial abscess

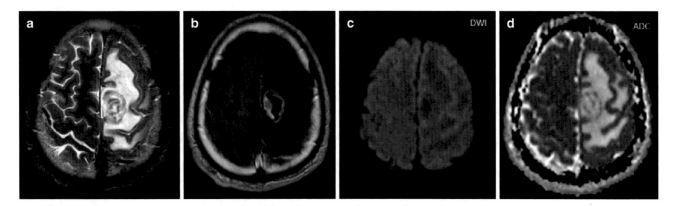

Fig. 8.21 Toxoplasmosis abscess in a 32-year-old HIV man. (**a**) Axial T2-weighted image, (**b**) axial contrast-enhanced T1-weighted image, (**c**) DWI, and (**d**) ACD map. There is a ring-enhancing (**b**) mass in the left superior frontal gyrus with surrounding oedema. T2W images demonstrate a "target sign." The lesion shows predominantly increased water diffusion (**c** and **d**). This is a toxoplasmosis abscess, which shows typically increased water diffusivity, as opposed to bacterial abscesses that show restricted water diffusion

8.9   Concluding Remarks

There are multiple tools for triangulating a short differential diagnosis list; and, it is important to use "pattern analysis" rather than simple "pattern recognition." Key features include lesion location, relative "volume effect"; secondary vasogenic edema; homogeneity or heterogeneity of the lesion; and patterns of contrast enhancement (homogeneous, patchy, closed or open ring). Multiple lesions usually represent a systemic process: inflammatory, toxic, metabolic, genetic, or, hematogenous dissemination. Extra-axial masses are non-glial, while intra-axial neoplasms may be metastatic from extra-CNS sources, or primary gliomas.

Take Home Messages
- Some of the primary gliomas have distinctive features, such as a T2-FLAIR mismatch in IDH mutant astrocytomas and calcification in oligodendrogliomas.
- Enhancement is not a reliable indicator for tumor grade.
- Primary CNS lymphomas have a different appearance in immunocompetent and immunocompromised patients.
- Extra axial lesions are commonly meningiomas, schwannomas, and congenital cysts but metastases, inflammatory lesions (e.g., sarcoidosis), and myeloma are in the differential diagnosis.
- Important non-neoplastic tumor mimics include tumefactive MS, ADEM, abscesses, and vascular lesions.

References

1. Smirniotopoulos JG, Murphy FM, Rushing EJ, Schroeder JW. Patterns of contrast enhancement in the brain and meninges. Radiographics. 2007;27(2):525–51.
2. Kim DS, Na DG, Kim KH, Kim JH, Kim EYBL, et al. Distinguishing tumefactive demyelinating lesions from glioma or central nervous system lymphoma: added value of unenhanced CT compared with conventional contrast-enhanced MR imaging. Radiology. 2009;251(2):467–75.
3. Suh CH, Kim HS, Jung SC, Choi CG, Kim SJ, Kim SJ. MRI findings in tumefactive demyelinating lesions: a systematic review and meta-analysis. AJNR Am J Neuroradiol. 2018;39(9):1643–9.
4. Suthiphosuwan S, Sati P, Guenette M, Montalban X, Reich DM, Bharatha A, et al. The central vein sign in radiologically isolated syndrome. AJNR Am J Neuroradiol. 2019;40(5):776–83.
5. Nussbaum ES, Djalilian HR, Cho KH, Hall WA. Brain metastases. Histology, multiplicity, surgery, and survival. Cancer. 1996;78(8):1781–8.
6. Hwang TL, Close TP, Grego JM, Brannon WL, Gonzales F. Predilection of brain metastasis in gray and white matter junction and vascular border zones. Cancer. 1996;77(8):1551–5.
7. Lyndon D, Lansley JA, Evanson J, Krishnan AS. Dural masses: meningiomas and their mimics. Insights Imaging. 2019;10(1):11.
8. Lee KJ, Joo WI, Rha HK, Park HK, Chough JK, Hong YK, et al. Peritumoral brain edema in meningiomas: correlations between magnetic resonance imaging, angiography, and pathology. Surg Neurol. 2008;69(4):350–5.
9. Osawa T, Tosaka M, Nagaishi M, Yoshimoto Y. Factors affecting peritumoral brain edema in meningioma: special histological subtypes with prominently extensive edema. J Neuro-Oncol. 2013;111(1):49–57.
10. Crisi G. H MR spectroscopy of meningiomas at 3.0T: the role of glutamate-glutamine complex and glutathione. Neuroradiol J. 2011;24(6):846–53.
11. D'Haese S, Parmentier H, Keppler H, Van Vooren S, Van Driessche V, Bauters W, et al. Vestibular schwannoma: natural growth and possible predictive factors. Acta Otolaryngol. 2019;139(9):753–8.
12. Andronesi OC, Rapilino O, Gerstner E, Chi A, Batchelor T. Detection of oncogenic IDH1 mutations using magnetic resonance spectroscopy of 2-hydroxyglutarate. J Clin Invest. 2013;123(9):3659–63.
13. Osborn AG, Louis DN, Poussaint TY, Linscott LL, Salzman KL. The 2021 World Health Organization classification of tumors of the central nervous system: what neuroradiologists need to know. AJNR. 2022;43(7):928–397.
14. Suh CH, Kim HS, Jung SC, Choi CG, Kim SJ. Imaging prediction of isocitrate dehydrogenase (IDH) mutation in patients with glioma: a systemic review and meta-analysis. Eur Radiol. 2019;29(2):745–58.
15. Eckel-Passow JE, Lachance DH, Molinaro AM, Walsh KM, et al. Glioma groups based on 1p/19q, IDH, and TERT promoter mutations in tumors. N Engl J Med. 2015;372(26):2499–508.
16. Pons-Escoda A, Naval-Baudin P, Velasco R, Vidal N, Majós C. Imaging of lymphomas involving the CNS: an update-review of the full spectrum of disease with an emphasis on the World Health Organization classifications of CNS tumors 2021 and hematolymphoid tumors 2022. AJNR. 2023;44(4):358–66.

Toxic and Metabolic Disorders

Sofie Van Cauter and Marco Essig

Abstract

Metabolic diseases are mostly congenital inborn errors leading to functional defects in metabolic pathways, whereas toxic and metabolic diseases in adults are usually acquired. MRI is the cornerstone in the assessment of these patients. The final diagnosis is often established in combination with laboratory findings and/or genetic analysis. Imaging patterns are almost invariably bilateral and often symmetric or nearly symmetric. The basal ganglia and thalami are often involved in acquired metabolic and toxic diseases. This chapter focuses on the most common inborn errors of metabolism that can present or persist into adulthood, as well as on the most common acquired metabolic and toxic disorders, relevant to daily clinical practice.

Keywords

Toxic encephalopathy · Metabolic disorders · Neuroimaging · MRI · Basal ganglia · Thalami · White matter

Learning Objectives

- To be familiar with the most common metabolic disorders presenting or persisting into adulthood.
- To evaluate the most common toxic encephalopathies, relevant to daily clinical practice.
- To recognize the typical imaging patterns of these disorders on MRI and be able to postulate a differential diagnosis.

Key Points

- MRI is the cornerstone in the assessment of CNS manifestations of toxic and metabolic diseases, in combination with laboratory and/or genetic testing.
- Imaging patterns are almost invariably bilateral and often symmetric or nearly symmetric. In acquired metabolic and toxic diseases, the basal ganglia and thalami are often involved.
- Adult-onset cerebral ALD accounts for about 5% of cases and presents typically with extensive symmetric white matter lesions displaying contrast enhancement in the regions of active demyelination.
- Metachromatic leukodystrophy is the most common hereditary leukodystrophy. Krabbe disease is a differential diagnosis.
- MELAS should be considered when stroke is encountered in adolescents, especially when there are multiple infarcts in different stages.
- Alexander disease presents with abnormalities in the lower brainstem.
- Wernicke encephalopathy typically presents with abnormalities around the midline organs in the diencephalon or mesencephalon.

S. Van Cauter
Department of Medical Imaging, Ziekenhuis Oost-Limburg Genk, Genk, Belgium
e-mail: Sofie.vancauter@zol.be

M. Essig (✉)
Max Rady College of Medicine, Radiology, Winnipeg, MB, Canada
e-mail: messig@exchange.hsc.mb.ca; messig@hsc.mb.ca

© The Author(s) 2024
J. Hodler et al. (eds.), *Diseases of the Brain, Head and Neck, Spine 2024-2027*, IDKD Springer Series,
https://doi.org/10.1007/978-3-031-50675-8_9

- Subacute combined degeneration is the only toxic-metabolic disease presenting with abnormalities in the medulla.
- Hypoglycemic encephalopathy presents with cytotoxic edema in the gray matter structures with typical sparing of the thalami.

9.1 Introduction

Metabolic diseases in children are mostly congenital inborn errors leading to functional defects in metabolic pathways, whereas toxic and metabolic diseases in adults are usually acquired.

Congenital metabolic disorders in children are a vast and highly specialized field, and the detailed knowledge of these belongs to the remit of tertiary referral centers.

This chapter focuses on the most common inborn errors of metabolism that can present or persist into adulthood, as well as on the most common acquired metabolic and toxic disorders, relevant to daily clinical practice [1].

The clinical presentation of these patients is often non-specific. Neuroimaging is the cornerstone in the workup of patients suspected of being affected by a toxic or metabolic disorder. The final diagnosis is most often reached in combination with laboratory analysis and genetic testing in case of congenital disorders.

Magnetic resonance imaging (MRI) is the preferential imaging modality to assess toxic and metabolic disorders in the brain due to its superior contrast resolution. Nonetheless, computer tomography (CT) has an added value in the detection of intracranial calcifications. Susceptibility-weighted imaging (SWI) is a valid alternative for detecting intracranial calcifications, especially when using phase information. Nonetheless, the accuracy is lower compared to CT.

The topographic distribution of brain pathology in toxic and metabolic disorders is a reflection of the metabolic pathways involved and the metabolic activity, often depending on age. Imaging patterns are almost invariable bilateral, often symmetrical or near-symmetrical. The basal ganglia and thalami are especially susceptible to injury due to their extensive energetic requirements related to the involvement in a myriad of processes related to the pyramidal and extra-pyramidal systems.

9.2 Most Common Congenital Metabolic Disorders Presenting or Persisting into Adulthood

9.2.1 X-Linked Adrenoleukodystrophy (ALD)

X-linked adrenoleukodystrophy is a disorder of peroxisomal fatty acid beta-oxidation leading to the accumulation of long-chain fatty acids, which can manifest itself in childhood (typically around 7 years of age) or in adult life. Adult-onset cerebral ALD accounts for about 5% of cases and usually presents with psychiatric symptoms, followed by dementia, ataxia, and seizures. As an X-linked disorder, ALD is more frequent in males. However, around 15–20% of heterozygote female carriers become symptomatic.

The typical MRI appearance is T2- and FLAIR-hyperintense white matter abnormalities starting in the parieto-occipital regions with early involvement of the splenium of the corpus callosum and corticospinal tracts. These signal abnormalities correspond to areas of demyelination. Active demyelination at the edge of the lesions is associated with contrast enhancement and restricted diffusion on diffusion-weighted imaging (DWI) (Fig. 9.1) [2].

Adrenomyeloneuropathy (AMN) is an adult phenotype with onset in the second decade to middle age, presenting with slowly progressive spastic paraparesis, bladder and bowel dysfunction, sexual dysfunction, and peripheral neuropathy, related to predominant involvement of the spinal cord. Typical imaging appearances include increased T2/FLAIR signal in the posterior limbs of the internal capsules, brainstem, and cerebellar white matter which may be followed by spinal cord atrophy.

9.2.2 Globoid Cell Leukodystrophy (Krabbe Disease)

Globoid cell leukodystrophy (GLD) has been linked to a mutation in the GALC gene on chromosome 14, leading to a deficiency of galactosylceramide β-galactosidase that causes accumulation of sphingolipids in the lysosomes. Late adolescent and adult forms (10%) present with slowly progressive gait abnormalities or spastic paresis. Other features include cognitive decline, seizures, and cortical blindness.

MRI shows predominantly posterior T2/FLAIR-hyperintense white matter changes with sparing of the

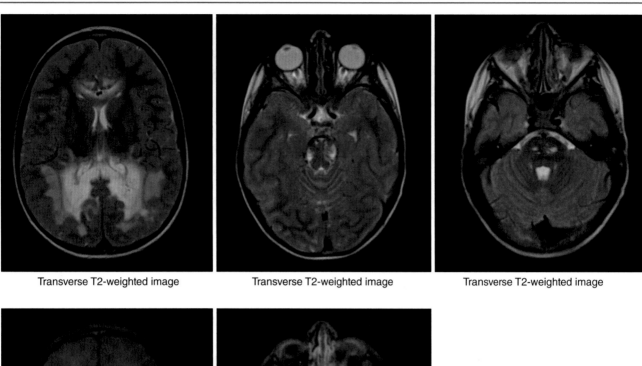

Transverse T2-weighted image Transverse T2-weighted image Transverse T2-weighted image

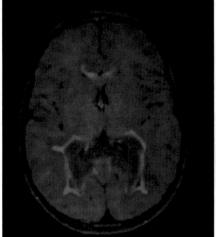

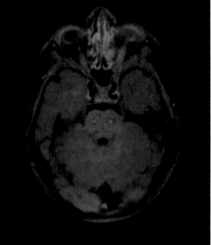

T1-weighted black blood image after T1-weighted black blood image after
gadolinium administration gadolinium administration

Fig. 9.1 A 16-year-old boy presented with progressive gait difficulties and behavioral disturbances. MRI shows extensive white matter lesions centered around the splenium of the corpus callosum, extending in the biparietal white matter. Similar but less pronounced abnormalities can be seen in the frontal lobes centered around the genu of the corpus callosum. Furthermore, there is hyperintensity on T2-weighted sequences along the corticospinal tracts. There is associated contrast enhancement in the areas of active demyelination. The diagnosis of X-linked adrenoleukodystrophy was confirmed on genetic testing. (**a**) Transverse T2-weighted image. (**b**) Transverse T2-weighted image. (**c**) Transverse T2-weighted image. (**d**) T1-weighted black blood image after gadolinium administration. (**e**) T1-weighted black blood image after gadolinium administration

U-fibers and involvement of the splenium of the corpus callosum, extending along the corticospinal tracts into the posterior limbs of the internal capsules and the pyramidal tracts. In some cases, there is a bilateral hyperdense signal on CT, corresponding to T1-hyperintense and T2-hypointense signal in the thalami. The affected areas do not show contrast enhancement.

Other lysosomal storage diseases, such as gangliosidoses and neuronal ceroid lipofuscinosis may also show the typical thalamic signal alterations. Metachromatic leukodystrophy is a differential diagnosis.

9.2.3 Metachromatic Leukodystrophy (MLD)

Several variants of metachromatic leukodystrophy have been described, all of which have deficient activity of arylsulfatase A, which results in defective degradation of sulfatides in the lysosomes and impaired myelination or dysmyelination. It is the most common hereditary leukodystrophy.

Approximately 20% of MLD patients have disease onset in adulthood, often with psychiatric symptoms, followed by spastic paraparesis, cerebellar ataxia, and cognitive decline.

MRI demonstrates symmetrical areas of confluent T2-hyperintense signal in the periventricular white matter with sparing of the subcortical U-fibers. Early involvement of the peritrigonal or periatrial white matter, corpus callosum, and cerebellar white matter is common, showing typically a "tigroid" pattern of radiating stripes. The white matter around the frontal horns is often affected to a lesser degree. As opposed to ALD, there is no contrast enhancement of the lesion edge. The lesions show restricted diffusion. Occasionally, multiple cranial nerve enhancement can be observed.

The main differential diagnosis is Krabbe disease, as the tigroid pattern has also been described in this disorder.

9.2.4 Mitochondrial Encephalomyopathy with Lactic Acidosis and Stroke-like Episodes (MELAS)

Mitochondrial encephalomyopathy with lactic acidosis and stroke-like episodes (MELAS) is a typical example of a mitochondrial disorder, with the involvement of multiple organs and often predominant manifestations in the central nervous system. About 40% of patients present in late childhood or early adulthood.

Clinical features are muscle weakness, extreme tiredness, and gastrointestinal symptoms such as vomiting and abdominal pain. Other features include seizures, hearing loss, and neuropsychiatric dysfunction.

MRI demonstrates a combination of infarcts in different stages, not confined to the major vascular territories. There is a predilection for the parieto-occipital regions and the cortical and deep gray matter. Vascular imaging is normal. The signal intensity of the lesions on T2/FLAIR-weighted sequences, diffusion-weighted imaging, and T1-weighted sequences with and without contrast depends on the time of onset.

9.2.5 Fabry Disease (Galactocerebrosidase Deficiency)

Fabry disease is a lysosomal storage disease related to a deficiency of a-galactosidase. It is an X-linked inherited disorder with varied clinical presentations and an estimated prevalence of 1 in 50,000. The deposition of globotriaosylceramide-3 in the endothelium and smooth muscles leads to the involvement of multiple organ systems, including the blood vessels, heart, and kidneys.

Macro- and microvascular complications are the leading CNS manifestations, with the first cerebrovascular event usually occurring around 40 years of age.

CT and MRI features are those of macrovascular disease (acute or chronic infarcts and parenchymal hemorrhage) and signs of microvascular disease (hyperintense foci in the periventricular and subcortical white matter and cerebral microhemorrhages).

Characteristic MRI features of Fabry disease are the uni- or bilateral T1 hyperintense signal in the pulvinar of the thalamus (the "pulvinar sign") and ectasia of the basilar artery on MR angiography, which has been found to be one of the best indicators of the presence of the disease in adults. Nonetheless, the incidence of the "pulvinar sign" is low, around 3%.

The main differential diagnosis is with the other lysosomal storage diseases.

9.2.6 Alexander Disease

Defects in the glial fibrillary acidic protein gene have been identified as the underlying cause of Alexander disease. Approximately 25% of patients present in adulthood, most commonly with bulbar dysfunction, pyramidal involvement, cerebellar ataxia, and sleep abnormalities.

In adult-onset disease, MRI findings consist of atrophy and abnormal T2-hyperintense signal within the medulla oblongata and upper cervical cord, which has been termed a "tadpole" appearance. The upper brainstem is almost never involved. Sometimes, there are periventricular white matter changes.

9.2.7 Primary Familial Brain Calcification (PFBC)

Primary familial brain calcification, formerly known as idiopathic basal ganglia calcification, bilateral strioapallidodentate or Fahr disease is a group of genetic disorders with currently 4 known mutations that are inherited in an autosomal dominant pattern. Symptomatic patients present in the late 40 s with a mostly Parkinsonian movement disorder, followed by cognitive decline, cerebellar features, and speech disorders.

Symmetrical calcification involving the lentiform nuclei, caudate nuclei, thalami (especially the posterolateral part), and dentate nuclei is mostly readily detected by CT. The cerebral and cerebellar cortex and the brainstem can be affected to a lesser degree. On MRI, the structures involved may show high signal on T1-weighted spin echo sequences and signal loss on susceptibility-weighted imaging. In some cases, there are additional confluent white matter lesions.

The differential diagnosis encompasses causes of secondary calcifications, primarily hypoparathyroidism.

9.3 Acquired Metabolic/Toxic Disorders

9.3.1 Wernicke Encephalopathy (WE)

Wernicke encephalopathy (WE) is caused by a deficiency of vitamin B1 (thiamine), which may be due to alcohol abuse, malabsorption, poor nutrition, increased metabolism, or iatrogenic elimination (hemodialysis). Thiamine depletion leads to failure of conversion of pyruvate to acetyl-CoA and α-ketoglutarate to succinate and the lack of Krebs cycle resulting in cerebral lactic acidosis with intra- and extracellular edema, swelling of astrocytes, oligodendrocytes, myelin fibers, and neuronal dendrites.

The classic clinical triad of ocular dysfunctions (nystagmus, conjugate gaze palsy, ophthalmoplegia), ataxia, and confusion is observed only in 30% of cases. Treatment consists of thiamine infusion, which can prevent progression to Korsakoff's dementia or death.

MRI shows T2/FLAIR hyperintensities in the periaqueductal and medial thalamic regions, mammillary bodies, hypothalamus, tectum, and cerebellum. The supratentorial lesions are most often symmetric. Contrast enhancement occurs most often in the mammillary bodies (80% of cases), often prior to T2 hyperintensities, or in the periaqueductal regions (50% of cases). The diffusivity of the lesions may vary.

Imaging abnormalities may regress with treatment. However, the prognosis is usually poor once there is cortical involvement or T1-hyperintense signal in the thalami and mammillary bodies indicating hemorrhage.

Chronic cases show atrophy of the mammillary bodies.

9.3.2 Subacute Combined Degeneration (SCD)

Subacute combined degeneration is a disorder of the spinal cord secondary to vitamin B12 deficiency, characterized by potentially reversible demyelination of the posterior and lateral columns. Clinical presentations are spastic paraparesis and spinal ataxia.

MRI demonstrates longitudinal, extensive T2 hyperintense signal in the posterior and lateral columns of the cervical spinal cord and to a lesser extent of the dorsal spinal cord. On transverse T2-weighted images, the pathological T2-hyperintense signal in the posterior spinal cord is called

the "inverted V-sign." Findings may regress after adequate B12 administration. Chronic non- or undertreated cases show spinal cord atrophy. Brain abnormalities in patients with SCD are rare. There are a few case reports of leukoencephalopathy with T2-hyperintense signal in the centrum semiovale and enhancement of the optic nerves.

9.3.3 Osmotic Demyelination Syndrome (ODS)

Osmotic demyelination syndrome includes central pontine myelinolysis (CPM) and extrapontine myelinolysis (EPM) and occurs in patients with hyponatremia that has been corrected too quickly.

The traditionally proposed pathophysiological mechanism is a disruption of the blood–brain barrier resulting in vasogenic edema, white matter compression, and myelinolysis. Additional implicated mechanisms are cerebral dehydration, intramyelinic edema, and oligodendrocyte degeneration. The most common damage is in the central pontine fibers. Extrapontine demyelination which may affect the basal ganglia, thalami, lateral geniculate nucleus, cerebellum, or cerebral cortex occurs in combination with CPM or in isolation in approximately 10% of cases.

Clinical symptoms of CPM include paralysis, dysphagia, dysarthria, and pseudobulbar palsy.

The typical feature of central pontine myelinolysis is T2/FLAIR-hyperintense signal in the central pons showing a symmetric "trident" or "bat-wing"-pattern, due to sparing of the peripheral fibers and the axons of the corticospinal tracts.

In the acute phase, there is restricted diffusion. This may occur within 24 h of symptom onset and precede the signal abnormalities on T2 or FLAIR-weighted sequences. The ADC values usually return to baseline within 3–4 weeks. CPM can appear moderately hypointense on T1-weighted sequences and rarely shows contrast enhancement [3].

If the patient survives the acute phase, the pontine lesions can cavitate and appear markedly hypointense on T1-weighted images.

9.3.4 Hepatic Encephalopathy

The term hepatic encephalopathy includes a spectrum of neuropsychiatric abnormalities in patients with liver dysfunction. Most cases are associated with cirrhosis and portal hypertension or portal-systemic shunts, but the condition can also occur in acute liver failure [4].

Classical MR abnormalities in chronic hepatic encephalopathy include high signal intensity in the globus pallidus on T1-weighted images, and less frequently, in the substantia nigra and the tegmentum of the midbrain, without corre-

Fig. 9.2 A 69-year-old
patient with chronic alcohol
abuse and liver cirrhosis
presented with a reduced level
of consciousness and delirium
MRI imaging findings present
typical intrinsic T1
hyperintense changes in the
basal ganglia, compatible
with hepatic encephalopathy.
No major atrophic changes
are noticed on the FLAIR-
weighted images. (**a**)
Transverse T1-weighted
image. (**b**) Sagittal
T1-weighted image. (**c**)
Transverse FLAIR-weighted
image. (**d**) Transverse
FLAIR-weighted image

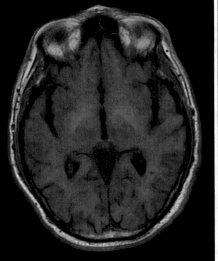
Transverse T1-weighted image

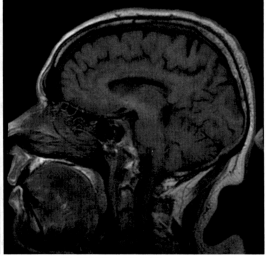
Sagittal T1-weighted image

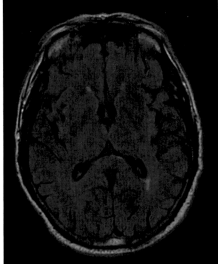
Transverse FLAIR-weighted image

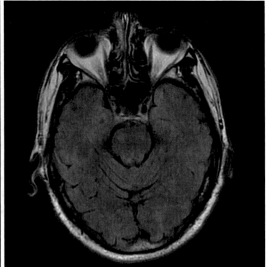
Transverse FLAIR-weighted image

sponding abnormalities on CT or T2-weighted imaging (Fig. 9.2). The accumulation of manganese is considered the cause of the signal alterations. Diffuse T2-hyperintense signal of the white may accompany the signal changes in the basal ganglia.

The signal alterations improve or disappear completely after restoration of the liver function.

On the contrary, in acute hepatic encephalopathy, there is a bilateral symmetric T2-hyperintense signal and swelling of the cortical gray matter, associated with restricted diffusion. Most commonly, the insula, thalami, the posterior limb of the internal capsule, and the cingulate gyrus are affected. In more severe cases, there may be additional involvement of the subcortical white matter, the remaining cortex, and the midbrain. These imaging abnormalities are thought to reflect cytotoxic edema secondary to acute hyperammonemia and are reversible with adequate therapy.

9.3.5 Hypoglycemic Encephalopathy

An acute decrease in serum glucose levels arises from an excess of exogenous or endogenous insulin or hypoglycemia-inducing drugs. This causes a decline in the function of the cell membrane ATPase pump and consequently a release of excitatory neurotransmitters such as aspartate. Patients present with coma.

CT can demonstrate enhancing hypodensities in the basal ganglia, cerebral cortex, hippocampus, and substantia nigra.

MRI is more sensitive and shows a T2-hyperintense signal as well as restricted diffusion in the posterior limb of the internal capsule, hippocampi, the basal ganglia, cortical areas, and splenium of the corpus callosum. These changes are likely to reflect cytotoxic edema, and extensive changes on DWI in the basal ganglia and deep white matter are associated with poor clinical outcomes.

The thalami are typically spared, and this allows a differential diagnosis with hypoxic ischemic encephalopathy where the thalami are most often involved.

9.3.6 Hyperglycemic Encephalopathy

Hyperglycemia occurs in uncontrolled diabetes mellitus and can lead to osmotic derangements in the basal ganglia and subthalamic region. The clinical presentation is fairly typical with hemichorea and hemiballismus, and the pathological process is hence described as non-ketotic hyperglycemia with hemichorea-hemiballismus.

Imaging findings on CT consist of a hyperdense signal in the putamen and caudate nucleus, typically contralateral to the side of the patient's symptoms. On MRI, there is a T1-hyperintense signal. The findings are almost invariably unilateral or with a striking asymmetry in rare bilateral cases.

After correction of blood glucose, the imaging abnormalities usually regress.

9.3.7 Hypoxic Ischemic Encephalopathy (HIE)

The pattern of brain injury in HIE depends on the level of brain maturation at the time of onset of the acute event and the severity and duration of the insult. HIE in adults results in symmetric involvement of the basal ganglia, thalami, and cortex and may be mild, moderate, or severe. The optimal time frame to image is 3–5 days after onset.

The affected areas show restricted diffusion on DWI. In the hyperacute events, reduced values on the ADC maps may be more pronounced than the hyperintensity on the b1000 maps. Afterwards, there is a corresponding hyperintense signal on T2- and FLAIR-weighted sequences and hypodense signal on CT, often accompanied by swelling of the injured gray matter structures. After 5 days, pseudonormalization of diffusivity occurs on the ADC maps.

The clinical context of HIE is mostly clear. However, in the unconscious patient of unknown etiology, a combined pathophysiology with a toxic cause or a differential diagnosis may be considered.

9.3.8 Drug-Induced Encephalopathy

Drug-induced changes to the brain result from acute intoxication or following long-term use of a number of drugs. Drug-induced encephalopathy is a disease entity that results from acute or chronic impaired cerebral metabolism, not causing focal but more diffuse structural brain lesions.

The imaging findings are very heterogeneous as are the drugs that can cause those changes. There is often a mix of acute and chronic changes present, including acute ischemic changes and others. Some drug-induced changes can result in not only diffuse but also focal structural lesions.

The list of drugs that can cause drug-induced encephalopathic changes is long and includes analgesics, antibiotics, neuromodulating medications, and chemotherapeutics.

More typical imaging changes reflect vasogenic and cytotoxic brain edema, posterior reversible leukoencephalopathy syndrome (PRES), leukoencephalopathy, and others.

9.4 Concluding Remarks

Toxic and metabolic diseases encompass a wide range of pathologies, often characterized by a specific pattern of findings. MRI is an important facet of the assessment, in combination with laboratory and/or genetic testing. Findings are almost invariably bilateral and often symmetric or nearly symmetric. In acquired metabolic and toxic diseases, the basal ganglia and thalami are often involved.

Most entities discussed in this chapter present a fairly specific imaging pattern. However, in congenital metabolic disorders presenting or persisting into adulthood, there may be overlap between entities and a differential diagnosis may be necessary in attendance of the results of genetic testing. In acquired metabolic-toxic disorders, clinical information and laboratory testing are warranted to aid in the final diagnosis.

Take-Home Messages
- Symmetric or nearly symmetric white matter lesions and/or pathologic changes in the basal ganglia and thalami are suspected of toxic-metabolic encephalopathy.
- The most common congenital leukodystrophies presenting or persisting into adulthood present with extensive lesions in the parieto-occipital white matter and involvement of the corticospinal tracts.
- Acquired metabolic-toxic disorders present with specific involvement of the basal ganglia and thalami, except for subacute combined degeneration, which is a disorder presenting with demyelination in the medulla.
- The pattern of brain injury in hypoxic ischemic encephalopathy depends on the severity and the duration of the event. Findings may be subtle.

References

1. Krishna SH, McKinney AM, Lucato LT. Congenital genetic inborn errors of metabolism presenting as an adult or persisting into adulthood: neuroimaging in the more common or recognizable disorders. Semin Ultrasound CT MR. 2014;35(2):160–91.

2. Ahmed RM, Murphy E, Davagnanam I, et al. A practical approach to diagnosing adult onset leukodystrophies. J Neurol Neurosurg Psychiatry. 2014;85:770–81.

3. Alleman AM. Osmotic demyelination syndrome: central pontine myelinolysis and extrapontine myelinolysis. Semin Ultrasound CT MR. 2014;35(2):153–9.

4. Alonso J, Córdoba J, Rovira A. Brain magnetic resonance in hepatic encephalopathy. Semin Ultrasound CT MR. 2014;35(2):136–52.

Imaging the Patient with Epilepsy or Seizures

10

Núria Bargalló and Timo Krings

Abstract

Neuroimaging plays an ever-increasing role in the workup of patients presenting with seizures, epilepsy, and, in particular in patients with medically refractory epilepsy. Abnormalities that may be amenable to surgery can be present in the latter group in up to 80% and thus the radiologist plays an important role in the interdisciplinary management of this patient population. In the current article, we are describing imaging protocols as well as typical pathologies and their imaging correlated to raise awareness of the spectrum of disorders typically encountered.

Keywords

Epilepsy · MRI · Hippocampal sclerosis · Malformation of cortical development

Learning Objective
- To understand the role of the radiologist in the diagnosis and management of patients with epilepsy.
- To describe the importance of a specific MR protocol in epilepsy patients, particularly if they are refractory to antiepileptic drugs.
- To describe typical pathologies and their imaging correlated to raise awareness of the spectrum of disorders typically encountered in epilepsy patients.

N. Bargalló (✉)
Neuroradiology Section, Radiology Department, Hospital Clinic de Barcelona, University of Barcelona, Barcelona, Spain
e-mail: bargallo@clinic.cat

T. Krings
Toronto Western Hospital and Joint Department of Medical imaging at the University Health Network, University of Toronto, Toronto, ON, Canada
e-mail: timo.krings@uhn.ca

It is estimated that up to 8–10% of the general population will experience a seizure during their lifetime [1]. Seizures may be defined as acute symptomatic or unprovoked. While acute symptomatic seizures occur at the time or near to a systematic insult, such cerebrovascular or traumatic brain injury, drug withdrawal, fever, sleep deprivation or metabolic insults, unprovoked seizures occurs without a precipitation factor [2]. Seizures can be focal or generalized [3]. Often, the initial imaging modality to study a patient with the first-ever seizures is an unenhanced CT head scan to exclude acute medical emergencies that can put the patient's life at risk, prior to a more extensive workup depending on clinical history and presentation. Potential epileptogenic lesions have been detected in about 30% of patients with first-ever seizures, being stroke, post-traumatic and neoplastic lesions the most common finding. Patients with epileptogenic lesions have a higher risk or seizure recurrence and therefore to develop epilepsy [4].

Approximately five millions of the general population will be diagnosed with epilepsy each year [5]. Epilepsy is defined by ILAE (International League Against Epilepsy) as at least two unprovoked (or reflex) seizures occurring >24 h apart [6], and there are several epilepsy types: focal epilepsy, generalized epilepsy, combined generalized and focal epilepsy, and also an unknown epilepsy group. The etiology of epilepsy can be classified in structural, genetic, infectious, metabolic, immune, and unknown [3]. Patients with focal epilepsy are more susceptible to have an epileptogenic lesion that irritates the brain and are more commonly present in structural etiology. This epileptogenic lesion can be identified on structural neuroimaging. Structural etiologies may be acquired such as stroke, trauma, and infection, or genetic such as many malformations of cortical development.

The vast majority of patients diagnosed with epilepsy can be treated satisfactorily with antiepileptic drugs. However, 0.4% of the general population will have recurrent and unprovoked seizures that do not respond to medication. These patients, defined as drug-resistant epilepsy patients are

© The Author(s) 2024
J. Hodler et al. (eds.), *Diseases of the Brain, Head and Neck, Spine 2024-2027*, IDKD Springer Series,
https://doi.org/10.1007/978-3-031-50675-8_10

potentially treatable with surgery, and surgical intervention is an appropriate consideration for 3% of people who develop epilepsy [6].

10.1 Image Indication and Epilepsy Dedicated MR Protocol

Indication for image evaluation in patients with epilepsy can be divide in four clinical scenarios: (1) evaluation of first-ever seizure when CT head usually is the first image modality; (2) status epilepticus, that should be evaluated by CT head in the emergency department including CT perfusion if it is available. MR exam should be indicated if the etiology remains unknown or the status is not controlled. (3) in epilepsy patients, ILAE stablish that all epilepsy patient need to have a neuroimage study, however it is strongly recommended to perform an MRI exam in these situations: Onset of partial seizures at any age, onset of generalized or unclassified seizures in the first year of life or in adulthood, evidence of a fixed deficit on neurological or neuropsychological examination, difficulty obtaining seizure control with first-line antiepileptic drugs (AED) and loss of seizure control, or change in the pattern of seizure [7]. (4) Finally, the last clinical scenario is when the epilepsy patients are AED resistant. In this case, the patients should be evaluated as possible candidates for surgical treatment.

In this chapter, we will focus on neuroimaging in this epilepsy patient population, as structural imaging will find a large proportion of abnormalities reaching up to 85% of patients. Lesions that are typically involved in medication refractory epilepsy are: mesial temporal lobe sclerosis (MTS) (primary or secondary to a long-standing seizure disorder), malformations of cortical development, certain epileptogenic tumors (e.g., dysembryoplastic neuroepithelial tumors (DNET), low grade temporal lobe glioma, or ganglioglioma), temporal lobe encephaloceles, vascular malformations, trauma, remote infection, and certain phakomatoses. Imaging findings in some of these conditions will be subtle which necessitates both a dedicated imaging protocol (as compared to a standard MR) and an "expert" experience in reading these types of scans. In a landmark study of von Oertzen et al. [8], the sensitivity of "non-expert" reports of standard MRI reports for focal lesions was 39%, while sensitivity of "expert" reports of standard MRI increased to 50%. "Expert" reports of epilepsy dedicated MRI further increased the sensitivity in detecting subtle lesions to 91%. Dedicated MRI showed focal lesions in 85% of patients with "non-lesional" standard MRI. Neuropathological diagnoses were predicted correctly in 22% of "non-expert" standard MRI reports but by 89% of dedicated MRI reports. Thus, the combination of dedicated MRI protocols and specialized radiologists trained in evaluating patients with medication refractory seizures

increases significantly the sensitivity of MRI in this subgroup of patients. A multidisciplinary approach that involves close communication between epilepsy neurologist, neuroradiology, EEG, nuclear medicine, neuropsychology, and neurosurgery is an important feature of modern management of the patient with seizures.

The necessity of expert MR reading with a dedicated imaging protocol is further highlighted by the fact that postsurgical seizure freedom is achieved significantly more often when a circumscribed, respectable epileptogenic lesion can be identified on MRI preoperatively compared to patients that are rated non-lesional [9]. As pointed out by Wellmer et al. in 2013 [10], the possible reasons for undetected epileptic lesions in standard outpatient MRI are insufficient clinical information from the referring clinician, routine MR protocols not optimized for the spectrum of epileptogenic lesions, and unfamiliarity with the spectrum of epileptogenic lesions. Wellmer pointed out that "because even the best focus hypothesis and most profound knowledge of epileptogenic lesions do not permit the detection of lesions when they are invisible on the MRI scan, the starting point for any improvement of outpatient MRI diagnostics should be defining an MRI protocol that is adjusted to common epileptogenic lesions."

Several recommendations for dedicated MR protocols in drug-resistant epilepsy patients have been published elsewhere, however, practices for the use of MRI are variable worldwide and may not harness the full potential of the MR to detect subtle epileptogenic lesions. In a recent consensus report from the International League Against Epilepsy Neuroimaging Task Force, Bernasconi et al. identified a set of sequences, with three-dimensional acquisitions at its core, the harmonized neuroimaging of epilepsy structural sequences—HARNESS-MRI protocol. As these sequences are available on most MR scanners, the HARNESS-MRI protocol is generalizable, regardless of the clinical setting and country [11]. Basically, the HARNESS-MRI protocol consists in these 3 core sequences: high resolution 3D T1-weighted MRI MPRAGE, with isotropic millimetric voxel resolution (voxel size, $1 \times 1 \times 1$ mm), high resolution 3D FLAIR (named CUBE, VISTA or SPACE, depending on the MR vendor) with isotropic millimetric voxel resolution (voxel size, $1 \times 1 \times 1$ mm), and high in plane resolution 2D coronal T2-weighted image acquired perpendicular to the long axis of the hippocampus (Fig. 10.1).

Wellmer et al. [10] reported the prevalence of epileptogenic lesions among 2740 patients and the following pathologies were found: mesial temporal lobe sclerosis (32%), tumors (including low and high grade tumors as well as malformative tumors and benign epilepsy associated tumors) in approximately 17% of patients, cortical dysplasias in 11%, glial scars (including post-traumatic, post-ischemic, post-hemorrhagic, postinfectious/abscess, ulegyria, and postsur-

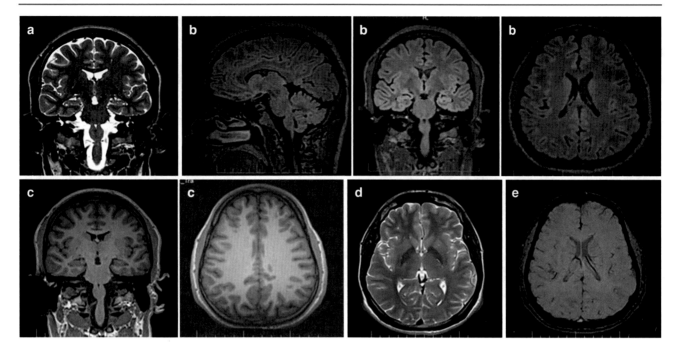

Fig. 10.1 MRI epilepsy protocol using hardness sequences: (**a**) T2 coronal perpendicular to log axis of the hippocampus with 2–3 mm of slices thickening, (**b**) 3DFLAIR acquired in sagittal (1 mm slice thickening) and posterior coronal and axial reconstruction, and (**c**) 3DMPRAGE T1 acquired in coronal (1 mm slice thickening). Other optional sequences: (**d**) T2 axial and (**e**) SWI

gical scars) in 11%, vascular diseases (cavernoma AVM, pial angiomatosis) in 5%, malformations of cortical development including nodular heterotopia, subcortical band heterotopia, polymicrogyria, lissencephaly, pachygyria, agenesis of corpus callosum, craniocephalic malformations, hemiatrophy, lobar dysgenesis, hemimegaloencephaly or hamartomas in 3%, and sequelae of encephalitis in 1% while in approximately 20% no lesion could be detected.

Lesion location—presumably related to the different epileptogenic potential in different brain regions—demonstrates preponderance for the temporal lobes (60%) followed by the frontal lobe (20%), the parietal lobe (10%) the periventricular white matter (5%) and the occipital lobe (5%).

In our own series [12]–being a tertiary epilepsy center, we recently reviewed 738 patients evaluated over a 13-year period in dedicated multidisciplinary epilepsy rounds and found mesiotemporal sclerosis in 132 (18%) of patients with 20 bilateral cases; concomitant mesiotemporal sclerosis with dual pathology in 64 (9%); encephalomalacia and gliosisin 79 (10%); focal cortical dysplasia in 47(6%); isolated enlargement of the amygdala in 40 (5%); tumors in 35 (5%) (including 18 DNET, 11 low-grade gliomas, 3 gangliolioma, 2 pleomorphic xanthoastrocytomas, 1 choroid plexus papilloma within the choroid fissure); cavernomas is 22 (3%), polymicrogyria in 14 (2%); and periventricular nodular heterotopic gray matter in 13 (2%). Rarer pathologies included subcortical nodular heterotopic gray matter, band heterotopia, ulegyria, perinatal hypoxic gliosis; temporal lobe encephaloceles, cortical siderosis, tuberous sclerosis; Rasmussen's encephalitis; neurocysticercosis, and closed-lip

schizencephaly. Exceedingly rare pathologies were pachygyria, hypothalamic hamartoma, Dandy-Walker variant, Dyke-Davidoff-Masson, diffuse axonal injury with cortical hemorrhage, hemimegalencephaly, limbic encephalitis, neurofibromatosis type I, and meningioangiomatosis.

The sensibility of the MR to detect abnormalities in temporal lobe epilepsy is about 90–97% [13]; however, this sensitivity drops in neocortical or extratemporal epilepsy, due to subtle epileptogenic abnormalities such as focal cortical dysplasia. In these cases, when the MR exam is negative, (no epileptogenic lesion detected), the use of quantitative imaging, or post-processing analysis such as voxel-based or surface-based machine-learning algorithm can increase the detection of subtle focal cortical dysplasia [14] Fig. 10.2.

In the future, the use of even higher field strengths (7 T) in clinical practice may increase the detection rate of epileptogenic substrates [15].

In presurgical evaluation, functional MRI (fMRI) can map eloquent cortex and provide information regarding language lateralization [16] Fig. 10.3, and the use of diffusion tensor imaging (DTI) and tractography may help to avoid injury to the optic radiation during temporal lobe resection [17].

Radionuclide imaging can add useful information in selected cases. Subtraction of ictal and interictal SPECT co-registered to MRI (SISCOM) can show a seizure–induced hyperperfusion (Fig. 10.4), whereas [18F]FDG–PET and PET co-registered to MR may show hypometabolism in the seizure onset zone. This is particularly useful in lateralization of temporal lobe epilepsy in the MR negative patient [18].

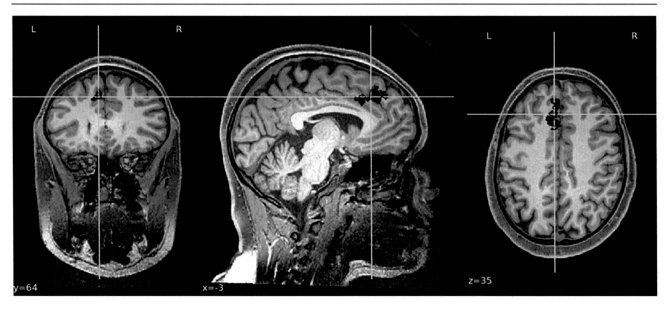

Fig. 10.2 Surface-based machine-learning algorithm (MELD-project) showing an abnormal cortical area in the left superior frontal gyrus in a patient with neocortical epilepsy and previous MR negative. https://meldproject.github.io//studies/MELD_FCD/

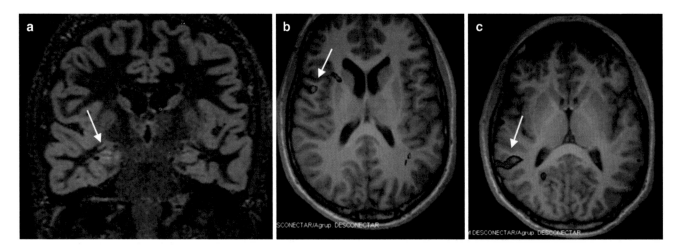

Fig. 10.3 Epilepsy patient with temporal lobe epilepsy and aphasia during the seizures. (**a**) Coronal FLAIR shows right temporal mesial sclerosis (arrow), (**b**) language fMRI with word naming paradigm demonstrates activation in the right inferior frontal gyrus (arrow). (**c**) Language MR with an auditive comprehension paradigm test demonstrating activation in the right posterior temporal gyrus (arrow). The language fMRI indicates that the language function is in the right hemisphere

Key Point
- In drug-resistant epilepsy patients, and patients with focal epilepsy, a dedicated imaging protocol with high resolution images will be necessary in order to find the epileptogenic lesion, and therefore have the potential of a surgical treatment. A variety of non-radiological adjunct tests are available that may help in the localization of the seizure focus and preferably these challenging cases are therefore discussed in multidisciplinary conferences.

In the following, we will discuss the imaging features of epileptogenic lesions highlighting imaging pearls and pitfalls.

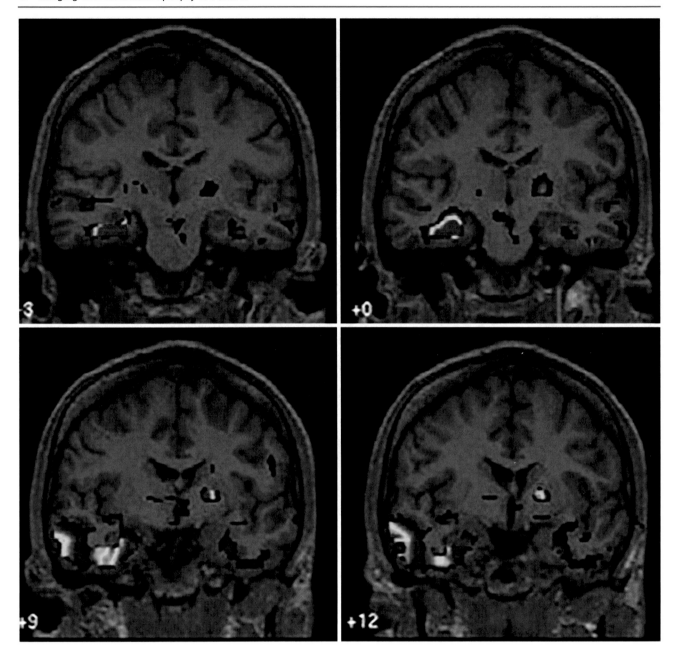

Fig. 10.4 SISCOM (subtracted ictal and interictal SPECT co-registered with MR) in an epilepsy patient with temporal lobe epilepsy demonstrates that there is hyperperfusion in the right hippocampus and anterior temporal lobe during the seizures, indicating the ictal onset zone

10.2   Mesial Temporal Lobe/Hippocampal Sclerosis

Most patients with mesial temporal sclerosis (MTS) present with complex partial seizures. These are characterized by seizure semiology that comprises déjà vu sensations, epigastric auras, lip smacking, or other oral automatisms and often have in their past medical history febrile seizures as a child with progressive worsening of seizure frequency and severity over time. MTS is characterized by sclerosis and volume loss in the hippocampus that often starting with loss of tissue in the stratum pyramidale in CA1 region [19]. The affected hippocampus will appear hyperintense on T2/FLAIR sequences due to the gliosis/sclerosis. The atrophy will lead to loss of the interdigitations of the head of the hippocampus, widening of the temporal horn, and atrophy of the white matter of the temporal lobe (Fig. 10.5). As a consequence of Wallerian degeneration, there may be atrophy of the projecting pathways of the hippocampus, including the Papez circuit, with atrophy of the ipsilateral fornix and the mammillary body. Importantly to

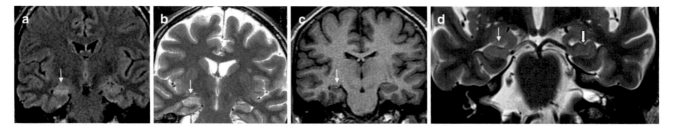

Fig. 10.5 Typical radiological findings in hippocampal sclerosis: (**a**) Coronal FLAIR, (**b**) coronal T2 demonstrates hyperintensity in the right hippocampus (white arrows), (**c**) coronal 3DMPRAGE shows better than T2 and FLAIR the atrophy in the right hippocampus (white arrow), (**d**) coronal T2 centered on the hippocampus shows loss of the interdigitation in the head of the right hippocampus (white arrow) with normal appearances in the left hippocampus (thick white arrow)

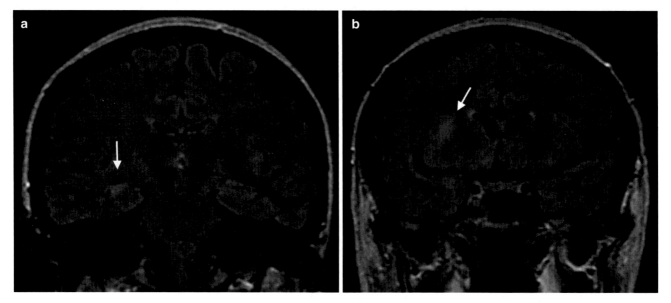

Fig. 10.6 Example of dual pathology in a patient with right hippocampal sclerosis and focal cortical dysplasia in the right inferior frontal gyrus. (**a**) Coronal FLAIR at the level of the hippocampi demonstrates the typical findings of HS with atrophy and hyperintensity within the right hippocampus (white arrow), (**b**) coronal FLAIR at the level of the frontal and anterior temporal lobes, showing blurring between gray and white matter in the right inferior frontal gyrus, consisting in focal cortical dysplasia (white arrow)

note, in nearly 20% of patients with MTS dual pathology is present with a second epileptogenic focus (Fig. 10.6). It is believed that in these cases, the other epileptogenic lesions triggered the mesial temporal lobe sclerosis (similar to febrile seizures as a child can trigger or "kindle" a mesial temporal lobe sclerosis). Dual pathology may also consist also of bilateral mesiotemporal lobe sclerosis as one hemisphere may trigger the other hippocampus to become sclerotic, thus constituting bilateral abnormalities. As the internal reference (i.e., the contralateral hippocampus) is similarly affected, comparison of the signal with other regions of 3-layered cortex, i.e., limbic structures can identify whether a mesial temporal lobe sclerosis is present bilaterally. Thus, if the T2/FLAIR signal of the hippocampus is bilateral symmetrical but higher as compared to the cingulum or insula one may consider bilateral mesial temporal lobe sclerosis (Fig. 10.7).

Key Point
- Mesial temporal lobe sclerosis is the most commonly seen cause for medication refractory epilepsy in temporal lobe epilepsy and is characterized by an indistinct gray–white matter differentiation, abnormal high signal on T2/FLAIR sequences, and atrophy. In up to 15–20% of cases, additional epileptogenic pathology is found in patients with mesial temporal lobe sclerosis.

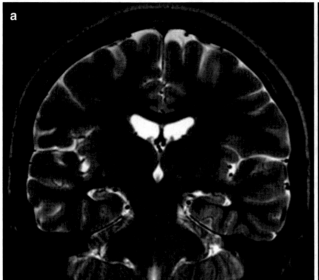

Fig. 10.7 Patient with bilateral hippocampi sclerosis. (**a**) Coronal T2 at the level of the body of the hippocampi demonstrates atrophy of both hippocampi, being difficult to distinguish abnormal signal because both are affected, (**b**) coronal FLAIR at the same level that T2 shows that both hippocampi are hyperintense (white arrows) in comparison with the insula (white thick arrow)

10.3 Malformations of Cortical Development

To understand the different types of malformations of cortical development (MCD), it is important to be aware of the embryology of cortical development: While during the seventh week of gestation neuronal proliferation in the subependymal germinal matrix occurs, at the eighth week of gestation, these cells migrate outward in multiple waves of radial outward migration aided by chemotaxis, i.e., radial glial cell guidance. In the last part of the cortical development, the lamination, cells are organized within different cortical layers in a process that is orchestrated by the subplate in the lowest layer of cortex. Chromosomal mutations, destructive events, or toxins may inhibit either of these three processes (proliferation, chemotaxis, or cortical organization) which will lead to abnormalities in stem cell development, migration, or lamination [20, 21].

Malformations related to abnormal stem cell development include focal or transmantle cortical dysplasias (balloon ell or type II FCDs) and the hemimegalencephalies.

Type II FCD is characterized by dysmorphic neurons with or without balloon cells in addition to cortical dyslamination and is identical to cortical hamartomas in tuberous sclerosis. The transmantle sign is a specific radiologic feature of FCD type II, which is more frequently detected in patients with FCD type IIb than FCD type IIa. Histologically, the transmantle sign reflects abnormal cells extending from the ventricle to the cortex manifesting as a linear T2-weighted or FLAIR hyperintensity from ventricle toward the cortex (the radial band or foot) can be seen in association with a subcortical FLAIR hyperintensity [14] (Fig.10.8).

There are MCD that predominantly or exclusively involve complete or substantial portion of one cerebral hemishere. There are disorders of neuronal proliferation and neuronal migration. It can occur as an isolated anomaly or in association with various neurocutaneous syndromes. There are two categories of hemispheric MCD: hemimegalencephaly and sublobar MCD, depending on the severity of the hemihere involvement. In hemimegalencephaly, a diffuse hamartomatous overgrowth as a result of abnormal stem cell proliferation is present resulting in broad gyri, shallow sulci, and a blurred gray–white matter junction. The ipsilateral ventricle is often enlarged and demonstrates an abnormal straight course of the frontal horn. In sublobar MCD, the affected hemisphere usually is not enlarged and the malformation may partially spare anterior or posterior regions of the affected hemisphere (Fig. 10.9). Clinically, patients present with macrocephaly, hemiplegia, developmental delay, and seizures. The affected hemisphere is non-functional, thus hemispherectomy can be proposed to these patients, if the contralateral hemisphere has no other epileptogenic lesions. Thus, pre-operative detailed clinical and radiologic assessments are required to determine if there are co-existing abnormalities in the contralateral hemisphere [22].

Lissencephalies, the agyria-pachygyria complex and heterotopia are malformations related to abnormal migration .

In the lissencephalies, there has been a global halt in the migration . An impaired last phase of neural migration will lead to paucity of the gyral and sulcal development with a

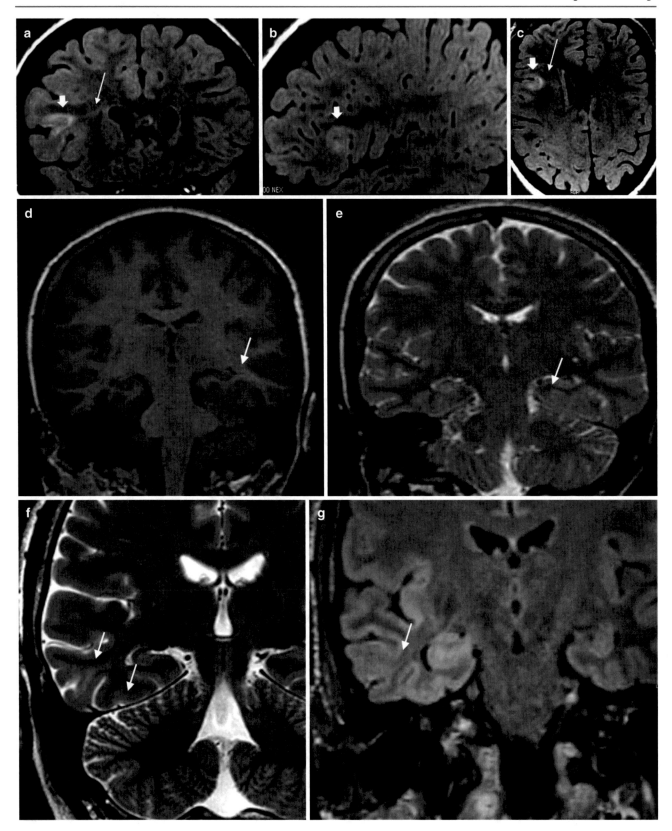

Fig. 10.8 Three cases of FCD type II. (**a**, **b**, **c**) patient 1; (**a**) 3DFLAIR with (**a**) coronal, (**b**) sagittal, and (**c**) axial, showing the typical signs of FCD type II, blurring between white and gray matter, juxtacortical (thick arrow), white matter hyperintensity, and the transmantle signs (arrow). (**d**, **e**) patient 2; (**d**) coronal 3DT1 (**e**) and coronal T2 show thickened cortex, blurring between gray and white matter in the left fusiform gyrus without transmantle sign (arrows) (**e**, **f**) patient 3, (**f**) coronal T2, and (**g**) coronal FLAIR shows juxtacortical white matter hyperintensity in the right inferior temporal gyrus and incomplete transmantle sign (arrow). The right hippocampus shows high signal on FLAIR indicating HS (dual pathology)

Fig. 10.9 Two cases of hemispheric malformation of cortical development. (**a**) Patient with hemimegalencephaly. Axial and coronal FLAIR showing the typical findings of enlargement of the affected hemisphere, diffuse thickening of the cortex with shallow sulci, blurred gray and white matter interface, heterotopic gray matter in the subcortical region, white matter increased volume with signal abnormalities, enlargement and abnormal configuration of the lateral ventricle, and dysplasia of subcortical gray matter structures. (**b**) Patient with sublobar FCD, coronal, and axial FLAIR showing similar findings than hemimegalencephaly but the abnormal hemisphere and the lateral ventricle are not enlarged, and the malformation spares the posterior region of the affected hemisphere

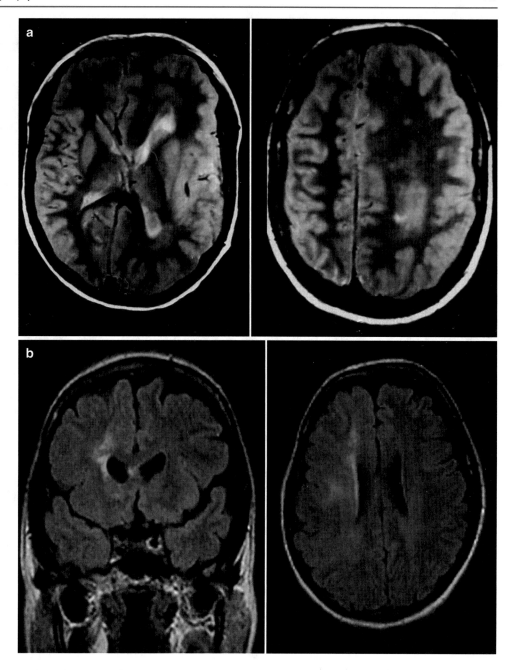

smooth brain surface and diminished white matter. Patients present with global developmental delay and seizures. Two different types of lissencephaly can be distinguished: the posterior agyria (related to an alteration on Chromosome 17) (Fig. 10.10) and the anterior agyria which is an X-linked disease.

Female carriers of the affected X-chromosome present with band heterotopias that is more present in the frontal lobes compared to the parietal lobes. Thus, if females present with band heterotopias, genetic counseling may be indicated. The band may be thin or thick depending on the amount of arrested migration. Patients with a thick band have less nor-

mal cortex (that can be thinned) and present with a more severe developmental delay.

In addition to the "band heterotopia," focal subcortical heterotopia can be present, On imaging, swirling, curvilinear bands of gray matter as well as thinned cortex, and paucity of the white matter are seen. The ipsilateral ventricle may be distorted, and there can be an associated callosal hypogenesis.

The third type of heterotopia is coined periventricular nodular heterotopia. On imaging an exophytic smooth ovoid mass in the residual germinal matrix, i.e., along the ventricular surface is seen. The periventricular nodular heterotopia may exhibit quite mild symptoms with normal development

Fig. 10.10 Patient with posterior lissencephaly. Axial 3DMPRAGE shows diffuse blurring between gray and white matter, cortical thickening, and abnormal gyral pattern in the posterior part of the brain

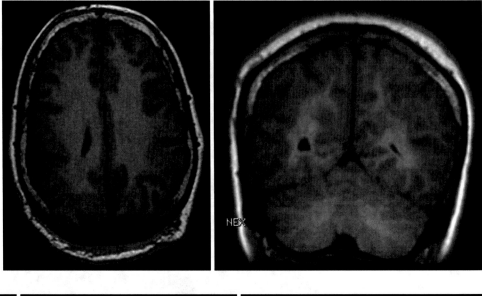

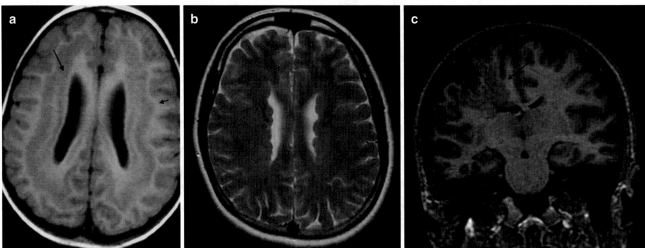

Fig. 10.11 Three examples of malformations related to abnormal migration: (**a**) T1 axial demonstrates typical band heterotopia (arrow), (**b**) T2 axial shows periventricular heterotopias involving both lateral ventricles (arrows), and (**c**) coronal T1 shows subcortical heterotopias extending from the subcortical white matter of the right lateral ventricle (arrow) and associated with abnormal gyral pattern and focal subarachnoid space enlargement

and late onset of seizures, if the amount of abnormal tissue is small. If the periventricular heterotopia completely lines the walls of both ventricles, a familiar form has to be considered, and in these cases developmental delay and seizure activity are typically more pronounced (Fig. 10.11).

Malformations related to abnormal cortical organization can be subdifferntiated into polymicrogyria, schizencephaly, and FCD type I (non-balloon cell). In polymicrogyria, neurons reach the cortex but distribute abnormally, thus multiple small gyri are formed. Polymicrogyria is most found around the posterior sylvian fissures when bilateral present in the perisylvian region patients who can present with pseudobulbar palsy (Fig. 10.12).

In open-lip schizencephaly, a cleft that is lined by gray matter reaches from the periphery to the ventricle while in the closed-lip schizencephaly, gray matter is reaching from the periphery to the ventricle and a dimple is seen in the ventricular wall. Schizencephaly can be multifocal and bilateral. The cortex lining the defect is polymicrogyria with ill-defined margins to the white matter. Disorders of lamination can be very subtle, and only mild focal blurring of the gray–white matter junction may be present.

Key Point
- Malformations of cortical development are commonly seen in pediatric patients with medication refractory epilepsy and usually are neocortical epilepsy. There malformations of cortical development depend on the embryological stage that they occur and can be very diffuse or very subtle.

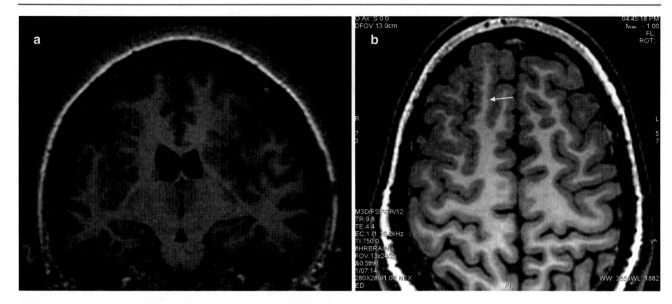

Fig. 10.12 Two patients with malformation of abnormal cortical organization. (**a**) coronal 3DMPRAGE demonstrates bilateral perirolandic bilateral polymicrogyria and abnormal and deep sulci. No dimple is seen in the lateral ventricles. (**b**) Axial 3DMPRAGE shows polymicrogyria in the right superior and middle frontal gyrus (arrow)

10.4 Epileptogenic Tumors

Nearly all brain tumors are epileptogenic, however, given their location, there are certain tumors that have a very high propensity of eliciting medication refractory seizures. Most of these are benign and just by means of location (i.e., within the cortical-white matter interface and with temporal lobe predilection) cause the seizures, these are often considered good candidates for surgery. As a general discussion of all tumors is beyond the scope of this chapter, we will focus only on three tumors that are commonly associated with epilepsy., Usually are slow growing tumors that appear during childhood or early adulthood and are defined as long-term epilepsy associated tumors (LEAT) [23]., The most common are (1) gangliogliomas, (2) DNETs, and (3) tuber cinereum hamartomas.

1. Gangliogliomas are cortically based, partly cystic tumors that may calcify and often harbor an enhancing nodule. Gangliogliomas occur in young adults and older children, when present under the age of 10, they are often larger with more cystic components. They are mainly located in the temporal lobes but can also occur in parietal and frontal lobes (Fig. 10.13).

2. DNETs are well demarcated, bubbly, intracortical masses that also are most common in the temporal, parietal, and frontal lobes. They may calcify but enhancement is very rare and if present should lead to more intensive follow-up as the enhancing portion of a DNET may recur following surgery (Fig. 10.14).

3. Tuber cinereum hamartoma present with the combination of gelastic seizures and precocious puberty. They are located at the floor of the third ventricle (i.e., the tuber cinereum) do not enhance and are isointense to cortex. They are non-neoplastic tumors with disorganized collection of neurons and glia (Fig. 10.15).

> **Key Point**
> • Long-term associated epilepsy tumors are usually low-grade tumors and usually appear in the infancy or early adulthood. Usually they involve the gray matter, and most commonly are located in the temporal and frontal lobes.

Fig. 10.13 Patient with temporal lobe epilepsy and ganglioglioma: (**a**) coronal FLAIR, (**b**) coronal T2, and (**c**) axial T2 demonstrate a heterogenous lesion in the right amygdala with a small cyst (arrow). (**d**) Post-contrast T1 shows a small enhancing nodule (arrow)

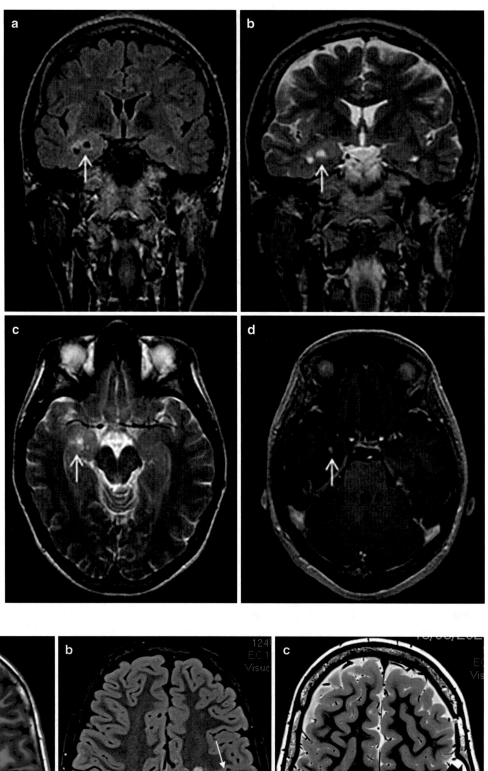

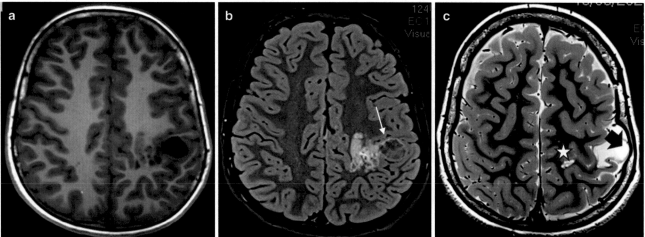

Fig. 10.14 DNET. (**a**) Axial 3DMPRAGE, (**b**) axial FLAIR, and (**c**) axial T2 showing a superficially multicystic lesion in the left parietal lobe with mixed signal of FLAIR (arrow), satellite cyst (star), and remodelling of the calvarium (thick black arrow)

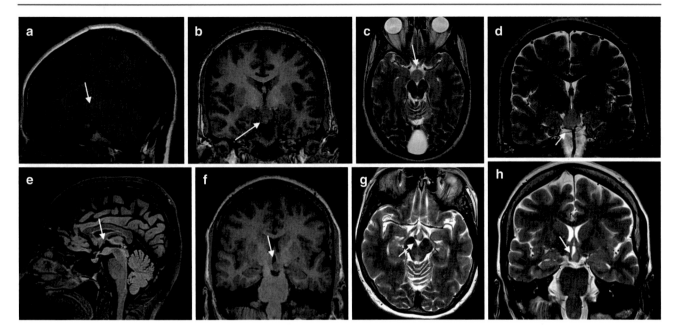

Fig. 10.15 Two epileptic patients with hamartomas of the tuber cinereum. The upper row shows a large tumor in the floor of the 3° ventricle extending into the suprasellar region with a similar signal to the hippocampus on T1 (**a, b**) and T2 sequences (**c, d**) (arrows). The patient has a retrocerebellar cyst. The lower row shows a small hamartoma inside the 3°ventricle with the same signal as the gray matter on sagittal FLAIR (**e**), coronal T1MPRAGE (**f**), and axial and coronal T2 (**g** and **h**) (arrows)

10.5   Other Causes of Focal Epilepsy

Many other pathologies can cause seizure. Similar to the previous paragraph, it is beyond the scope to in detail describe imaging features of vascular malformations, infections, or trauma that can go along with seizures, and most of the entities are described in other chapters of this syllabus. We therefore only want to highlight few epilepsy-relevant facts and features of these conditions.

Vascular malformations can cause seizures due to previous hemorrhage and scarring, hemosiderin deposition (especially when close to the cortex), or gliosis. AVMs in the temporal lobe have a higher likelihood of producing seizure due to interference of the normal blood supply and drainage of potentially epileptogenic structures such as the hippocampus.

Cavernous malformations that are cortically located and have hemosiderin staining reaching the cortex, and in particular the mesial temporal lobe structures, are very often associated with seizures as the hemosiderin stain is believed to have a strong irritative potential for neurons. They are best visualized on T2 gradient echo or SWI sequences where they demonstrate with the classical blooming artifact (Fig. 10.16).

Patients with previous trauma can experience post-traumatic seizure disorder, especially after having sustained contusional hemorrhages of their temporal lobes as gliosis and hemosiderin staining can cause irritation of the surrounding cortex.

Neonatal anoxic ischemia or hypoxemia can cause ulegyria—i.e., a scar/defect of the cerebral cortex that mainly involves the cortex in the depth of the sulcus, whereas the cortical crowns remain relatively unaffected [24].

If the perinatal ischemia has only involved one hemisphere (perinatal stroke), a Dyke-Davidoff-Masson syndrome will ensue where stable hemiatrophy is present with hypertrophy of the skull and the sinuses, paucity of white matter, ventricular enlargement, and mild gliosis (Fig. 10.17).

Virtually any infection (bacterial, fungal, parasitic) can produce epileptogenic lesions, and worldwide infections are the leading cause of epilepsy (Fig. 10.18). A typical example is neurocysticercosis which is a very common cause of focal epilepsy in the developing world.

Antero-basal temporal lobe encephaloceles are lesions that are either related to a congenital defect of the bone or to previous trauma. Brain tissue can extend into the pterygopalatine fossa through the bony defect at the base of the greater sphenoid wing in the region of the foramen rotundum and pterygoid process. The herniated brain demonstrates high T2/FLAIR signal and is believed to be the epileptogenic focus (Fig. 10.19). Following resection of the abnormal brain tissue seizure freedom can be obtained in a very large proportion of cases.

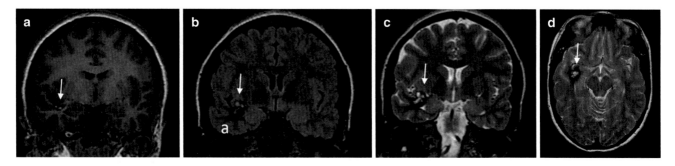

Fig. 10.16 Patient with temporal lobe epilepsy, showing a typical cavernoma finding with (**a**) popcorn appearances on T1 coronal, and surrounded by hemosiderin in the white matter seen on (**b**) coronal FLAIR, (**c**) coronal T1, and (**d**) axial T2 sequences. Note that the right amygdala and hippocampus are normal

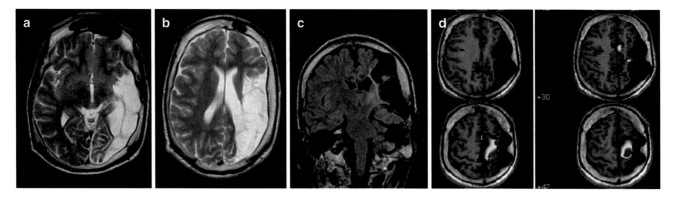

Fig. 10.17 A 16-year-old boy with perinatal vascular injury and epilepsy and right hemiparesis. A large porencephalic cyst that involves the part of the left middle cerebral artery territory. The cyst shows some septa and contacts with the ependyma of the left lateral ventricle. There is an abnormal signal in white matter indicating gliosis and Wallerian degeneration. Note the hypertrophy of the left side of the skull and asymmetric enlargement of the frontal sinus (**a, b**) axial T2WI; (**c**) coronal FLAIR. (**d**) SISCOM indicates that the seizure onset zone is in the midsagittal cortex near the porencephalic cyst

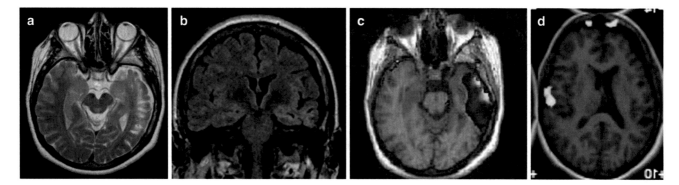

Fig. 10.18 A 35-year-old female with a previous history of meningitis and epilepsy. MRI (**a**) axial T2WI (**b**) coronal FLAIR shows atrophy of the left temporal lobe with white matter hyperintensity associated with left HS (arrow). (**c**) SISCOM images indicate that the ictal onset zone initiates in the left neocortical temporal lobe. (**d**) Language fMRI demonstrates activation of the right hemisphere during an auditive comprehension paradigm, indicating that the language function has been transferred to the other hemisphere

Rasmussen's encephalitis is a presumably autoimmune-mediated chronic inflammation of the brain that presents with progressive gliosis and volume loss. Patients experience seizures and a progressive hemiparesis (Fig. 10.20).

> **Key Point**
> - Many other pathologies including vascular malformations, phakomatoses, or remote infections or trauma can cause medication refractory epilepsy, particularly if they involve the gray matter.

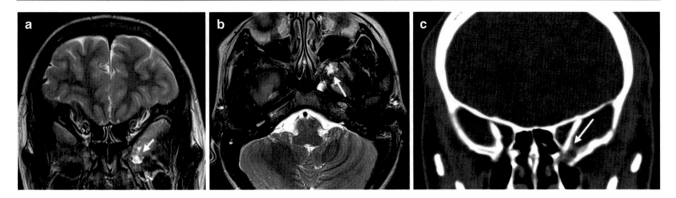

Fig. 10.19 Patient with temporal lobe epilepsy. MRI exam (**a**) T2 coronal and (**b**) axial T2MRI show the left temporal pole extending into the pterygopalatine fossa throughout a small defect of the left greater sphenoid wing seen on (**c**) coronal CT (arrows)

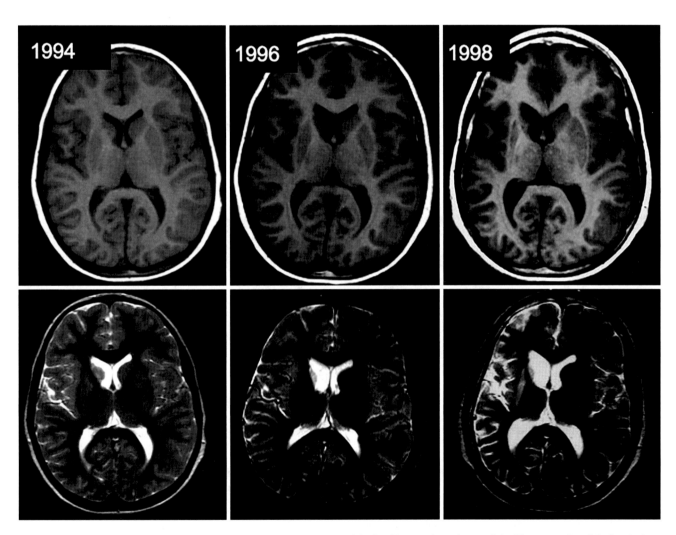

Fig. 10.20 A 9-year-old patient with continuous partial seizures arising from the right hemisphere, progressive cognitive deterioration, and left hemiparesis. MRI studies over time show progressive atrophy of the right lentiform and caudate nuclei with progressive right hemisphere atrophy. (Axial 3DT1 upper row, axial T2 lower row)

10.6   Concluding Remarks

Neuroimaging in patients with medication refractory epilepsy should identify clinically relevant abnormalities in a high percentage of cases and therefore the radiologist plays a crucial role in the identification of epileptogenic lesions and their possible surgical removal. A dedicated epilepsy protocol is necessary to identify these lesions, and the MR should be interpreted and multidisciplinary rounds with radiological input are paramount to manage these challenging patients.

> **Take-Home Messages**
> - When evaluating a dedicated seizure protocol MR, a structured approach is helpful that includes a detailed assessment of (a) the hippocampus and mesial temporal lobe structures, (b) the ventricular outline, and (c) the gyral and the sulcal anatomy.
> - Particular emphasis should be paid upon the T2/FLAIR signal within the cortex and hippocampus, its similarity to other regions of neo- and archicortex, the internal architecture of the hippocampus, the indentations of the head of the hippocampi, the fornix and mammillary bodies, and the gray–white matter interface of the neocortex (blurring, gray matter thinning, or thickening).
> - The malformations of cortical development can be differentiated into disorders of neuronal proliferation, migration, and cortical organization and can be diffuse or very subtle. There are slow growing tumors, usually neuroglial lineage that are associated with chronic epilepsy.

References

1. Gavvala JR, Schuele SU. New-onset seizure in adults and adolescents: a review. JAMA. 2016;316(24):2657–68.
2. Hauser WA, Beghi E. First seizure definitions and worldwide incidence and mortality. Epilepsia. 2008;49(Suppl 1):8–12.
3. Scheffer IE, et al. ILAE classification of the epilepsies: position paper of the ILAE Commission for Classification and Terminology. Epilepsia. 2017;58(4):512–21.
4. Ho K, et al. Neuroimaging of first-ever seizure: contribution of MRI if CT is normal. Neurol Clin Pract. 2013;3(5):398–403.
5. Organization, W.H. Epilepsy: a public health imperative. Geneva: CC BY-NC-SA 3.0 IGO; 2019.
6. Fisher RS, et al. ILAE official report: a practical clinical definition of epilepsy. Epilepsia. 2014;55(4):475–82.
7. Epilepsy, C.o.N.o.t.I.L.A. Recommendations for neuroimaging of patients with epilepsy. Commission on Neuroimaging of the International League Against Epilepsy. Epilepsia. 1997;38(11):1255–6.
8. Von Oertzen J, et al. Standard magnetic resonance imaging is inadequate for patients with refractory focal epilepsy. J Neurol Neurosurg Psychiatry. 2002;73(6):643–7.
9. Téllez-Zenteno JF, et al. Surgical outcomes in lesional and non-lesional epilepsy: a systematic review and meta-analysis. Epilepsy Res. 2010;89(2–3):310–8.
10. Wellmer J, et al. Proposal for a magnetic resonance imaging protocol for the detection of epileptogenic lesions at early outpatient stages. Epilepsia. 2013;54(11):1977–87.
11. Bernasconi A, et al. Recommendations for the use of structural magnetic resonance imaging in the care of patients with epilepsy: a consensus report from the International League Against Epilepsy Neuroimaging Task Force. Epilepsia. 2019;60(6):1054–68.
12. Hainc N, et al. Imaging in medically refractory epilepsy at 3 tesla: a 13-year tertiary adult epilepsy center experience. Insights Imaging. 2022;13(1):99.
13. Lee DH, et al. MR in temporal lobe epilepsy: analysis with pathologic confirmation. AJNR Am J Neuroradiol. 1998;19(1):19–27.
14. Urbach H, et al. MRI of focal cortical dysplasia. Neuroradiology. 2022;64(3):443–52.
15. van Lanen RHGJ, et al. Ultra-high field magnetic resonance imaging in human epilepsy: a systematic review. NeuroImage Clin. 2021;30:102602.
16. Bauer PR, et al. Can fMRI safely replace the Wada test for preoperative assessment of language lateralisation? A meta-analysis and systematic review. J Neurol Neurosurg Psychiatry. 2014;85(5):581–8.
17. Piper RJ, et al. Application of diffusion tensor imaging and tractography of the optic radiation in anterior temporal lobe resection for epilepsy: a systematic review. Clin Neurol Neurosurg. 2014;124:59–65.
18. von Oertzen TJ, et al. SPECT and PET in nonlesional epilepsy. Clin Epileptol. 2023;36(2):104–10.
19. Howe KL, et al. Histologically confirmed hippocampal structural features revealed by 3T MR imaging: potential to increase diagnostic specificity of mesial temporal sclerosis. AJNR Am J Neuroradiol. 2010;31(9):1682–9.
20. Barkovich AJ, et al. A developmental and genetic classification for malformations of cortical development: update 2012. Brain. 2012;135(Pt 5):1348–69.
21. Severino M, et al. Definitions and classification of malformations of cortical development: practical guidelines. Brain. 2020;143(10):2874–94.
22. Sato N, et al. Aberrant midsagittal fiber tracts in patients with hemimegalencephaly. AJNR Am J Neuroradiol. 2008;29(4):823–7.
23. Urbach H. Long-term epilepsy-associated tumors. In: Barkhof F, et al., editors. Clinical neuroradiology: the ESNR textbook. Cham: Springer International Publishing; 2019. p. 951–63.
24. Colombo N, Bargalló N, Redaelli D. Neuroimaging evaluation in neocortical epilepsies. In: Barkhof F, et al., editors. Clinical neuroradiology: the ESNR textbook. Cham: Springer International Publishing; 2018. p. 1–35.

Found Down

Imaging Evaluation of the Patient Found Unconscious

11

Christopher P. Hess and James G. Smirniotopoulos ·

Keywords

Unconscious · Coma · Emergency · Trauma · Hypoxia
Hydrocephalus · Herniation · Ischemia · Stroke · Seizure
Overdose · Metabolic · Infection

Learning Objectives
- To understand the spectrum of disorders that may cause a patient to become unconsciousness.
- To appreciate the central role of imaging in the evaluation of patients found unresponsive.
- To recognize key imaging findings that define diagnosis, drive treatment, and predict outcome in the unconscious patient.

Consciousness is believed to arise from two inter-related brain functional states: *wakefulness*, reflecting an individual's level of arousal and response to external stimuli, and *awareness*, representing the content of one's conscious experience and the ability to interact with the external environment. Disruption to either or both states may result in a patient being "found down." The inability to take an accurate medical history, the limitations of physical examination in the obtunded patient, and the need to rapidly make treatment decisions position imaging centrally within the evaluation of most of these patients. Radiologists should be prepared to help decide on an appropriate imaging strategy, suggest a limited differential diagnosis as to root causes for the patient's condition, identify problems that mandate emergent medical or surgical intervention and, in some cases, assist in defining short- and long-term prognosis.

Any disruption to the normal brain chemistry, structure, metabolism, or function may cause a patient to become unconscious. Because the brain has a remarkable ability adapt to chronic stress, disorders of arousal usually come as the result of acute rather than longstanding disease. Acute trauma (known or occult) and cardiorespiratory failure are the most frequent causes. In one study of seven major centers, roughly one third of patients found down were initially triaged for trauma, and two thirds were triaged for medical illnesses [1]. The majority (74.1%) underwent head CT at some point during their treatment, typically during initial assessment but also later during their hospitalization. The delayed use of imaging derived in part from the fact that nearly half (47.7%) of patients suffered from comorbid traumatic and medical illness.

Given the frequency of traumatic injury in patients found down, it is convenient to divide causes for unconsciousness into traumatic and non-traumatic. In both cases, the brain may be involved either from a primary insult or from secondary dysfunction due to other systemic disorders such as sepsis, metabolic derangement, toxic exposure, hypotension, or hypertension (Table 11.1). Among primary brain abnormalities, diseases caused by diffuse neuronal dysfunction should be distinguished from diseases that disproportionately involve the individual anatomic structures that contribute to consciousness (Table 11.2) [2]. We highlight several important diagnoses with actionable findings that may be identified in imaging studies of patients who are found down.

C. P. Hess (✉)
Department of Radiology and Biomedical Imaging, University of California, San Francisco, San Francisco, CA, USA
e-mail: christopher.hess@ucsf.edu

J. G. Smirniotopoulos
MedPix® Medical Image Database, National Library of Medicine, Bethesda, MD, USA
e-mail: james.smirniotopoulos@nih.gov

© The Author(s) 2024
J. Hodler et al. (eds.), *Diseases of the Brain, Head and Neck, Spine 2024-2027*, IDKD Springer Series,
https://doi.org/10.1007/978-3-031-50675-8_11

Table 11.1 General differential considerations in the imaging evaluation of patients found down

| Acute traumatic brain injury |
| Acute vascular abnormalities |
| Hypoxia and hypoperfusion |
| Seizures |
| Elevated or low intracranial pressure |
| Herniation syndromes |
| Viral encephalitis |
| Acute necrotizing encephalopathy . |
| Toxic exposures, for example: |
| *Carbon monoxide* |
| *Methanol* |
| *Ethylene glycol* |
| *Organophosphates* |
| Metabolic abnormalities, for example: |
| *Hypoglycemia and hyperglycemia* |
| *Hyponatremia and hypernatremia* |
| *Uremia* |
| *Hyperammonemia* |
| *Wernicke's encephalopathy* |
| *Osmotic demyelination* |

Table 11.2 Anatomic brain structures contributing to the conscious state

| Brainstem (especially nuclear components of the reticular activating system) |
| Hypothalamus (especially midline paraventricular nuclei) |
| Anterior striatum |
| Claustrum |
| Thalamus (especially central nuclei) |

11.1 Structural and Vascular Abnormalities

Traumatic axonal injury (TAI), a severe form of traumatic brain injury that often renders patients' unconscious, represents up to half of all brain injuries after severe trauma in the United States [3]. High-speed motor vehicle accidents, shake injuries to infants, fall from heights—any major traumatic mechanism associated with rapid acceleration-deceleration of the brain relative to the skull can lead to TAI. Exposed to mechanical shear, structures within the brain with different tensile strength, viscosity, and microscopic architecture suffer from stretch or tear injuries of axons, cell bodies and myelin, disruption of normal chemical processes, and abnormal cellular function. Although all areas of the brain may be involved, TAI most often affects the corpus callosum, the brainstem (especially the dorsal midbrain), and cortical gray-white interfaces. Findings are evident on CT only in the most severe injuries, in which tiny foci of parenchymal hemorrhage are observed. Susceptibility-sensitive and diffusion-weighted MRI are usually necessary to detect and characterize the extent of TAI and show multiple focal areas of signal abnormality in typical brain areas (Fig. 11.1).

After trauma, hypoxic insults from cardiac or respiratory failure, as may result from cardiac arrest, shock, choking, or drug overdose, represent the most common cause for diffuse brain injury in the patient found down. The degree to which the brain is injured depends upon the severity and duration of deprivation of oxygen and/or reduced perfusion, which is required to make glucose that supplies the brain's energy. Complete anoxia, even for short periods, usually involves the entirety of the brain. When oxygen in the blood is insufficient to support energy production, the most metabolically active areas of the brain are disproportionately affected. The hippocampus, basal ganglia, thalami, and cerebellum are most often involved in adults suffering from global hypoxic and ischemic injuries. Importantly, the imaging appearance of hypoxia also depends on the timing of imaging relative to the injury. Swelling and loss of normal gray-white differentiation in the acute phase progresses to atrophy in chronic stages, and white matter abnormalities are delayed with respect to those in gray matter. Early evidence of hypoxic injury on both CT [4] and MRI [5] have been advocated as useful markers to predict clinical outcome.

Low cerebral perfusion pressure due to systemic hypotension or intracranial hypertension, which occurs together with hypoxia, may also cause patients to become acutely unconscious (Fig. 11.2). In this scenario, it is the border-zone or "watershed" areas of the brain—in-between vascular territories—that are most impacted. Reduced cerebral blood flow not only causes cellular ischemia, but also results in platelet microemboli that lodge preferentially within end arteries, especially the leptomeningeal arteries that overlie arterial border zones [6]. The degree of injury may be most severe in vascular territories that lie distal to pre-existing arterial stenosis, for example, distal to from carotid or intracranial atherosclerosis. Hypoperfusion injury is diagnosed when wedge-shaped areas of injury are evident between affected arterial territories or in a linear "string of pearls" pattern paralleling the lateral ventricles.

Although CT can detect watershed injury in the patient found down, MRI is usually necessary to characterize the severity and extent of injury. This is especially the situation for micro-occlusive disease, such as occurs in thrombotic microangiopathy. Here, low cerebral perfusion pressure occurs in the microcirculation of the brain because of in situ occlusions within capillaries, arterioles, and sometimes venules from cerebral vasculitis, intravascular lymphoma, disseminated intravascular coagulation, or thrombocytopenia, for example [7]. This diagnosis is particularly challenging to make in the unconscious patient and relies on the MRI observation of multiple tiny foci of susceptibility signal change scattered throughout the brain, often together with edema and punctate foci of reduced diffusion.

Diffuse brain disease can be distinguished from other disorders that directly impact the brain areas that are responsible

Fig. 11.1 Diffuse brain injury. (**a**) Axial T2*-weighted gradient echo MRI shows diffuse axonal injury, with multiple foci of susceptibility in a patient found unconscious after high-speed motor vehicle. (**b**) Axial diffusion-weighted MRI in a patient after global hypoxia, with relatively symmetric involvement of the basal ganglia. (**c**) Axial unenhanced CT 4 h following cardiac arrest, with diffuse parenchymal swelling and loss of gray-white differentiation. (**d**) Axial unenhanced CT showing reversal of normal gray and white matter density in a patient 6 days after being found unresponsive

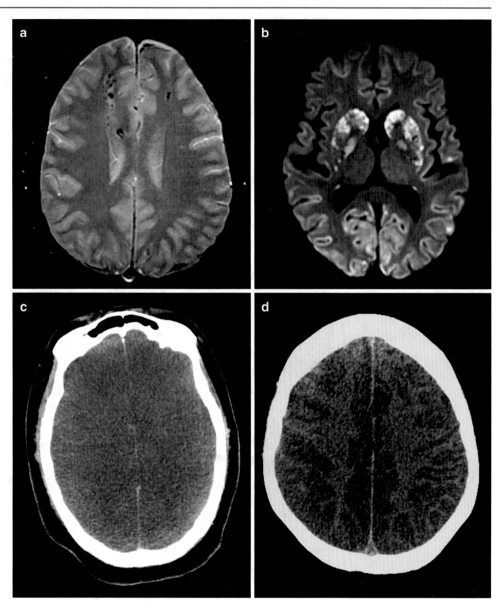

Fig. 11.2 Hypoperfusion injury. (**a**) Axial diffusion trace MRI showing watershed injury after acute aortic dissection, with wedge-shaped infarcts in the junctional zones of the right anterior and middle cerebral arteries and the right middle and posterior cerebral arteries. (**b**) Axial susceptibility-sensitive MRI in a patient with autoimmune hemolytic anemia and diffuse thrombotic microangiopathy, showing innumerable foci of intravascular susceptibility and associated edema

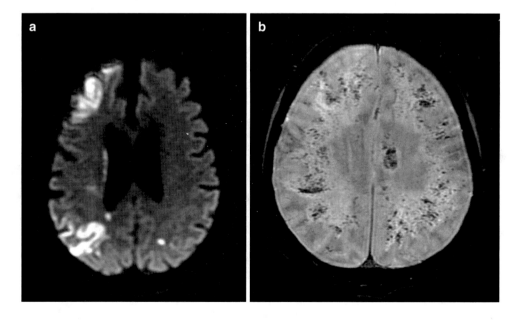

Fig. 11.3 Localized brain abnormalities. (**a**) Axial unenhanced CT showing hyperdense basilar artery from thrombotic occlusion. (**b**) Axial unenhanced CT with internal cerebral venous thrombosis, seen as hyperdense internal cerebral veins with venous edema in the thalami and basal ganglia. (**c**) Axial T2 FLAIR MRI in a comatose patient with Japanese encephalitis. (**d**) Axial T2-weighted MRI in a child found unresponsive after febrile illness, diagnosed with acute necrotizing encephalopathy

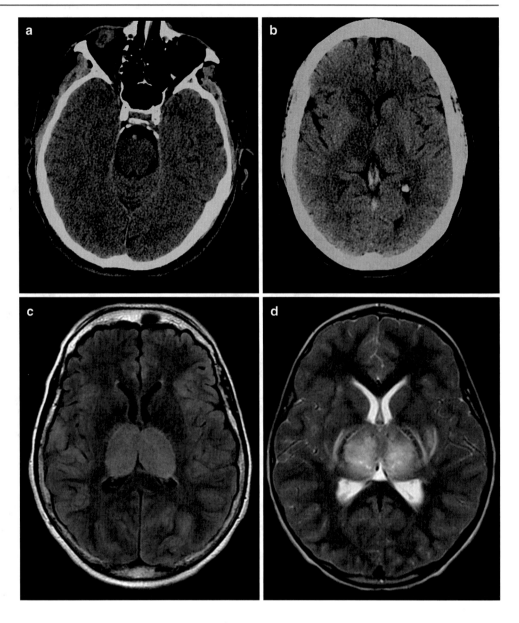

for maintaining the brain's conscious activity (Fig. 11.3). Insults to the thalamus, hypothalamus and brainstem may cause patients to become unresponsive. Interruption of the arterial supply or venous drainage of the thalami and brainstem, especially from basilar artery thrombosis or internal cerebral venous thrombosis, are critical abnormalities to identify on CT examinations of patients found down. Certain viral illnesses, such as West Nile virus, Japanese encephalitis, Murray Valley encephalitis, Eastern equine encephalitis, and influenza A, also have a predilection for selective involvement of the thalami and brainstem. Acute necrotizing encephalopathy (ANE), a para-infectious disorder that follows acute viral illness, is also associated with symmetric abnormalities of the thalami. In contradistinction to direct viral infection, ANE results from delayed immune-mediated injury to these structures [8]. The disease is more common in genetically susceptible individuals.

> **Key Point**
> • Loss of consciousness may result from any process that structurally involves the entire brain or specifically impacts the brainstem, the hypothalamus, or the thalamus. MRI is typically more sensitive for most disorders, especially early following the onset of hypoxia, hypoperfusion, or ischemia.

11.2 Intracranial Pressure and Herniation Syndromes

Intracranial pressure (ICP) normally ranges from 7 to 15 mm Hg in supine adults and increases or decreases in response to changes in volume of the structures contained within the rigid skull—brain, blood, and cerebrospinal fluid (CSF). ICP is distributed relatively equally within the cranium, including the intra- and extra-ventricular CSF spaces and across the different intracranial compartments defined by bony boundaries and by the rigid falx and tentorium cerebelli. Patients may lose consciousness because of abnormally increased or decreased ICP, when the pressure gradients across intracranial compartments give rise to herniation and brain compression syndromes, and when elevated intraventricular pressure causes hydrocephalus. In each scenario, the mechanical distortion of the brain and/or associated reduction in its normal perfusion disrupts brain function, causing the patient to fall unconscious.

Diffuse brain swelling, space-occupying lesions, and hydrocephalus all cause elevated ICP. Hypertension, metabolic derangements, hypoxia, ischemia, meningitis, traumatic injury, and other disorders may be sources of life-threating diffuse swelling (Fig. 11.4). Although mild swelling can be difficult to recognize on imaging studies, more severe swelling is associated with significant narrowing of convexity sulci, ventricular compression, and effacement of the normal CSF cisternal spaces (e.g., peri-mesencephalic and suprasellar cisterns). Its diagnosis relies on the observation of diffusely diminished CSF spaces, venous dural sinus narrowing, and flattening of the posterior sclera, enlargement and tortuosity of the optic nerve sheath, and protrusion of the optic papilla (an imaging correlate to papilledema) [9]. Intracranial hemorrhage and tumors of a

Fig. 11.4 Brain swelling and herniation. (**a**) Axial unenhanced CT showing diffuse brain swelling in the setting of severe hyponatremia, with diffuse effacement of sulci and ventricular compression. (**b**) Axial unenhanced CT showing right holohemispheric subdural hematoma with leftward midline herniation in an elderly patient on anticoagulants. (**c**) Midline sagittal T2 FLAIR MRI showing findings of intracranial hypotension. (**d**) Axial unenhanced CT with hydrocephalus due to third ventricular colloid cyst

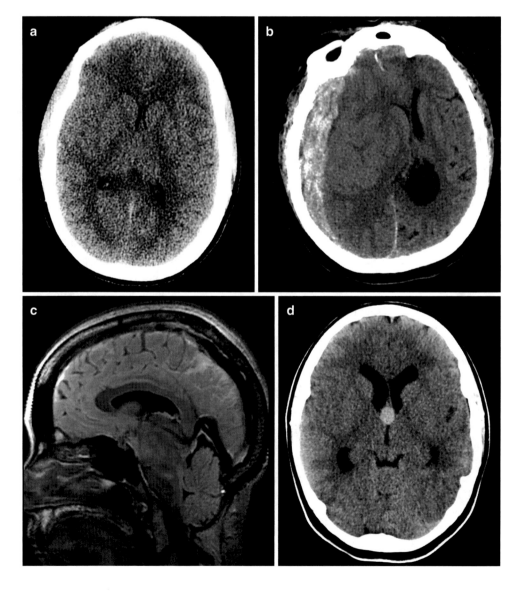

sufficient size in any intracranial compartment can displace normal brain structures and produce herniation syndromes that cause a patient to become unconscious. Similarly, any obstruction to normal CSF flow that leads to acute hydrocephalus can lead to obtundation. Among the many causes for acute hydrocephalus, various infections, intraventricular hemorrhage, and tumors such as colloid cysts and pineal neoplasms are most common.

Low ICP of sufficient degree may also cause patients to become unresponsive. Intracranial hypotension is caused by low CSF volume, typically from CSF leakage from the thecal sac in the spine (e.g., from a ruptured root sleeve or avulsion). Positional headache, cognitive difficulty, and neck pain are more typical of this disorder than frank unconsciousness, but extremely low CSF volume causes coma in some presenting patients when there is severe anatomic distortion of the brainstem, downward transtentorial or cerebellar tonsillar herniation, alternations in cerebral perfusion, and/or unilateral or subdural hematoma in profound intracranial hypotension. Findings of cerebellar tonsillar descent, brainstem sag, enlargement of the pituitary gland, and engorged appearing dural sinuses on are diagnostic for intracranial hypotension and should prompt spinal MRI to identify the site of CSF leak for targeted treatment.

> **Key Point**
> - Alterations in intracranial pressure cause widespread electrochemical neuronal dysfunction and/or mechanical deformations of the brain that can result in unresponsiveness.

11.3   Seizures

Seizures causing unconsciousness may occur in the setting of chronic epilepsy or as a symptom of another underlying neurologic or systemic illness. Tumors, vascular lesions, infections, and other acute and chronic brain injuries and many anatomic abnormalities can cause seizures. In most patients undergoing imaging after a single first seizure, however, an anatomic substrate for the seizure is not found. Instead, another metabolic or systemic illness is responsible for provoking the seizure. Even in cases without a structural brain lesion, both focal and generalized seizure activity may be associated with peri-ictal imaging abnormalities. These findings can be helpful to suggest that a seizure led to the patient being found down.

After a seizure, CT may be normal, or may show focal swelling of involved brain areas (Fig. 11.5). MRI, which is far more sensitive than CT, often depicts swelling, abnormal diffusion, and/or T2 signal in one or both hippocampi, sometimes with more broad involvement of multiple limbic system structures or other cortical gray matter areas. Occasionally, the thalamus also appears abnormally swollen and hyperintense on T2, particularly after prolonged uncontrolled seizures or status epilepticus [10]. On both CT and MRI perfusion studies, hypoperfusion that extends across normal vascular territories may be a clue that a seizure has occurred [11]. It is particularly important to differentiate the swelling and abnormal perfusion caused by post-ictal changes from what is seen in stroke, particularly in patients with who have focal neurologic deficits such as aphasia, motor weakness, or impaired consciousness after a seizure (Todd's paralysis).

White matter abnormalities are less common peri-ictal changes after seizures, except in patients whose seizures are provoked by underlying hypertension and loss of normal cerebrovascular autoregulatory function. In this subgroup of patients found down, imaging is necessary to make the diagnosis of posterior reversible encephalopathy syndrome (PRES). In contrast to other causes for seizures, PRES causes swelling and vasogenic edema that predominates within the juxtacortical white matter, particularly within brain regions supplied by the posterior circulation (occipital lobes, brainstem, and cerebellum), a location that has been linked to a relative deficiency of sympathetic innervation within these vessels. Reduced diffusion and hyperperfusion within the cortex overlying the involved white matter are often present on MRI [12]. Both peri-ictal imaging changes and findings of PRES are transient and resolve over a period of days to weeks after the underlying cause for seizures is removed. Severe prolonged seizures, however, frequently cause permanent injury, evident as atrophy of the involved structures.

> **Key Point**
> - Most seizures are not associated with discrete brain lesions on imaging after a single first seizure. Post-ictal changes characteristically cause gyral swelling with disproportionate gray matter signal abnormalities, especially in limbic or epileptogenic brain areas. PRES, in which white matter abnormalities predominate, is one important exception.

Fig. 11.5 Peri-ictal imaging abnormalities. (**a**) Axial unenhanced CT and (**b**) corresponding axial CT mean transit time (MTT) perfusion map illustrating localized right parietal swelling and increased MTT crossing different arterial territories in a patient found down with right hemiparesis. (**c**) Coronal T2 MRI with bilateral hippocampal swelling and hyperintensity in a child found unresponsive after grand mal seizure. (**d**) Axial unenhanced CT showing bilateral medial occipital low density from PRES in a hypertensive patient found down. All findings resolved on follow-up imaging

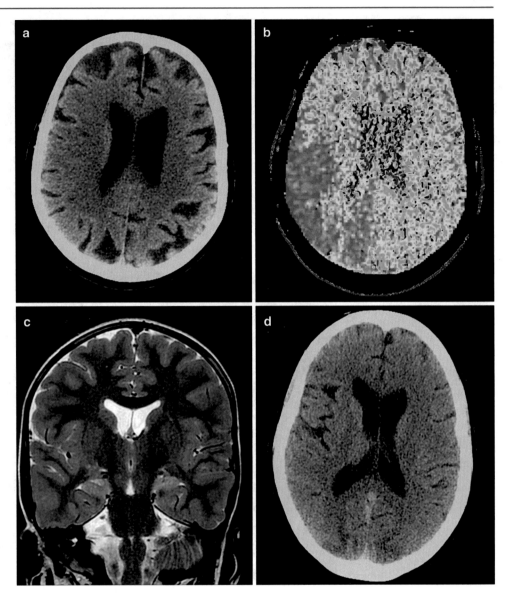

11.4 Toxic Exposures and Metabolic Abnormalities

A variety of medications, toxic exposures, and metabolic disturbances can cause a patient to become unconscious. Some may cause cardiorespiratory failure, reducing oxygen concentration and blood flow in the brain and leading to some of the imaging findings previously described with hypoxic and ischemic injuries. Other substances are directly neurotoxic, including certain medications and by-products of metabolism that accumulate in the setting of organ failure. An important clue to the presence of one of both toxic and metabolic conditions affecting the brain is the observation of bilateral symmetrical imaging abnormalities, particularly within susceptible brain structures. Several of these disor-

ders have characteristic findings that are important to recognize, as the radiologist may be the first to suggest an underlying exposure that requires urgent treatment.

Acute carbon monoxide (CO), methanol, and ethylene glycol poisoning all symmetrically involve the basal ganglia. As a potential exhaust product from heating systems, CO is the most frequent among these three exposures (Fig. 11.6). CO dissolved in blood binds to hemoglobin and displaces normal oxygen, in the most severe cases resulting causing hypoxic patterns of injury. Unlike typical hypoxic insults, however, the CO poisoning has a propensity to cause symmetric necrosis of the internal globus pallidus. Delayed effects of CO exposure also include diffuse white matter abnormalities, with demyelination induced by endothelial cell dysfunction, release of nitric oxide, and consequent for-

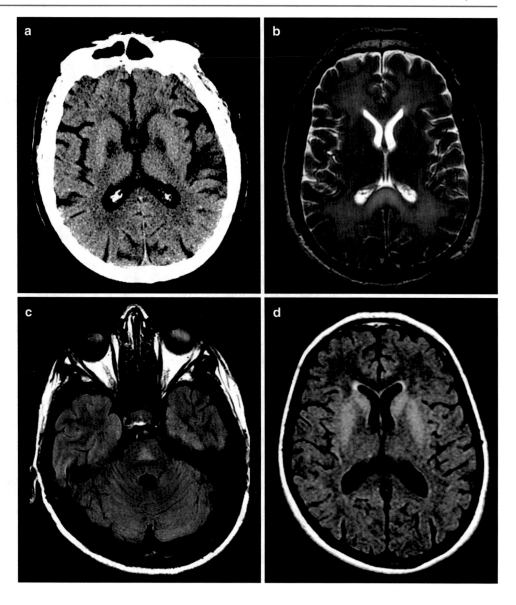

Fig. 11.6 Carbon monoxide poisoning and osmotic demyelination. (**a**) Axial unenhanced CT in acute CO poisoning, with symmetric low density within the globus pallidus bilaterally. (**b**) Axial T2-weighted MRI with diffuse white matter signal abnormality due to delayed leukoencephalopathy occurring 15 days after hypoxic event. (**c**) Axial T2-weighted MRI showing hyperintensity in the central pons in a "trident" configuration, caused by central pontine myelinolysis. (**d**) Axial T2 FLAIR MRI showing extra-pontine myelinolysis, with abnormal symmetric hyperintensity of the basal ganglia

mation of oxygen free radicles and lipid peroxidation [13]. This delayed white matter injury, or delayed toxic leukoencephalopathy, typically occurs several weeks following CO exposure or hypoxic insult. Ingestion of ethylene glycol, a common ingredient in antifreeze, characteristically involves the globus pallidus, together with the thalami, hippocampi, and brainstem [14]. Finally, brain injury due to methanol localizes more frequently to the putamina or lentiform nuclei, may involve subcortical white matter, and is often associated with basal ganglionic hemorrhage [15].

As enumerated in Table 11.1, multiple metabolic derangements can lead to loss of consciousness. The adverse effects on brain function come about as the result of shifts in serum osmolarity, electrochemical instability, seizures, and/or disruption of normal neurotransmitter activity. Like toxic exposures, metabolic disturbances are frequently symmetric on imaging and involve specific brain structures, reflecting the selective vulnerability of neurons in particular areas of the

brain. Inborn errors of metabolism are a rare cause of disrupted brain metabolism; more often in adults these abnormalities come about through hepatic, renal, or pituitary insufficiency or as toxic side effects of medications. As characteristic examples, hypo- and hypernatremia cause brain swelling and contraction, respectively. The consequent alterations in brain volume, especially when taking place over a short period of time, cause headaches, altered mental status, and unconsciousness. Corrected too rapidly, especially in patients with hyponatremia and comorbid alcohol use disorder, liver transplants, or malnutrition, shifts in osmotic pressure can result in demyelination. The central pons is most susceptible to osmotic myelinolysis, causing coma and quadriparesis in affected patients, but involvement of extrapyramidal structures including the basal ganglia and cortex may also be seen.

Hypoglycemic encephalopathy and hyperglycemia merit particular discussion given the frequency of these conditions

Fig. 11.7 Metabolic derangements. (**a**) Axial diffusion-weighted MRI showing high signal in the posterior internal capsule and corona radiata bilaterally in a patient with hypoglycemia. (**b**) Axial unenhanced CT several weeks after profound hyperglycemia, with relatively hyperdense left striatum consistent with diabetic striatopathy. (**c**) Axial diffusion-weighted MRI in hyperammonemia, with symmetric high signal in the insula and cingulate cortices. (**d**) Axial unenhanced CT in uremic encephalopathy, as manifest by swollen, hypodense lentiform nuclei bilaterally

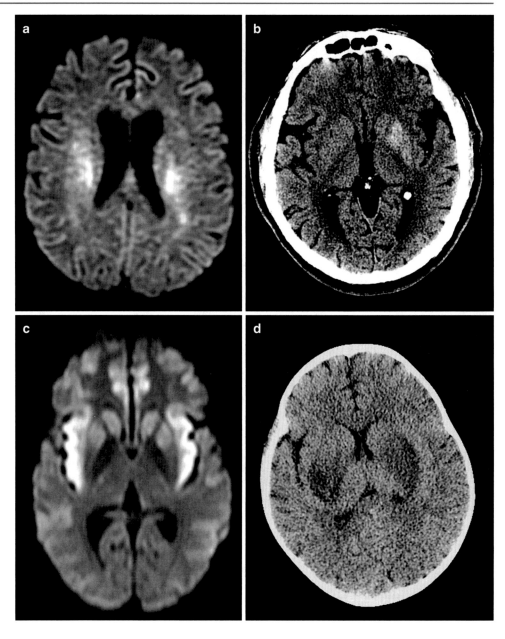

in diabetic populations (Fig. 11.7). Both are now diagnosed easily by laboratory or point-of-care testing, but their effects on the brain should be recognized by radiologists as loss of consciousness in these patients often leads to imaging. Brain injuries due to prolonged or profoundly low blood sugars typically result from excessive administration of hypoglycemic agents. Best seen on diffusion and T2-weighted MRI, imaging abnormalities in hypoglycemia symmetrically involve the white matter in the posterior limb of the internal capsule, corona radiata, centrum semiovale, and callosal splenium and gray matter in the basal ganglia, insula, hippocampus, and hemispheric cortex [16]. The effects of acute hyperglycemia, in contrast, are not typically observed on CT or MRI. Diabetic striatopathy, with asymmetric changes in the putamen and/or caudate, is an uncommon late imaging finding in patients that present with hemiballismus and hemi-

chorea after seizures or coma from severe non-ketotic hyperglycemia.

Finally, accumulation of ammonia in patients with hepatic failure and of uremic toxins in patients with renal failure both may lead to unconsciousness and have characteristic imaging. When ammonia, produced by the digestion of proteins and metabolism of bacteria in the gut, fails to be eliminated by the liver, it is metabolized by astrocytes into glutamine. In excess, this important precursor of the neurotransmitters glutamate and GABA can produce symmetric abnormalities of the insula, cingulate cortex, and in more severe cases, the subcortical white matter, basal ganglia, thalami, and brainstem [17]. In the case of renal failure, uremic toxins and metabolic acidosis cause disruptions in the normal excitatory-inhibitory amino acid balance and metabolic acidosis. Symmetric swelling of the basal ganglia and insula is the most common imaging finding in severe uremia although this is sometimes accompanied by posterior abnormalities patterns typical for PRES given concomitant hypertension usually present in these patients [18].

> **Key Point**
> - Both toxic exposures and metabolic disturbances are associated with relatively symmetric involvement of selectively vulnerable brain structures, and may co-exist with post-ictal, hypoxic, intracranial pressure-related or other findings depending on the underlying cause.

11.5   Concluding Remarks

Imaging serves as cornerstone to the evaluation and management of most patients found down, as almost all patients who present with this scenario undergo some sort of imaging during their hospitalization. Both CT and/or MRI may show findings related to different primary brain abnormalities or to characteristic secondary effects of systemic illness. CT is faster and can be useful to exclude diseases that require urgent or emergent surgery. However, MRI is far more sensitive and is more commonly warranted in patients with prolonged issues with coma or loss of consciousness. Across different categories of issues that can be seen as a cause for or a response to unconsciousness, a subset of causes exhibits diffuse brain abnormalities on imaging and another group is characterized by strategic insults to the brain areas that most important to maintaining consciousness.

> **Take-Home Messages**
> - Patients may be found unconscious after any injury that diffusely disrupts brain function or selectively affects specific brain areas responsible for maintaining consciousness.
> - Imaging is performed in most patients found down at some point during their hospitalization, typically during the initial triage for acute medical and surgical emergences.
> - The most frequent findings in patients discovered unconscious are related to traumatic injury and/or cardiorespiratory failure. Overlapping physiology may result in more than one imaging abnormality.
> - Hypoxic-ischemic injuries, seizures, electrolyte disturbances, toxic exposures, and altered intracranial pressures have characteristic imaging findings that can assist in their diagnosis.

References

1. Howard BM, et al. The found down patient: a Western trauma association multicenter study. J Trauma Acute Care Surg. 2015;79:976–82.
2. Zhao T, et al. Consciousness: new concepts and neural networks. Front Cell Neurosci. 2019;13:1–7.
3. Meythaler JM, et al. Current concepts: diffuse axonal injury-associated traumatic brain injury. Arch Phys Med Rehabil. 2001;82:1461–71.
4. Kim SH, et al. Early brain computed tomography findings are associated with outcome in patients treated with therapeutic hypothermia after out-of-hospital cardiac arrest. Scand J Trauma Resusc Emerg Med. 2013;21:57.
5. Gonzalez RG, et al. Diffusion-weighted MR imaging: diagnostic accuracy in patients imaged within 6 hours of stroke symptom onset. Radiology. 1999;210:155–62.
6. Torvik A, Skullerud K. Watershed infarcts in the brain caused by microemboli. Clin Neuropathol. 1982;1:99–105.
7. Ellchuck TN, et al. Suspicious neuroimaging pattern of thrombotic microangiopathy. AJNR Am J Neuroradiol. 2011;32:734–8.
8. Vanjare HA, et al. Clinical and radiologic findings of acute necrotizing encephalopathy in young adults. AJNR Am J Neuroradiol. 2020;41:2250–4.
9. Passi N, et al. MR imaging of papilledema and visual pathways: effects of increased intracranial pressure and pathophysiologic mechanisms. AJNR Am J Neuroradiol. 2013;34:919–24.
10. Cianfoni A, et al. Seizure-induced brain lesions: a wide spectrum of variably reversible MRI abnormalities. Eur J Radiol. 2013;82:1964–72.
11. Gelfand JM, Wintermark M, Josephson SA. Cerebral perfusion-CT patterns following seizure. Eur J Neurol. 2010;17:594–601.
12. Wakisaka K, et al. Epileptic ictal hyperperfusion on arterial spin labeling perfusion and diffusion-weighted magnetic resonance images in posterior reversible encephalopathy syndrome. J Stroke Cerebrovasc Dis. 2016;25:228–37.
13. Lo C-P, et al. Brain injury after acute carbon monoxide poisoning: early and late complications. AJR Am J Roentgenol. 2007;189:W205–11.
14. Malhotra A, et al. Ethylene glycol toxicity: MRI brain findings. Clin Neuroradiol. 2017;27:109–13.
15. Hoang TN, et al. Characteristics of brain magnetic resonance imaging in acute methanol intoxication: report of 3 cases. Radiol Case Rep. 2023;18:4414–8.
16. Ma JH, et al. MR imaging of hypoglycemic encephalopathy: lesion distribution and prognosis prediction by diffusion-weighted imaging. Neuroradiology. 2009;51:641–9.
17. U-King-Im JM, et al. Acute hyperammonemic encephalopathy in adults: imaging findings. AJNR Am J Neuroradiol. 2011;32:413–8.
18. Kim DM, et al. Uremic encephalopathy: MR imaging findings and clinical correlation. AJNR Am J Neuroradiol. 2016;37:1604–9.

Evaluation of Patients with Cranial Nerve Disorders

12

Jan W. Casselman, Alexandre Krainik, and Ian Macdonald

Abstract

Neurologists, neurosurgeons, ENT and maxillofacial surgeons, ophthalmologists, and others often detect cranial nerve deficits in their patients but remain uncertain about the underlying cause. It is the radiologist's task to identify the causative disease, including inflammatory, infectious, vascular, traumatic, tumoral, and neurodegenerative etiologies. To detect this pathology, the neuroradiologist or head and neck radiologist must have a detailed knowledge of the anatomy of the 12 cranial nerves and available MR techniques. Furthermore, selecting the optimal sequences significantly depends on access to the patient's history, clinical and biological data. In this chapter, emphasis will be put on employing the certain imaging techniques best suited to detect pathologies on the different parts/segments of the cranial nerves: intraaxial, extraaxial intracranial, skull base, and extracranial.

Keywords

Cranial nerves · Cranial nerve diseases · Cranial nerve disorders · Cranial nerve tumours, benign · Cranial nerve tumours, malignant · Perineural tumour spread · Cranial nerve injuries · Cranial nerve V · Cranial nerve VII · Magnetic resonance imaging · Computed tomography

Abbreviations

ADC	Apparent diffusion coefficient
BB	Black blood
CN	Cranial nerve
CNs	Cranial nerves
CPA	Cerebellopontine angle
CSF	Cerebrospinal fluid
CT	Computed tomography
CTA	Computed tomography angiography
DWI	Diffusion weighted images
FS	Fat-saturated
IAC	Internal auditory canal
ICA	Internal carotid artery
MR	Magnetic resonance
MRA	Magnetic resonance angiography
MRN	Magnetic resonance neurography
MS	Multiple sclerosis
NF1	Neurofibromatosis type 1
NF2	Neurofibromatosis type 2
NMOSD	Neuromyelitis optica spectrum disorders
NVC	Neurovascular conflict
NVCS	Neurovascular compression syndrome
PD	Proton density
SWI	Susceptibility weighted images
T1W	T1 weighted
T1WI	T1 weighted images
T2W	T2 weighted
T2WI	T2 weighted images
TN	Trigeminal neuralgia
TOF	Time of flight
TZ	Transition zone

J. W. Casselman (✉) · I. Macdonald
Department of Neuroradiology & Head and Neck Radiology, Dalhousie University, Halifax, NS, Canada
e-mail: jan.casselman@nshealth.ca; Ian.Macdonald@dal.ca

A. Krainik
Department of Neuroradiology, University Hospital of Grenoble, Grenoble, France
e-mail: akrainik@chu-grenoble.fr

© The Author(s) 2024
J. Hodler et al. (eds.), *Diseases of the Brain, Head and Neck, Spine 2024-2027*, IDKD Springer Series, https://doi.org/10.1007/978-3-031-50675-8_12

Learning Objectives
- To understand that lesions can be found on the different anatomical segments of the cranial nerves: intraaxial–extraaxial–skull base–extracranial.
- To be aware that the MR technique must be adapted for each of these anatomical segments to detect all pathologies.
- To be familiar with the imaging appearance of the most frequent cranial nerve pathologies.

Key Points
- MR anatomy, from brainstem nuclei to extracranial cranial nerve segments, is fundamental to identify disease.
- Available clinical history, clinical presentation, and laboratory tests are crucial to make the correct diagnosis on imaging.
- MRI is the preferred technique to detect CN disorders.
- To be aware of the latest MRI techniques to visualize cranial nerve anatomy and pathology.

12.1 Introduction

The anatomy of the 12 paired cranial nerves (CNs) is complex and their origin, in the brain (CN I and II) or the brainstem (CN III–XII) as well as further intracranial and extracranial courses must be known. Moreover, it is technically challenging to cover the complete courses of the different CNs during imaging as well as to choose the right sequences on magnetic resonance imaging (MRI).

There are a wide variety of diseases that can cause cranial nerve (CN) disorders and imaging is needed to depict the causative pathology, for therapy planning and to assess response. The clinical examination, medical history, laboratory, and neurophysiological tests will all aid the radiologist to select the correct imaging modality or technique and use the best adapted protocol.

The first goal of CN imaging is to find the exact location of the disease: intraaxial (within the brain or the brainstem), extraaxial intracranial (outside the brain but inside the skull), skull base (in foramina, fissures, or canals of the skull base), extracranial (outside the skull). The tumoral, inflammatory, infectious, traumatic or dysfunctional disorders occurring along the different CN segments differ. Therefore, once imaging can link the lesion to one of these segments, a more precise and refined differential diagnosis is possible.

In this chapter, the most frequent pathologies involving the different CNs will be discussed [1–8] with emphasis on the MR techniques that should be used to visualize these lesions at the different CN segments.

12.2 Anatomy

In most anatomy and clinical papers, 12 pairs of CNs are mentioned; however, CNs I and II are extensions of the brain and are therefore not true CNs. This also explains why schwannomas do not occur along the olfactory tract and bulb or on the optic nerve. Hence, only 10 pairs of real CNs exist, and these nerves III–XII have their nuclei and origin in the brainstem.

Both the olfactory (CN I) and optic nerve (CN II) become discernible at the basal forebrain and leave the anterior cranial fossa through the cribriform plate and optic canal, respectively. The ten other CNs originate from the brainstem: the oculomotor (CNIII) and trochlear (CN IV) nerves exit from the midbrain, the trigeminal nerve (CN V) from the pons, while the abducens (CN VI), facial (CN VII), and cochleovestibular (CN VIII) nerves leave the brainstem at the medullopontine sulcus. The glossopharyngeal (CN IX), vagus (CN X), accessory (CN XI), and hypoglossal (CN XII) nerves become apparent at the level of the medulla oblongata. Nerve XII is present anterior to the olivary bodies at the pre-olivary sulcus while nerves IX–XI are posterior to the olivary bodies at the post-olivary sulcus. Cranial nerves III–VI pass through the foramina/fissures of the middle cranial fossa. Cranial nerves VII–XII leave the posterior cranial fossa through the internal auditory canal (CN VII–VIII), jugular foramen (CN IX–XI), and hypoglossal canal (CN XII).

Therefore, the location of the causative lesion, in the anterior fossa close to CN I–II, middle cranial fossa close to CN III–VI, or posterior cranial fossa close to CN VII–XII, will correlate with the presenting cranial nerve symptoms. Furthermore, lesions on distal extracranial branches most frequently will result in specific CN deficits, while proximal intracranial lesions (e.g. the brainstem) can result in deficits of multiple CNs in combination with other central neurological symptoms.

In practice, the optimal imaging techniques must be used to investigate CN impairments caused by (1) intraaxial lesions, affecting the CN nuclei and "fascicular segment" or segment of the nerve inside the brainstem, (2) extraaxial intracranial lesions compromising the cisternal CN fibres, (3) skull base lesions involving the CN segment at the skull base foramina/fissures and canals, and (4) extracranial lesions affecting the CN segments in the head and neck.

Knowing the complex CN anatomy and function is mandatory to study CN disorders in an adapted manner (Table 12.1). More anatomical and functional CN details can be found in CN textbooks [3–6].

Table 12.1 Cranial nerves disorders and apparent routes

CN name	Main dysfunctions	CNS coverage	Skull base coverage	Face and neck coverage
I: Olfactory	Anosmia	Basal forebrain: olfactory tracts, bulbs, and striae. Uncus, parahippocampal and cingular gyri	Anterior skull base: cribriform plate	Nasal mucosa
II: Optic	Vision loss. Prechiasmatic: unilateral anop(s)ia Chiasmatic: bitemporal hemiano(s)pia Retrochiasmatic: homonymous hemianop(s)ia	Basal forebrain: optic radiation, chiasma, lateral geniculate bodies, occipital calcarine sulci	Anterior skull base: optic canal	Orbit: eye ball retina
III: Oculomotor	Oculomotor palsy, ptosis, mydriasis	Midbrain: interpeduncular fossa	Middle skull base: cavernous sinus, superior orbital fissure	Orbit: oculomotor m. (superior, medial, inferior recti, inferior oblique), levator palpebrae m., ciliary m.
IV: Trochlear	Trochlear palsy	Midbrain: tectum	Middle skull base: cavernous sinus, superior orbital fissure	Orbit: superior oblique m.
V: Trigeminal	Facial anaesthesia-numbness Trigeminal neuralgia	Pons: anterolateral	Middle skull base: cavernous sinus; V_1: superior orbital fissure V_2: f. rotundum V_3: f. ovale	Face V_1: forehead V_2: upper cheek V_3: lower jaw, sensory tongue (2/3 ant.)
VI: Abducens	Abducens palsy	Medullopontine s. (ant.)	Middle skull base: basilar plexus, cavernous sinus, superior orbital fissure	Orbit: lateral rectus m.
VII: Facial	Facial palsy. Hemifacial spasm	Medullopontine s. (lat.)	Posterior skull base: internal auditory canal, facial nerve canal, stylomastoid f.	Face m., lacrimal and salivary glands
VIII: Cochleovestibular	Hearing loss, tinnitus, dizziness	Medullopontine s. (lat.)	Posterior skull base: internal auditory canal	Inner ear: cochlea and semicircular canals
IX: Glossopharyngeal	Ageusia, dysphagia, throat anaesthesia. Glossopharyngeal neuralgia.	Medulla: retroolivary s.	Posterior skull base: jugular foramen	Stylopharyngeus m.; sensory tongue (1/3 post)
X: Vagus	Dysphagia, dysphonia	Medulla: retroolivary s.	Posterior skull base: jugular foramen	Pharyngeal m.
XI: Accessory	Impairment of head rotation, scapula elevation	Medulla: retroolivary s., lateral cervical cord	Posterior skull base: jugular foramen	Sternocleidomastoid, trapezius m.
XII: Hypoglossal	Palsy of the tongue	Medulla: pre-olivary s.	Posterior skull base: hypoglossal canal	Tongue muscles

m. muscle, *s.* sulcus, *ant.* anterior, *lat.* lateral, *post* posterior

Courtesy to: A. Krainik, J.W. Casselman, Imaging evaluation of patients with cranial nerve disorders. In: Hodler J, Kubik-Huch R, Von Schulthess G (Eds) Diseases of the Brain, Head and Neck, Spine 2020–2023, IDKD Springer, Cham, Switzerland, 2020, pp. 143–161. https://doi.org/10.1007/978-3-030-38490-6_12

12.3 Imaging Technique

12.3.1 Imaging Technique: General Considerations

Computed tomography (CT) is valuable in the detection of bone lesions and calcifications. Strengths of CT are that it is fast, immediately available and that monitored/unstable patients can be examined in a non-magnetic safe environment. Therefore, CT is often the first technique used in trauma patients, patients with inflammation or infection/abscess and in patients with compromised airways.

MRI provides superior tissue contrast to noise and is the method of choice to investigate CN disorders. As already mentioned, MRI protocols must be adapted to the regional CN anatomy, based on the available clinical information.

This allows selection of the optimal adapted sequences and field of view for this anatomical region [2, 8]. The use of intravenous contrast media must be justified and will depend on the clinical presentation, the initial imaging findings, and the potential lesions on the differential (Table 12.2).

Evaluation of the size and density/signal intensity of CNs is easiest when the affected nerve can be compared with the normal contralateral CN. This is best achieved on coronal images for CNs I–VI as these nerves run in a postero-anterior direction. The axial plane is best suited for CNs VII–VIII as these nerves run in a slightly oblique axial plane in postero-medial to anterolateral direction.

In many cases, nerve enhancement is the only imaging finding in cranial nerve disorders and consequently the use of intravenous gadolinium (Gd) contrast enhancement is highly recommended in almost all cases.

Phased array head coils are anatomically suited to image the 12 CNs in their course down to the level of the mandible and hyoid. Study of the lower cranial nerves in the infrahyoid neck or upper mediastinum (CN X) requires the use of an additional dedicated neck coil.

12.3.2 Imaging Technique: New Techniques

Over the years, new MRI techniques have been developed and many of these have proven utility in clinical CN imaging.

High-angular resolution diffusion weighted imaging (at least 32 directions) allows cranial nerve tractography based on diffusion tensor imaging. Postprocessing however is crucial and routine software provided by MR vendors will in most cases be insufficient for cranial nerve tractography. Even with the best available techniques and postprocessing, currently only the larger isolated cranial nerves, II, III, V, VI, VII, and VIII can be adequately studied [9] (Fig. 12.1a). Apart from studying the course of the cranial nerves, for instance, the relation of the facial nerve to an VIIIth nerve

Table 12.2 Technical recommendations to investigate CN disorders

CN nuclei and segments	Brainstem: nuclei and intramedullary fibres	Cisternal segment	Segments surrounded by venous plexus—intraforaminal fibres	Extracranial nerves—face, neck, mediastinum
Sequences	T2W/PD (2D) DWI (2D) m-FFE/medic/merge(2D)-nuclei	b-FFE XD (3D) DRIVE TSE T2 (3D) MRA (3D) unenhanced	T1W TSE HR (2D) FFE (3D) Black blood TSE T1 (3D)	T1W TSE HR (2D) T2W TSE HR (2D) Neurography (3D)
Plane	Axial	3D sequences, isotropic. Measured in the axial plane, reformatted in any other plane	Cavernous sinus: coronal Basilar plexus: axial Jugular foramen: axial > coronal Hypoglossal canal: axial > coronal 3D sequences: reformatted any plane	Axial + coronal Neurography: axial 3D isotropic
Resolution ($X \times Y \times Z$ in mm)	T2W/PD: 0.70 × 0.88 × 3.00 DWI: 1.40 × 1.42 × 3.00 m-FFE: 0.65 × 0.87 × 2.00	b-FFE XD: 0.5 × 0.5 × 0.5 mm DRIVE T2: 0.46 × 0.46 × 0.50 mm MRA: 0.69 × 0.70 × 0.70 mm	T1W TSE HR: 0.40 × 0.45 × 2.30 mm FFE: 0.60 × 0.59 × 1.20 mm Black blood: 0.55 × 0.55 × 0.55 mm	T1W TSE HR: 0.40 × 0.45 × 2.3 mm T2W TSE HR: 0.60 × 0.53 × 3.3 mm Neurography: 0.89 × 0.90 × 0.90 mm
Range	T2W/PD: 60 mm DWI: 128 mm m-FFE: 48 mm	b-FFE XD: 80 mm DRIVE T2: 36 mm MRA: 120 mm	T1W TSE HR: 69 mm FFE: 59 mm Black blood: 39 mm	T1W TSE HR: 69 mm T2W TSE HR: 106 mm Neurography: 90 mm
Acquisition time	T2W/PD: 2 min 31 s DWI: 2 min 21 s m-FFE: 14 min 46 s	b-FFE XD: 4 min 43 s (CS 10) DRIVE T2: 2 min 47 s (CS 3.3) MRA: 6 min 50 s (CS 3)	T1W TSE HR: 7 min 30 s (S 1.5) FFE: 4 min 8 s (S 1.4) Black blood: 5 min 5 s (CS 4)	T1W TSE HR: 7 min 30 s (S 1.5) T2W TSE HR: 3 min 15 s (CS 2.5) Neurography: 8 min 17 s (CS 3)

2D two dimensional, *3D* three dimensional, *b-FFE* balanced fast field echo, *CN* cranial nerve, *CS* compressed sense factor, *DRIVE* driven equilibrium, *DWI* diffusion weighted imaging, *FFE* fast field echo, *medic* multi-echo data image combination, *merge* multiple echo recombine gradient echo, *m-FFE* merged fast field echo, *HR* high resolution, *MRA* magnetic resonance angiography, *PD* proton density, *S* sense factor, *T2W* T2 weighted, *TSE* turbo spin echo

Courtesy to: A. Krainik, J.W. Casselman, Imaging evaluation of patients with cranial nerve disorders. In: Hodler J, Kubik-Huch R, Von Schulthess G (Eds) Diseases of the Brain, Head and Neck, Spine 2020–2023, IDKD Springer, Cham, Switzerland, 2020, pp. 143–161. https://doi.org/10.1007/978-3-030-38490-6_12

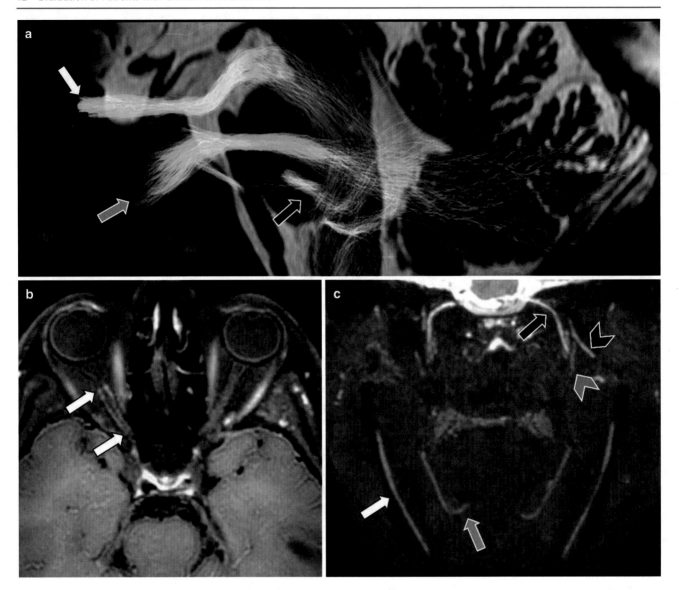

Fig. 12.1 New imaging techniques for cranial nerves (CNs): (**a**) Tractography of CNs III (white arrow), V (grey arrow), VII and VIII (black arrow) in a normal volunteer (courtesy of Dr. T. Jacquesson and A. Attayé, CHU Grenoble, France). (**b**) Contrast-enhanced axial 3D black blood image showing enhancement of the optic nerve sheath in the posterior half of the orbit (arrows) in a patient with optic perineuri-

tis. (**c**) Coronal 3D cranial nerve imaging (3D CRANI) showing the normal anatomy of the extracranial CNs: inferior alveolar nerve in the mandible (white arrow), distal end of the lingual nerve inside the anterior 2/3 of the tongue (grey arrow), vagus nerve (grey arrowhead), accessory nerve (black arrowhead), and hypoglossal nerve (black arrow)

schwannoma or parotid tumour, global tractography is also efficient in mapping cranial nerve ischaemia [10]. Future faster imaging acquisition techniques and more refined post-processing software will further elevate this CN imaging technique in routine clinical practice [9, 11–13].

In recent years, 3D black blood (BB) MRI is increasingly used in the neuroradiological and Head and Neck fields. The major advantage of this technique is that the vessels remain dark on the contrast-enhanced images and therefore do not mask pathology. The general background tissue also remains hypointense, and therefore the sequence is very sensitive for enhancement (Fig. 12.1b). Hence, enhancing cranial nerve

lesions are easier to depict and can be distinguished from surrounding vessels. Furthermore, it is a 3D T1 weighted (T1W) TSE technique, resulting in almost no susceptibility artifacts, important at the level of the skull base. As it is a 3D sequence, excellent multiplanar reconstructions can be made in any desired plane.

MR neurography (MRN) techniques were further optimized during recent years. They use a contrast-enhanced black blood (BB) 3D STIR TSE sequence preceded by an MSDE (motion-sensitized driven equilibrium) pulse in combination with a pseudo-steady-state sweep and compressed sensing [14, 15]. Compressed sensing was needed to acquire these high-resolution isotropic images in an acceptable time. This technique is very sensitive to detect neuritis, neuropathy, nerve transection, etc. of the extracranial segments of the CNs, pathologies that were often not detectable with standard sequences [16]. Furthermore, this allows visualization of the extracranial segments of the CNs, down to the level of the hyoid and tongue (Fig. 12.1c) [17]; however, higher resolution sequences and improved neck coils that are available today will be needed to follow these nerves in the infrahyoid neck and upper mediastinum.

12.4 Cranial Nerve Lesions

12.4.1 Intraaxial Cranial Nerve Lesions

The nuclei and fascicular segment of the CNs III–XII are located in the brainstem. Involvement of these intraaxial CN structures will result in complex clinical presentations, consisting of multiple CN impairments, hemiplegia, hemiparesis, internuclear ophthalmoplegia, extrapyramidal syndrome, awareness impairment, nausea, etc. Cranial nerves I and II also have their "intraaxial" tract/cortical areas; therefore, lesions affecting these structures will result in cranial nerve I and II deficits.

Lesions in the brainstem are best studied with selective T2 weighted (T2W) and Proton Density (PD) images or mFFE/Merge/Medic images. These images should be 3 mm or less to avoid partial volume effects which can limit visualization of lesions. In the acute setting, diffusion weighted images (DWI) should be added to exclude recent infarctions and unenhanced T1 weighted images (T1WI), magnetic resonance angiography (MRA), and susceptibility weighted images (SWI) are useful in trauma patients and patients with vascular malformations or ischaemic lesions. Gd-enhanced T1WI should be added when tumour or infection is suspected.

Stroke and demyelinating disease are the most frequent intraaxial causes of CN involvement.

12.4.1.1 Ischaemic Stroke

Occlusion of the basilar artery, its perforating arteries, the distal portion of the vertebral arteries and the posterior-inferior cerebellar arteries can result in brainstem stroke and neurologic deficits with secondary CN disorders.

Unenhanced CT and T1W, T2* or SWI images can be used to exclude haemorrhage. DWI, T2 FLAIR images and perfusion MR or CT can be used to confirm the acute nature of the stroke (Fig. 12.2a) and to detect a penumbra, indicating that viable brainstem tissue around the irreversibly damaged ischaemic core can be saved by intravenous thrombolysis [18]. Mechanical thrombectomy for vertebral and basilar artery occlusions is a promising approach with initial studies

demonstrating the potential of this intervention to benefit these patients. Finally, CT angiography and MR angiography (MRA) can be used to confirm vessel occlusion or stenosis.

The nuclei of CN III, IV, VI reside in proximity of the medial longitudinal fasciculus and therefore in case of stroke, the resulting nerve deficit is most often associated with internuclear ophthalmoplegia (Fig. 12.2a).

12.4.1.2 Demyelinating Disease

Multiple sclerosis (MS), neuromyelitis optica spectrum disorders (NMOSD) with anti-MOG or anti-AQP4 antibodies, etc. are a heterogeneous group of inflammatory disorders [19]. Lesions located in the cranial nerve nuclei or fascicular segments of the cranial nerves will cause related CN symptoms. The trigeminal nerve is the most frequently involved CN and trigeminal neuralgia (TN) is the most frequent symptom (Fig. 12.2b). Patients with MS have a 20-fold increased risk in developing TN, and it affects 1.9–4.9% of MS patients. Conversely, MS is detected in 2–4% of patients with TN [20]. MS lesions are best seen on T2 weighted images (T2WI) or PD images, and the diagnosis is often already established clinically or confirmed by the typical supratentorial, infratentorial or medullary location, and morphology of the lesions.

Central pontine myelinolysis is another demyelinating disease mostly affecting the central pons and occurring primarily in alcoholic or malnourished patients complicated by hyponatraemia. The rapid correction of hyponatraemia has been recognized as the cause of the demyelination. Patients present with subacute progressive quadriparesis with lower cranial nerve involvement. It is usually fatal but can be mitigated by gradual correction of the electrolyte disturbance.

12.4.1.3 Trauma

High velocity trauma or trauma with a major impact on the brain can cause diffuse axonal injuries secondary to structural neural shearing. These focal lesions are hyperintense on T2WI, hypointense on T2* images or SWI and can be hyperintense on unenhanced T1WI in the acute phase and result in CN impairment when located in CN nuclei or the fascicular course. Acceleration–deceleration trauma can also result in injury of the posterior midbrain due to impact with the tentorium, causing oedema or superficial haemorrhage with consequent cranial nerve III or IV involvement.

12.4.1.4 Vascular Malformations

Cavernous haemangiomas are the most frequent vascular malformations found in the brainstem. They are best detected on T2* images or SWI and have a popcorn-like hyperintense centre on unenhanced T1WI which can slightly enhance after Gd administration. They can suddenly increase in size with spontaneous bleeding resulting in localized haemor-

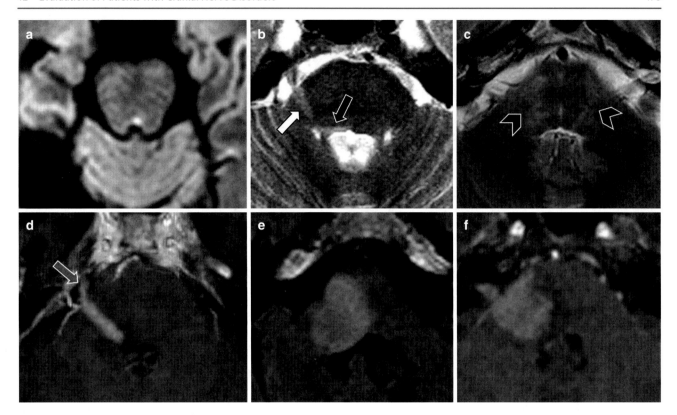

Fig. 12.2 Intraaxial lesions with CN disorders: (**a**) DWI image with acute infarct at the site of the left nucleus of CN IV and the left medial longitudinal fasciculus (MLF) causing a right superior oblique muscle palsy and internuclear ophthalmoplegia (INO). (**b**) MS patient with right trigeminal neuralgia with demyelinating lesions on the fascicular segment of the right trigeminal nerve (white arrow) and in the sensory and motor nucleus (black arrow) seen as hyperintensities on T2W imaging. (**c**) Neuroborreliosis rhombencephalitis with diffuse high signal intensity changes on T2W imaging in a patient presenting with falls and VIIIth nerve (vertigo) symptoms. (**d**) Covid-19 patient presenting with right Vth nerve neuropathy and neuralgia showing enhancement along the cisternal (arrow) and fascicular segment and in the brainstem nuclei on contrast-enhanced T1W (courtesy Dr. G. Hespel, AZ Zeno, Knokke-Heist, Belgium). (**e**) FLAIR image showing a low-grade glioma of the brainstem in a patient presenting with a right facial nerve palsy due to involvement of the right nucleus and fascicular segment of this nerve. (**f**) Contrast-enhanced T1W showing lymphoma in the right pons, cerebellopontine angle, and interna auditory canal in a patient presenting with deafness and dysequilibrium (CN VIII) and a grade 2 facial nerve palsy (VII) due to involvement of the nuclei, fascicular, and cisternal segments of these nerves

rhage. This can then result in cranial nerve impairment, often improving and eventually resolving as the haemorrhage resorbs. Fistulas and arteriovenous malformations are less frequent causes.

12.4.1.5 Infectious Diseases

Listeria rhombencephalitis is caused by the Listeria monocytogenes anaerobic bacterium. This septicaemia occurs after oral contamination of infected fresh products. It is the most frequent cause of rhombencephalitis, and patients develop a spectrum of symptoms related to the brainstem involvement. Multiple cranial nerve palsies occur in 75% of the patients. The lesions are best seen on MR and are hyperintense on T2 and FLAIR (Fig. 12.2c) with linear CN enhancement and heterogeneous (diffuse inflammation) or ring enhancement (abscess) on the contrast-enhanced T1WI. The survival is only 50% and depends on the timely use of antibiotics. The presence of small foci of diffusion restriction indicates a worse outcome.

Some viruses like the cytomegalovirus can manifest in immunocompromised patients and cause encephalitis and involvement of the CN nuclei. Other viruses like the herpes simplex, herpes zoster and corona (COVID 19) virus can have a neurotropic behaviour. They can follow the cranial nerves into the brainstem where they follow the fascicular segment and even the course of the nuclei. High signal intensity can be seen on T2WI and FLAIR images along these structures and enhancement is possible on the contrast-enhanced T1WI (Fig. 12.2d).

12.4.1.6 Tumours

Midline infiltrating glioma of the pons and other tumours that can infiltrate the brainstem like metastases, CNS lymphoma, ependymomas, and medulloblastomas can all cause cranial nerve deficits, especially when growth is rapid. The lesions have a high signal intensity on T2WI and FLAIR images and heterogenous enhancement on post-contrast T1WI, except for lymphoma which has a homogeneous enhancement (Fig. 12.2e, d).

12.4.2 Intracranial Extraaxial Cranial Nerve Lesions

The intracranial extraaxial segment or cisternal segment of the cranial nerves course between the brainstem and the skull base neuroforamina and fissures. They are surrounded by cerebrospinal fluid (CSF), and therefore submillimetric heavily T2WI are optimal to demonstrate the nerves as grey/black surrounded by high signal intensity white CSF. Submillimetric 3D-DRIVE/FIESTA/SPACE T2WI can be used for this purpose but their range is limited, and thus difficult to cover the desired field of view. The 3D balanced-FFE sequence can acquire submillimetric isotropic images with a high resolution and a large range, covering all the CNs in an acceptable acquisition time. This sequence is however more sensitive to banding artifacts and motion. The banding artifacts result in black lines running through the high signal intensity fluid of the orbits, semicircular canals, cochlea, and CSF surrounding the olfactory bulbs. Hence, these peripheral regions and structures are better examined with 3D TSE T2W sequences. Another drawback of the 3D b-FFE sequence is that the pulsation of the basilar artery can cause dephasing or loss of the high signal intensity in the CSF surrounding this artery and in turn will frequently cause non-visualization of the abducens nerve. Visualization of this nerve can be accomplished with 3D TSE T2WI. A recent improvement of 3D b-FFE T2W sequence to 3D b-FFE XD T2W sequence eliminates these banding artifacts and therefore this new sequence can be used in all areas, including olfactory bulbs, inner ear, orbits, and for the abducens nerve. Gadolinium-enhanced T1WI or black blood (BB) images are used to detect abnormal nerve enhancement and are the most sensitive images to detect pathology on the cisternal segment. However, it should be cautioned that 3D T1W gradient-echo sequences are less sensitive to gadolinium enhancement and that subtle/weak enhancement can be missed on these images. TSE, SE and BB sequences, 3D or 2D, are more sensitive for gadolinium enhancement with the BB sequence being the most sensitive.

Intracranial extraaxial CN lesions like nerve sheath tumours and neuritis can involve the CN itself, or these CNs can be compressed/displaced by skull base, meningeal or vascular lesions as well as even normal vascular structures. The resulting CN symptoms and the patient's history are helpful to localize and determine size of lesions. In the event of negative imaging studies, CSF sampling via lumbar puncture is needed to further evaluate these patients. CT can be used in the emergency setting to exclude intracranial hypertension prior to lumbar puncture and can also be used to exclude bone metastases. However, in most cases MR is needed to further characterize CN lesions [2, 8, 21, 22].

12.4.2.1 Tumours/Cysts/Cyst-Like Lesions

Nerve Sheath Tumours

Schwannomas are the most frequent CN tumours and develop from the Schwann sheath of these nerves. Schwannomas of CN I and II do not exist as they are extensions of the brain, thus do not possess Schwann cells. However, the nerve fibres that connect the olfactory bulb with the olfactory mucosa in the upper nasal meatus have Schwann cells along their course below the cribriform plate. Schwannomas developing at this site are called "olfactory schwannomas", but they do not develop from CN I itself. Schwannomas can occur on all other cranial nerves and are most frequent on the vestibular branches of CN VIII and CN V. They are rare on the pure motor CNs IV, VI, XI (Fig. 12.3a). Schwannomas can be found in isolation or can involve multiple CNs. In the latter case, this is often in the context of Neurofibromatosis type 2 or schwannomatosis. The genes associated with these disorders are located on chromosome 22 but in schwannomatosis, there is incomplete penetrance with lower risk of its transmission to the offspring. Furthermore, these patients with schwannomatosis do not typically develop vestibular schwannomas [23]. Schwannomas are sharply delineated and have a homogeneous enhancement on contrast-enhanced T1WI. However, cystic degeneration and haemorrhage can occur when they become larger. The haemorrhages are best recognized on T2* images or SWI. The most frequent location of schwannomas is on the vestibular nerves, at the site of the ganglion of Scarpa. This ganglion can routinely be seen as a nodular thickening on the superior vestibular nerve on high-resolution T2WI at 3T MRI. However, it is impossible to tell whether a normal ganglion or a schwannoma is causing this nodular thickening and hence the use of gadolinium is crucial to exclude an early schwannoma at this site. Sometimes it is difficult to recognize in which direction CN VII is displaced by the cochleovestibular schwannoma and in these cases, CN tractography can provide this crucial information to the surgeon (Fig. 12.3b).

Neurofibromas are less frequent encapsulated nerve sheath tumours. The major difference on imaging is that instead of a rounded morphology, they typically appear elongated in appearance, following the course of the nerves, and show no or only weak gadolinium enhancement. These nerve sheath tumours must be distinguished from other tumours. When solitary they must be differentiated from neuromas, which develop on the CNs secondary to a trauma or insult, and haemangiomas [21, 22, 24].

The most frequent causes of bilateral enhancement of multiple CNs are metastasis, lymphoma, and leukaemia. Unfortunately, they have overlapping imaging characteris-

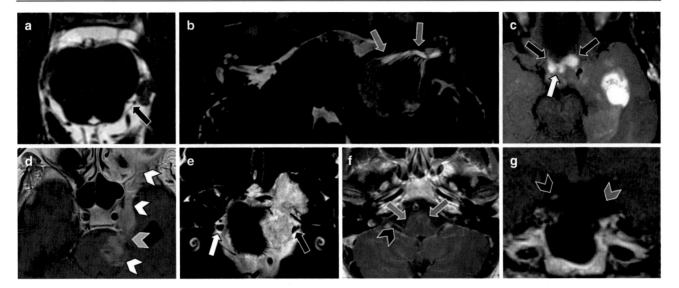

Fig. 12.3 Intracranial extraaxial CN lesions: (**a**) Heavily T2W DRIVE image showing a schwannoma in the ambient cistern on the course of the IVth nerve (arrow) in a patient with left superior oblique muscle palsy. (**b**) High-angular resolution DWI tractography confirming anterior displacement of the facial nerve (arrows) by a cochleovestibular schwannoma. (**c**) Left temporal glioblastoma, with perineural tumour spread along the optic chiasm (white arrow) and intracranial optic nerves (black arrows). In the past, perineural extension was not typically seen in the context of glioblastoma as survival was very short, however, is now increasingly depicted as novel therapies result in longer survival. (**d**) Axial contrast-enhanced T1W showing a recurrent sarcoid carcinomatous tumour of the left maxillary sinus with extension along the maxillary nerve in the parasellar region and into the brainstem (white arrowheads), also involving the cisternal segment of the trigeminal nerve (grey arrowhead) in a patient presenting with left CN V neuropathy and acute right hemiparesis. (**e**) Coronal T2 weighted DRIVE

images showing lower signal intensity inside an epidermoid tumour in the left cerebellopontine angle compared with CSF. The patient presented with trigeminal neuropathy with the cisternal segment of the left trigeminal nerve laterally displaced and flattened (black arrow) compared to the normal contralateral nerve (white arrow). (**f**) Axial contrast-enhanced T1W in a patient presenting with multiple bilateral CN deficits. Enhancement of the lower cranial nerves on the right side (arrowhead) and multiple other CNs (not shown) was seen and were associated with leptomeningeal enhancement around the brainstem (arrows), pathognomonic for sarcoidosis. (**g**) Patient presenting with diplopia and ptosis following a trauma. Coronal contrast-enhanced T1W shows enhancement of the cisternal segment of the right oculomotor nerve 1 month after the trauma, representing post-traumatic enhancement caused by contusion and/or elongation of the nerve. (Courtesy Dr. D. Vanneste, Hospital Geel-Mol, Belgium)

tics and thus, the clinical history, CSF sampling, biochemistry, further whole-body imaging and pathology are typically needed to narrow the diagnosis. Also, metastases from primary brain neoplasms like glioblastoma (Fig. 12.3c), medulloblastoma, ependymoma, and germinoma can be found on the CNs and finally perineural spread of head and neck tumours can reach the cisternal segment of the cranial nerves and can eventually reach the brainstem (Fig. 12.3d).

Meningiomas

Meningiomas are common tumours, can be isolated or multiple, and can displace and even follow CNs. They are isointense with grey matter on all MRI sequences and enhance homogeneously, and classically often have a dural tail enhancement. Olfactory groove meningiomas can cause olfactory symptoms like anosmia. Meningiomas of the planum sphenoidale frequently reach the optic nerves and can even follow these nerves in the optical canal and orbit, with visual impairment and potential eventual blindness as a result. Therefore, early diagnosis and treatment of meningiomas at this location is crucial. At the level of the internal

auditory canal (IAC) and cerebellopontine angle (CPA), meningioma is the most common differential diagnosis for schwannoma. CT can help in the differential diagnosis by demonstrating the presence of calcifications and hyperostosis of the adjacent bone and even pneumosinus dilatans of the adjacent sinuses in the context of meningiomas, while schwannomas typically displace adjacent bone. On MRI, meningiomas can be distinguished from nerve sheath tumours due to broad base contact with the meninges, a course along the walls of the IAC rather than the nerves in the centre, and often a lateral border in the IAC running perpendicular to the VIIIth nerve, while schwannomas follow the course of the nerve. Petro clival meningiomas and posterior fossa meningiomas can also cause trigeminal and lower cranial nerve symptoms, and these meningiomas can also follow CN V_3 and CNs IX, X, XI outside the skull although this occurs less frequent than for CN II.

Other Tumours, Cysts/Cyst-Like Lesions

Epidermoid cysts are well-defined lesions with inclusion of ectodermal epithelial elements, they can be thought of as "skin in the wrong place". They are often an incidental finding but can cause CN symptoms when they become large. They are isodense with CSF on CT and isointense with CSF on most MR sequences and do not enhance. However, they have a typical hyperintensity on b-1000 DWI images and show diffusion restriction on the apparent diffusion coefficient (ADC) map. Submillimetric heavily T2W 3D gradient-echo images (e.g. balanced-FFE) are ideally suited to make the diagnosis and evaluate the exact extension of the lesions. On these images, the epidermoid has a low signal intensity and can easily be distinguished from CSF (Fig. 12.3e), which is not the case on heavily T2W TSE images. Treatment consists of surgical decompression.

Subarachnoid CSF encapsulation or cyst formation can also cause displacement of or compression on CNs. They are isointense to CSF on all sequences, including DWI and 3D T2W GE sequences. On heavily T2W 3D sequences, the typically thin wall of the cyst can be demonstrated, confirming the diagnosis, and resolving the cyst dimensions. Surgical cyst fenestration is performed in cases of causative CN or other neurological symptoms.

Pituitary adenomas and craniopharyngiomas can compress the optic chiasm and cause bitemporal hemianopsia. Rathke cleft cysts are most often an incidental finding but may rarely cause vision loss.

Pineal tumours and cysts can cause compression on the dorsal midbrain with a Parinaud syndrome as consequence. The syndrome consists of upgaze palsy, convergence retraction nystagmus, and pupillary hyporeflexia.

Dermoid cysts, lipomas, and neurenteric cysts less frequently cause CN disorders, but surgical decompression or partial resection can be considered for symptom management.

12.4.2.2 Vascular Diseases

The cisternal segment of the CNs pass through the CSF spaces around the brainstem, where they are in the close vicinity of the posterior circulation vessels, with a potential nerve–vessel conflict (NVC) as a result.

Neurovascular Compression Syndromes

Arteries and veins can directly compress and displace the cisternal segment of the CNs, resulting in a neurovascular compression syndrome (NVCS). Arteries elongate and become more tortuous as patients get older and this can increase compression. The relation between the anatomical NVC and the resulting NVCS is most reliable for conflicts with CN V—resulting in trigeminal neuralgia, CN VII—causing hemifacial spasm, CN VIII—provoking vestibular paroxysmia, and CN IX—generating glossopharyngeal neuralgia. Indeed, only a minority of neurovascular contacts are symptomatic and therefore the relationship with patients' symptoms remains controversial. The challenge is to recognize which NVC could be symptomatic and in this context, four characteristics of the NVC should be considered. First, the NVC should be at the short 1–2 mm long vulnerable transition zone between the central myelin that originates from oligodendrocytes and covers the proximal intracisternal portion of the CN and the more distal peripheral myelin from Schwann cells. These transition zones are located 4 mm, 2 mm, 10 mm, and less than 2 mm distal to the location where CN V, CN VII, CN VIII, and CN IX leave the brainstem, respectively [25]. Second, venous conflicts exist but arterial conflicts result more frequently in a NVCS. Third, conflicting arteries crossing the CNs in a perpendicular fashion are more prone to provoke a NVCS. Fourth, displacement of the involved CN is probably the most important predictor of a clinically significant NVC.

MR is the method of choice to demonstrate these conflicts and unenhanced 3D TOF MRA images can visualize the arteries, heavily T2W TSE or GE images can demonstrate the nerves and post-contrast submillimetric 3D T1WI are able to depict the veins. Hence, all involved anatomical structures are visualized and fusion software with selective colour coding for each anatomical structure makes the diagnosis easier, especially after decompression surgery when a recurrent NVCS is suspected and the position of the interposed surgical material (e.g. Teflon) must be assessed.

Aneurysm and Arterial Dissection

In patients presenting with painful unilateral CNs, aneurysm and arterial dissection should be considered. Aneurysms on the medial wall of the internal carotid siphon, on the posterior communicating artery and proximal part of the posterior cerebral artery can push on the superior to superomedial border of the oculomotor nerve (CN III), resulting in complete intrinsic and extrinsic oculomotor nerve palsy. Pupillary function loss is seen in 14% of these patients and is explained by compression on the preganglionic parasympathetic pupillomotor fibres to the ciliary ganglion which are located on the superior medial surface of CN III. However, CN III palsy is in most cases limited to extrinsic oculomotor function which is caused by ischaemia of the central motor fibres. This is also the mechanism leading to diabetic ophthalmoparesis, counting for 25% of all ocular motor nerve palsies. Imaging remains negative in these cases and should therefore be judicious when the clinical context is obvious [26].

CTA and MRA are both able to visualize aneurysms and arterial dissections and FS T1W TSE images can also detect the high signal intensity of methaemoglobin in the wall of the artery in case of dissection. Black blood images with and without gadolinium are also very sensitive.

12.4.2.3 Infectious Diseases

Viral neuritis with enhancement of the cisternal segment of the CNs is most frequently seen along the cisternal segment of CN II, III, V, VI and is best depicted on contrast-enhanced coronal high-resolution T1WI. The enhancement of the cisternal segment of CN VII in case of Bell's palsy is limited to the fundus of the IAC and is best seen on axial post-contrast T1WI. Additionally, in these patients the CSF around the facial nerve at the fundus of the IAC disappears, and this area becomes hypointense and blunted. However, the most important enhancement can be seen inside the facial nerve canal, and this will be discussed in Sect. 12.4.3 on the "skull base" segment/course of the CNs.

The main differential diagnosis is varicella zoster virus infection affecting the sensory fibres of both the cochleovestibular nerve and facial nerve causing sensorineural hearing loss and facial palsy. This is accompanied clinically by an external vesicular rash with burning ear pain, fever, vertigo, and nausea and is called "Ramsey Hunt syndrome". The role of MR is to demonstrate CN VII and CN VIII enhancement in the fundus of the IAC to confirm the diagnosis, especially when the CN symptoms precede the other clinical symptoms, and the diagnosis is still uncertain.

As already mentioned, neurotropic viruses like herpes zoster and corona virus (COVID-19) can follow the cisternal segment of the CNs into the brainstem and even brainstem nuclei.

CN disorders may be the first signs of underlying meningeal disease. Often multiple CNs are involved on both sides, but it can also be an isolated nerve, for example, non-specific abducens palsy (CN VI). The meningeal enhancement is difficult to detect on 3D T1WI as all meninges show enhancement even in normal patients and is even more difficult to see on post-contrast CT. 3D FLAIR is more sensitive but today post-contrast 3D BB imaging is the sequence of choice. In normal patients, no meningeal enhancement is seen on these images, making it easy to identify abnormal meningeal enhancement in the case of meningitis. In leptomeningitis, the leptomeninges, on the surface of the brain and the brainstem, are thickened and enhancing. In pachymeningitis, the thickened enhancing meninges are contiguous to the skull. Pyogenes and tuberculous meningitis are two common causes of the brainstem and skull base leptomeningitis.

12.4.2.4 Non-infectious Inflammatory Diseases

Neurosarcoidosis is the most common cause of non-infectious leptomeningitis leading to CN disorders. All CNs can be involved but the most frequent affected nerve is the facial nerve, which can even be involved bilaterally. As mentioned, leptomeningeal enhancement is best detected on post-contrast 3D FLAIR and 3D BB images (Fig. 12.3f). Additionally, diabetes insipidus also causes thickening of the pituitary stalk and disappearance of the high signal intensity spot in the neurohypophysis. Non-infectious leptomeningitis can also be seen in Granulomatosis with Polyangiitis (PGA),

formerly Wegener's disease, and in Langerhans cell and non-Langerhans cell histiocytosis.

12.4.2.5 Trauma

The most frequently involved CN in trauma is CN I. Anosmia can occur after a frontal or occipital trauma or acceleration-deceleration trauma with contusion of the olfactory bulbs, best seen on coronal T2W TSE images, and olfactory fibre shearing at the level of the cribriform plate. Acceleration-deceleration trauma can also result in a fracture of a CN. The CNs with the longest cisternal segment, for example, CN IV, and those with a vulnerable anatomical location, for example, CN VI with a long course between pons and clivus, are most prone to injury. A fracture of the cisternal segment of a CN can be seen on submillimetric heavily T2W TSE images and sequelae of elongation of the CNs can sometimes be seen in the acute and subacute phase as CN enhancement on the coronal and/or axial contrast-enhanced T1WI (Fig. 12.3g). Further post-traumatic oedema of the brain can result in brain herniation and secondary CN disorders. CN III and CN IV can be involved in cases of transtentorial herniation of the internal temporal gyrus. The lower CNs IX–XI and CN XII can be involved in case of herniation of the cerebellar tonsils through the foramen magnum.

Repetitive trauma with bleeding can also result in meningeal superficial siderosis. This haemosiderin deposition occurs also on the CNs and can result in degeneration and disorders of the involved CN. CN VIII is most frequently involved with resulting sensorineural hearing loss. The haemosiderin deposit can be seen as a hypointense rim around the CN on T2* images or SWI and atrophy can be visualized on submillimetric heavily T2WI (e.g. DRIVE, b-FFE). Similar siderosis can also be caused by haemorrhagic surgery, subarachnoid haemorrhage, slow growing tumours and in cerebral amyloid angiopathy.

12.4.3 Skull Base Cranial Nerve Lesions

The CNs must pass through the skull base once they leave the intracranial CSF spaces. They can achieve this by running through foramina, fissures and canals, routes which are also used by traversing arteries and veins. In the parasellar region, CNs even first course through a venous space, the cavernous sinus, before traversing the skull base. These foramina, fissures and canals can be visualized on CT but the nerves, except for the olfactory bulb and optic nerve, cannot be visualized. Widening of the foramina, canals, and fissures or bone destruction are an indirect sign of CN involvement or pathology. MR is better suited to visualize the cranial nerves themselves in the foramina, fissures, and canals. They are visible on unenhanced T1WI with surrounding fat or fatty marrow in bone. However, many of the nerves and especially those running in the cavernous sinus, can only be depicted as dark spots surrounded by hyperintense enhancing veins on contrast-enhanced T1W images. Therefore, high-resolution imaging is critical to visualize many of these small CNs or CN branches. Contrast-enhanced 3D BB images are very sensitive for the detection of CN nerve enhancement in foramina, fissures, and nerve canals. Alternatively contrast-enhanced 3D T1WI (e.g. thrive, vibe, SPGR) with fat suppression can be used.

Lesions involving the optic canal, facial nerve canal, and hypoglossal canal will result in isolated disorders of CN II, CN VII, and CN XII. However, pathology at the level of the superior orbital fissure and cavernous sinus can affect multiple CNs (CNIII, IV, V, and VI), and the same is true for jugular foramen lesions that result in combined CN IX, X, and XI disorders.

Most of the causes that affect the intracranial extraaxial CN segments can also affect the skull base segments. To avoid repetition, the focus in this chapter will be on pathology specific to the skull base and the CNs at this site.

12.4.3.1 Trauma

CNs are very vulnerable for trauma in their course through the skull base. Sharp fracture edges, loose bone fragments, and bullet fragments in case of a gunshot trauma can damage the nerves inside their foramen, fissure, or canal. CN II inside the optic canal is most frequently involved followed by CN VII in the facial nerve canal, CN XII in the hypoglossal canal, and the lower cranial nerves at the level of the jugular foramen. CT with bone window setting is employed to detect fractures and demonstrate potential nerve conflicts, but only MR can confirm injury to the nerves themselves.

Acute and subacute contusion of the optic nerve can result in high signal intensity of the nerve on STIR or 3D FLAIR images and can show contrast enhancement on 3D BB images, while contrast-enhanced 3D T1WI is less sensitive. The smaller the calibre of the CNs, the more difficult it will become to see these relevant signal changes.

The tympanic segment and geniculate ganglion fossa are the most frequently fractured parts of the facial nerve canal. However, the nerve can also be contused without associated fracture, and this will cause swelling of the nerve. When this occurs in the labyrinthine segment of the facial nerve, where the nerve occupies 95% of the space inside the canal, nerve ischaemia, and necrosis can occur as the swollen nerve can completely occlude feeding vessels at this site. This can be detected as enhancement of the labyrinthine segment on 3D BB or 2D/3D T1WI in the acute and subacute phase. Depending on the severity and evolution of the facial nerve palsy as well as experience of the surgeon, nerve decompression at the labyrinthine segment can be considered a safe and effective management approach.

12.4.3.2 Neuritis

Peripheral facial nerve palsy or Bell's palsy, caused by the herpes simplex virus, is one of the most frequent reasons to perform CN imaging. In most cases, the palsy spontaneously disappears in less than 2 months. Imaging is requested when the Bell's palsy persists, recurs or in cases of atypical clinical presentation. Imaging can confirm the diagnosis when gadolinium enhancement is seen along the facial nerve at the fundus of the IAC or along the labyrinthine segment on thin post-contrast T1WI and 3D-FLAIR images. Enhancement at these locations is always abnormal. Enhancement of the geniculate ganglion, tympanic and mastoid segment of the facial nerve are unreliable as these nerve segments are surrounded by veins and arteries which of course also enhance in normal circumstances. This can be solved by using contrast-enhanced submillimetric 3D BB sequence as flow and enhancement inside the vessels are suppressed on these images, showing selectively the nerve enhancement in the geniculate ganglion, tympanic and mastoid nerve segments as well (Fig. 12.4a–c). Comparison with the contralateral nerve facilitates the diagnosis [5, 27, 28]. Neuritis with nodular enhancement in the geniculate ganglion must be differentiated from a facial nerve schwannoma and haemangioma. On CT, schwannomas enlarge the geniculate fossa while in haemangiomas, honeycomb calcifications are seen in the centre of the fossa. In cases of neuritis, the geniculate fossa retains its normal anatomical shape without any central calcifications.

Neuritis of CNs III, IV, VI, and V_1 in the cavernous sinus are best seen on contrast-enhanced high-resolution coronal submillimetric T1WI. The in-plane resolution of these 2D images must be very high to identify these small nerves in the parasellar area. In this context, the slice thickness must be at least under 3 mm, without gap between the slices. Optimal visualization of these nerves and their enhancement, in cases of neuritis, is more confidently identified once the slice thickness is lower than 2.5 mm.

12.4.3.3 Skull Base Infections and Tumours

Unilateral involvement of several CNs is suggestive of skull base disease. CT and contrast-enhanced MR together with the clinical history and laboratory data are used to obtain the correct diagnosis. In case of osteomyelitis, the infectious cause must be sought in the paranasal sinuses, middle ear and/or mastoids with different CNs affected, depending on where the infection is located. Cranial nerve VI runs in Dorello's canal passing through the venous basilar plexus behind the clivus. Aggressive fungal infections originating in the sphenoid sinus can destroy the posterior wall of the sinus and enter this plexus, thus provoking a unilateral abducens palsy. In this case, CN VI will enhance and no longer be visible as a black dot inside the enhancing basilar plexus on axial high-resolution post-contrast T1WI.

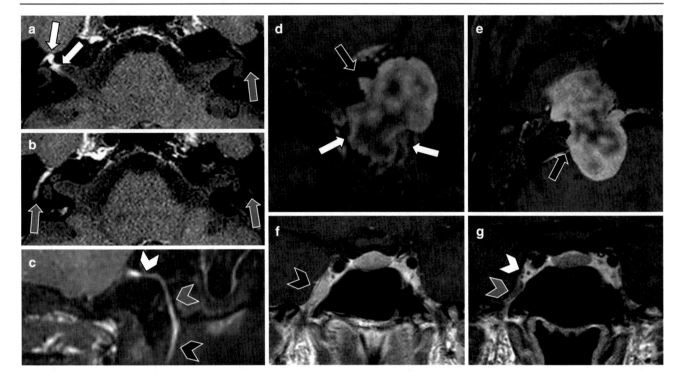

Fig. 12.4 Skull base CN lesions: (**a–c**) Patient presenting with right Bell's palsy assessed with contrast-enhanced 3D BB images. (**a**) Abnormal nerve enhancement can be seen at the fundus of the internal auditory canal, labyrinthine segment, and geniculate ganglion (white arrows). The normal tympanic segment of the left facial nerve is not enhancing and no vascular enhancement is seen on this axial BB image (grey arrow). (**b**) At a slightly lower level, the enhancing tympanic segment of the right CN VII is seen while the normal posterior part of the tympanic segment on the left side is not enhancing (arrows). (**c**) Reconstruction of the enhancing abnormal labyrinthine (white arrowhead), tympanic (grey arrowhead), and mastoid (black arrowhead) segment of the right facial nerve. (**d, e**) Chondrosarcoma of the

petro-occipital fissure in a patient presenting with vertigo and lower cranial nerve deficits on the right side. Coronal (**d**) and axial (**e**) contrast-enhanced 3D BB images showing the enhancing mass with extension in the internal auditory canal (black arrows) and in the jugular foramen (white arrows). (**f, g**) Patient presenting with suspected Tolosa-Hunt syndrome but eventually diagnosed having IgG4 disease. Pre-therapy (**f**) and post-therapy (**g**) contrast-enhanced coronal high resolution T1W images. At presentation, the cavernous sinus was thickened and nerves V_1 and V_2 could no longer be distinguished (black arrowhead). Complete recovery after 4 weeks of steroid treatment with reappearance of the ophthalmic nerve (white arrowhead) and maxillary nerve (grey arrowhead)

Skull base tumours can displace, compress, or encase CNs with fibrous dysplasia, chordoma, chondrosarcoma (Fig. 12.4d, e), and metastasis as the most frequent etiologies. A combination of T2W, unenhanced and contrast-enhanced T1W and DWI sequences help in the characterization of these lesions. Detailed anatomical delineation of the tumour is best obtained on contrast-enhanced 3D images and 3D T1W BB images, reconstructed in the axial, coronal, and sagittal planes.

Meningiomas can follow the CNs in their course through the skull base. They most frequently follow CN II, CN V3, and CN IX–XII. Most of these meningiomas originate in the posterior fossa and then follow the nerves more peripherally. Rarely, these neoplasms develop in the jugular foramen itself and additionally, are then difficult to distinguish from other calcified tumours like chondrosarcomas. The isointensity with grey matter, homogeneous enhancement, intact cortex of the jugular foramen walls, and dural tail enhancement all aid to facilitate the correct diagnosis.

Nonetheless, the most frequent lesions found in the jugular foramen are schwannomas of the lower CNs and paragangliomas with both presenting with dysfunction of the lower CNs [29]. Distinguishing between these on CT relies on the fact that schwannomas enlarge the foramen with intact cortical walls, while paragangliomas permeate into the bone and result in a moth-eaten appearance. Unenhanced MRA will show the feeding vessels inside the paragangliomas as high signal intensity spots, and these are absent in case of a schwannoma. Furthermore, a salt (hyperintensities on T1) and pepper (hypointensities on T2) appearance is characteristic for a paraganglioma.

Metastases can be found anywhere in the skull base and can cause CN dysfunction. A common location is the hypoglossal canal and the most frequent diagnosis in case of an isolated hypoglossal nerve palsy is a skull base metastasis.

12.4.3.4 Cavernous Sinus

Cranial nerves III, IV, and V_1 are located in the wall of the cavernous sinus and CN VI is located deeper inside the cavernous sinus. Hence enhancing schwannomas and neuritis of these nerves can be found in the cavernous sinus. In this anatomical region, schwannomas most frequently involve the trigeminal nerve. Schwannomas in Meckel's cave can become quite large and will then also extend towards the posterior fossa, giving them a classic dumbbell appearance. Schwannomas on the maxillary and mandibular nerves will eventually enlarge the round and oval foramen, respectively. Perineural tumour spread along the CNs and metastases in the cavernous sinus are important differential diagnoses when enhancing lesions or nerves are identified in this location.

Aneurysms of the parasellar ICA can also be responsible for palsies of CNs III, IV, V_1, and VI. However, due to its location deep in the cavernous sinus, the abducens nerve is often the first to be affected by these aneurysms. The same is true for pituitary adenomas and craniopharyngiomas that extend in the parasellar region. Although the overall most frequently involved CN inside the cavernous sinus, regardless of the cause, is CN III followed by CN VI.

Idiopathic non-neoplastic non-infectious granulomatous inflammation of the cavernous sinus and orbital apex is called "Tolosa-Hunt Syndrome". The patients present with periorbital and frontal pain and CNs II, III, IV, V_1, and VI, can be involved. Several days of headache are followed by diplopia and ptosis, almost always unilateral. On contrast-enhanced coronal T1WI, strong enhancement of all structures inside the cavernous sinus including all CNs, and lateral bulging of the enlarged cavernous sinus, can be seen. The headache disappears typically over the course of days and the ophthalmoplegia within 2 weeks following corticosteroid treatment. Follow-up MR at 6 months will demonstrate a complete normalization of the cavernous sinus, confirming the diagnosis [30].

IgG4 is a rare autoimmune disease which can also involve the cavernous sinus and its cranial nerves in a similar way as Tolosa-Hunt syndrome (Fig. 12.4f, g). The combination with bilateral lacrimal gland, CN and especially infraorbital nerve, pituitary infundibulum, and salivary gland involvement leads to a preferred diagnosis of IgG4 [31].

12.4.4 Extracranial Cranial Nerve Lesions

Primary extracranial CN diseases are rare and most of the extracranial CN disorders are caused by lesions of the surrounding structures that may insult the nerves. Most often, the symptoms are unilateral.

CN I dysfunction caused by ethmoidal and nasal lesions will result in anosmia.

Orbital diseases can cause partial or complete monocular visual loss when the optic nerve (CN II) is involved. CN III,

IV, and VI dysfunctions will lead to diplopia. Miosis and mydriasis occur when the inferior branch of CN III and its side branch with the ciliary ganglion are affected at the orbital apex.

Facial lesions can result in CN V neuropathy with unilateral hypoesthesia, numbness, or burning pain when extracranial branches of the trigeminal nerve are involved. These symptoms can be restricted to the territory of one branch, V_1, V_2, or V_3, depending on the location of the lesions. Numbness, motor weakness, and progressive CN V symptoms are the most reliable clinical signs of a trigeminal lesion and frequently correlate with positive imaging findings; however, the more frequent non-specific facial pain usually does not have a culprit-associated lesion.

Isolated peripheral CN VII dysfunction, with intact lacrimal function and stapes reflex and taste in the anterior 2/3 of the tongue, may be provoked by parotid and peri mastoid lesions.

At the suprahyoid level, CNs IX–X course next to each other and are often injured together. Patients can then present with dysphagia, uvula deviation, absent gag reflex, hoarseness, vocal cord palsy, loss of taste to the posterior 1/3 of the tongue, otalgia, and tachy- or bradycardia. Inability to raise the arm and a shoulder drop indicate a CN XI palsy. Deviation of the tongue to the side of the lesion and tongue muscle atrophy are the signs of a CN XII palsy.

Only CN X continues at the infrahyoid level, and when injured at this level, endolaryngeal symptoms (hoarseness, vocal cord palsy, and taste loss in posterior 1/3 of the tongue) is found.

Muscle atrophy or dystrophy are helpful signs on imaging to confirm injury to motor CNs and should always be verified [32].

The method of choice to study extracranial nerves is MRI. For many years, high-resolution T2W, unenhanced T1W and fat-saturated Gd-enhanced T1W images were the primary sequences to visualize the extracranial nerves and to characterize associated lesions. Later, diffusion and perfusion MRI further advanced characterization of these lesions. However, many of the nerve branches and associated pathology remained below the limits of resolution. In recent years, MRN was optimized for CN imaging and slightly different techniques are used for MR systems of different vendors [14–17, 33]. This technique was described above in Sect. 12.3.2. In the infrahyoid neck, only part of the vagus nerve can be visualized with this technique. Yet CN X continues into the thorax and lesions along the course of the recurrent laryngeal branches, down to the clavicle on the right and down to the aorta-pulmonary window on the left. At this level, CT is the modality of choice as the neck and thorax can be studied together in a fast single scan with better visualization at the thoracic level in comparison with MR.

It is beyond the current scope to cover all extracranial pathology that can cause CN dysfunction, only the most frequent and important causes are highlighted.

12.4.4.1 Vascular Lesions

In the orbit, CN II dysfunction can be caused by cavernous haemangiomas and venous varices. Cavernous haemangiomas are round to ovoid sharply delineated homogeneous enhancing lesions that can compress the optic nerve. Venous varices can enhance, demonstrate flow voids as well as increase in size with prone positioning.

Cranial nerve IX–XII dysfunction can be caused by ICA dissection or aneurysm resulting in compression of the cranial nerves inside the carotid space. Damage of the lower CNs can also be iatrogenic during endarterectomy.

Finally, aortic arch aneurysms can narrow the aortic-pulmonic window with compression on the recurrent laryngeal nerve resulting in left vocal cord palsy [33].

12.4.4.2 Infectious Diseases

Aggressive bacterial and fungal infections of the sinuses and temporal bone can lead to extracranial CN involvement. Fungal infections can be recognized by their low signal intensity on T2WI while abscess formation in aggressive bacterial infections shows diffusion restriction on DWI. Aspergillus and especially mucormycosis can destroy the sinus walls thereby directly affecting the adjacent cranial nerves. Vulnerable locations are the frontal sinus (for CN V_1), ethmoid and sphenoid sinus (CN II, III, IV, V_1, V_2, VI in the orbital apex and superior orbital fissure), and temporal bone (CN VII). MRI can visualize the thickened and enhancing cranial nerves while both CT and MRI can demonstrate late-stage infection surrounding and eventually encasing involved CNs.

Dental periapical and periodontal disease of the upper and lower jaw can result in V_2 and V_3 neuropathy, respectively. The resulting CN changes, oedema-demyelination-Wallerian degeneration, can only be visualized with new MRN techniques like 3D-CRANI and optimized 3D-FISP sequence. On these post-contrast images, the nerves are thickened, irregular, and have a high signal intensity compared to the normal contralateral nerves [15–17, 33]. These neuropathies could not be confirmed or visualized before the advent of these new MRN techniques and thus facilitates timely use of appropriate therapies (Fig. 12.5a).

Malignant otitis externa, a pseudomonas aeruginosa infection affecting immunocompromised or diabetic patients, can lead to CN VII dysfunction.

Osteomyelitis (Fig. 12.5a) and osteoradionecrosis can cause dysfunction of the lower CNs IX–XII at the level of the skull base and can irritate the inferior alveolar nerve, with resulting pain and numbness, at the level of the mandible. Both pathologies cause loss of the high signal intensity of the bone marrow on unenhanced T1WI and show bone marrow

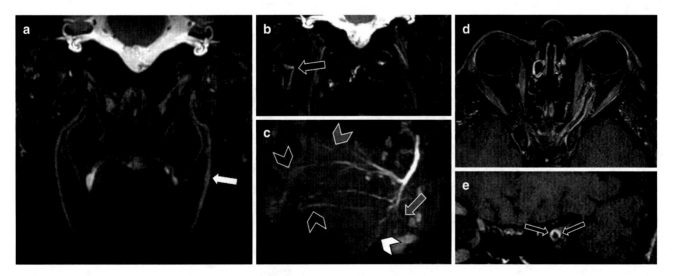

Fig. 12.5 Extracranial CN lesions: (**a**) Coronal contrast-enhanced 3D CRANI sequence with paracoronal MIP reconstruction in a patient presenting with numbness of the left chin and dysesthesia in the left inferior alveolar nerve territory following osteomyelitis of the left mandible. The left inferior alveolar nerve is thickened, irregular and hyperintense (arrow), compatible with neuropathy. (**b**, **c**) Contrast-enhanced 3D CRANI with coronal MIP reconstruction (**b**) and 3D MIP reconstruction with lateral view (**c**) in a patient with right Bell's palsy. The hyperintense and thickened nerve branching inside the right parotid gland can be seen (black arrow) and even the peripheral hyperintense zygomatic branch (grey arrowhead), buccal branches (black arrowheads), mandibular branch (white arrowhead) and cervical branch (grey arrow) can be followed. (**d**, **e**) Axial (**d**) and paracoronal (**e**) contrast-enhanced 3D BB images of a left optic nerve meningioma. The tram track sign can be followed in detail from intracranial to the distal part of the left optic nerve. The coronal reconstruction shows that the meningioma surrounds the optic nerve over 270° (arrows)

enhancement on the post-contrast T1WI. CT is best suited to distinguish both entities and can demonstrate the characteristic bone sequestration, lytic defects in the cortical bone and periosteal new bone formation in case of osteomyelitis. The resulting CN changes are in most cases only recognizable on MRN images.

Viral neuritis of extracranial CNs or of their branches was not resolvable on MR even a couple of years ago. Today, the new MRN sequences allow the visualization of the inflamed distal CN branches of the facial and trigeminal nerve (Fig. 12.5b, c).

12.4.4.3 Non-infectious Inflammatory Diseases

Demyelinating Diseases
Spontaneous vision loss in young and middle-aged adults is often due to optic neuritis, frequently in the context of multiple sclerosis (MS) and neuromyelitis optica spectrum disorders (NMOSD) with anti-AQP4 or anti-MOG antibodies. The optic nerve lesions are best identified on 3D FLAIR and T2 STIR images. In most cases, post-contrast T1WI are negative and when contrast is used the more sensitive 3D BB sequence should be used. MR imaging of the brain and spine can be used to confirm the diagnosis of MS and to distinguish the demyelinating disease subtypes [19]:

MS
(a) Unilateral optic neuritis, short segment involving the middle portion of the nerve.
(b) Scattered demyelinating lesions in the brain.
(c) Lesions in the upper half of the spinal cord, lesions are shorter than two vertebral levels and involve less than 50% of the cord diameter.

Anti-AQP4+
(a) Bilateral optic neuritis, long segment involving the posterior portion of the nerves with chiasmatic extension.
(b) Predominantly periventricular demyelinating lesions.
(c) Lesions in the upper half of the spinal cord, extending over more than three vertebral levels and more than 50% of the cord diameter.

Anti-MOG+
(a) Bilateral optic neuritis, long segment involving the anterior portion of the nerves.
(b) Brain lesions more frequently found in the basal ganglia, thalamus, and pons.
(c) Lesions located in the lower half of the spinal cord, extending over more than three vertebral levels and more than 50% of the cord diameter.

Vision loss with optic nerve signal changes on MR can also be seen in case of inflammatory neuritis or ischaemia.

The above-mentioned associated brain and spinal cord changes can help to distinguish these etiologies from demyelinating disease. The clinical history, biochemical data and follow-up are needed to distinguish the three entities when the brain and spine imaging are normal.

Granulomatous Diseases
In sarcoidosis, an inflammatory granulomatosis, optic nerve involvement occurs in 1–5% of the patients. The differential diagnosis, which includes optic nerve meningioma, can be difficult to elucidate but the MR demonstration of involvement of both optic nerves, complete optic nerve enhancement from globe to the chiasm, bilateral enlarged parotid and lacrimal glands, leptomeningeal enhancement and infundibular thickening all support the diagnosis of sarcoidosis.

Extracranial manifestations of granulomatosis with periangiitis, Langerhans cell, and non-Langerhans cell histiocytosis can also insult the optic nerves besides their orbital and nasosinusal involvement. The nearby maxillary nerve is also prone to be involved and intracranial extension along the involved nerves has been described [1, 2, 5, 7].

Graves' Orbitopathy
Graves' disease is an autoimmune condition of the thyroid involving the orbit in 25% of patients. The resulting ophthalmopathy is caused by extraocular muscle hypertrophy and adipogenesis leading to increased ocular pressure and proptosis, diplopia, and vision loss due to CN II compression and/or elongation.

Orbital Pseudotumor
Patients with orbital pseudotumor present with vison loss (CN II), ophthalmoplegia (CN III, IV, VI), sudden painful proptosis and uveitis, and retinal detachment. Infections and neoplasms must be excluded before this diagnosis can be made and rapid improvement with corticosteroid treatment can confirm the diagnosis. An ill-defined enhancing pseudo mass in the orbit, orbital apex, and superior/inferior orbital fissures can be seen on post-contrast FS T1W images. A useful imaging sign is that although the pseudo-mass can be large, the surrounding anatomical structures are not displaced accordingly.

12.4.4.4 Tumours

Primary Nerve Lesions
Esthesioneuroblastoma develops from the neurosensory receptor cells in the olfactory epithelium in the upper nasal meatus. They are typically centred on the anterior skull base, with often a dumbbell mass extending upward in the anterior fossa and downward in the nasal cavity, ethmoid and sphenoid sinuses. The extension of the mass, which can have cysts at the periphery, can best be delineated on MR. The

destruction of the cribriform plate and anterior skull base is best depicted on CT. The intracranial component can involve CN I with anosmia as a result while the nasosinusal component causes nasal obstruction, rhinorrhoea, and epistaxis.

Optic nerve glioma, usually pilocytic astrocytoma, is the primary tumour of CN II and presents under the age of 20 years. On MRI and CT, these lesions follow the optic nerve in a fusiform way, cause kinking of the optic nerve, and may extend to the optic chiasm. On MRI, they have a typical high signal intensity on T2 and variable enhancement. Optic gliomas can be associated with neurofibromatosis I (NFI) and this is more likely with bilateral involvement, when they are not cyst-like, and do not extend to the optic chiasm, in contrast to the non-NFI-associated optic gliomas [34].

Nerve Sheath Tumours

The olfactory tracts and bulbs as well as the optic nerves are extensions of the brain and have no Schwann cells. However, the olfactory filia which connect the olfactory bulbs with the olfactory mucosa in the upper nasal meatus do have Schwann cells. Therefore, olfactory schwannomas exist but are not related to the olfactory tracts and bulbs themselves.

The intraorbital optic nerve has a meningeal sheath, and this explains the presence of meningiomas along CN II. Most of the meningiomas are isointense with grey matter, are fusiform, and enhance homogeneously with a "tram track" sign. This enhancement is best seen on contrast-enhanced 3D BB images as this sequence is more sensitive for contrast enhancement and less affected by susceptibility artifacts than post-contrast 3D T1WI (Fig. 12.5d, e).

All other CNs, except for CN VIII, have an extracranial course with a Schwann cell sheath on which schwannomas, neurofibromas, and rarely malignant tumours can arise. It is more likely to find schwannomas and neurofibromas on the extracranial end branches of CN V than on the short intraorbital branches of CN III, IV, and VI [32]. Regardless, intracranial CN schwannomas are far more frequent than extracranial CN schwannomas.

Nerve sheath tumours along the intraparotid branches of CN VII can occur but schwannomas/neurofibromas on the mastoid segment of the facial nerve with extension into the parotid gland are far more frequent.

Schwannomas can develop on the extracranial segment of all four lower cranial nerves but are most frequent on CN X. Extracranial schwannomas of CN XII can most often be followed into the hypoglossal canal and intracranial subarachnoid space. Extracranial nerve sheath tumours of cranial CNs IX and XI are rare.

On MRI, schwannomas are well-circumscribed, fusiform and have an intense enhancement. However, cystic, fatty, and haemorrhagic changes can occur resulting in an inhomogeneous lesion and/or inhomogeneous enhancement. Multiple extracranial CN schwannomas are most often found in

patients with autosomal dominant neurofibromatosis type 2 (NF2), and bilateral vestibular schwannomas are even pathognomonic for NF2.

Extracranial CN neurofibromas are found in younger patients (20–30 years old), enhance weakly or not at all, and present as thickening of longer nerve segments. Nevertheless, they are sometimes difficult to distinguish from schwannomas. Most neurofibromas occur isolated, but the presence of multiple extracranial CN neurofibromas or a plexiform neurofibroma strongly suggests the diagnosis of NF1.

Secondary Nerve Involvement

Head and Neck Malignancies and Perineural Tumour Spread

All head and neck malignancies can displace or invade extracranial CNs. Squamous cell carcinomas, adenoid cystic carcinomas, adenocarcinoma, lymphomas, melanomas, retinoblastomas, esthesioneuroblastomas, rhabdomyosarcomas, malignant parotid gland tumours, thyroid malignancies, etc. can all affect the extracranial CNs, and which nerve is affected often depends on the typical location where some of these tumours arise. Tumoral infiltration of extracranial CNs is difficult to visualize although the use of diffusion tractography is promising for demonstrating nerve displacement and suggesting tumoral infiltration [11].

Adenoid cystic carcinoma, squamous cell carcinoma, and lymphoma are the most frequent malignant head and neck lesions with perineural spread although other malignant tumours also have the potential to follow the cranial nerves [35]. The most frequently involved nerves are V_1 (skin and lacrimal malignancies), V_2 (skin, oral and nasal cavity, and sinus malignancies), V_3 (oral cavity-sublingual and submandibular gland and masticator space malignancies) [36], VII (parotid malignancies), and rarely CN XII.

Perineural spread can be seen as an abnormal enhancement and thickening of the involved nerves on post-contrast FS T1WI. Comparison with the contralateral nerve facilitates the diagnosis. It is crucial to detect intracranial CN extension as it limits therapeutic options, thereby avoiding potentially futile interventions, and results in a poorer prognosis.

CN V and VII have several connections which allow perineural tumoral spread along both nerves and their branches. The connection between the maxillary nerve (V_2) and Vidian nerve (VII) at the level of the pterygopalatine fossa is most frequently involved. Hence, the pterygopalatine fossa should always be assessed in detail as involvement often heralds intracranial extension along these nerve branches.

Paragangliomas

The imaging characteristics of paragangliomas were already discussed in Sect. 12.4.3.3. Extracranially, they arise from glomus bodies located along the carotid bulb and vagus nerve inside the carotid space. Jugular foramen paraganglio-mas can also extend caudally in these carotid spaces where they can compress the four lower CNs. Intracranial extension should always be assessed prior to surgery.

Metastases

Hematogenous metastases to the head and neck region can involve all extracranial nerves with secondary CN deficits. Breast, kidney, lung, and prostate tumours as well as mela-noma are the most frequent primary tumours that metastasize to the head and neck region. In the orbit, metastases from breast carcinoma are most frequent and involvement of CN II is more often caused by nerve compression by the orbital metastasis than by direct metastasis to the nerve itself. The extracranial CNs III–XII can be directly affected by all the above-mentioned metastases or indirectly by associated ade-nopathies. Metastatic extracranial CN involvement is best seen on post-contrast FS T1WI in the axial and coronal plane.

12.4.4.5   Trauma

Facial fractures can damage the extracranial CNs. The frac-tures and displaced bone fragments are best seen on CT, with contusion or shears, and oedema of the CNs best studied on MRI with 3D FLAIR and STIR images (Fig. 12.6a, b). One of the most frequently damaged nerves is the V_2 branch. Its

course along the floor of the orbit makes it vulnerable in cases of orbital floor, orbital blow out and tetrapod fractures. Also, the V_1 branch can be damaged in cases of orbital roof fractures and the fractures can even reach the optic nerve (CN II) in the centre of the orbit. However, more frequently CN II involve-ment represents contusion (Fig. 12.6a, b) with nerve transec-tion being relatively rare. Mandibular fractures can damage the V_3 branch and/or the inferior alveolar nerve. CN disorders may also be iatrogenic and CN II, III, IV, and VI can be dam-aged during sinonasal and periorbital surgery. CN V_3 can be injured during mandibular and tooth implant surgery while CN VII can be injured during parotid surgery, etc. One of the best-known iatrogenic CN traumas is contusion or transection of the lingual nerve, a branch from CN V_3, during wisdom tooth extraction. Previously imaging was unable to demon-strate lingual nerve injury, but this is now possible with new dedicated MRN sequences (e.g. 3D CRANI) [37]. Lower cra-nial nerve deficits are most often caused by neck dissections or by surgery of the lower neck with recurrent laryngeal nerve damage and consequent vocal cord palsy one of the best-known examples [38]. Surgery can also cause scar formation around the extracranial CNs, replacing the usual fat around the nerves on unenhanced T1WI and enhancing in the early post-surgical period. Finally, neuromas can develop on extracranial CNs in cases of chronic trauma. Visualization of these neuro-

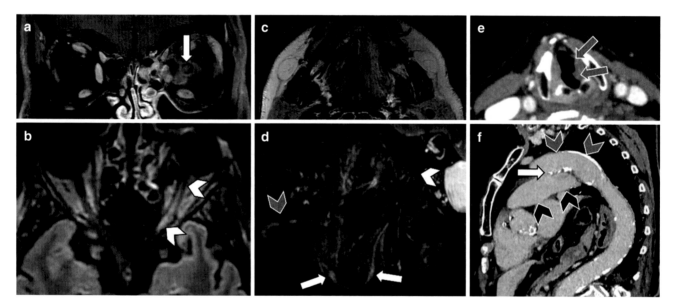

Fig. 12.6 Extracranial CN lesions: (**a**, **b**) Post-traumatic CN II contu-sion with visual loss. (**a**) Coronal contrast-enhanced high-resolution T1W image with fat suppression showing oedema of the optic nerve (arrow) and the oedematous changes of the optic nerve sheath and sur-rounding retro-ocular fat. (**b**) Axial 3D FLAIR image shows the extent of nerve contusion, reaching the optic canal (arrowheads); (**c**, **d**) Intensive care patient with left hypoglossal nerve palsy following a 3-month intubation. (**c**) Atrophy and fatty degeneration of the tongue muscles on the left side can be recognized on this axial T2W TSE image and confirms left hypoglossal nerve palsy. (**d**) Contrast-enhanced 3D CRANI image with parasagittal MIP reconstruction shows two neuro-mas on the inferior bend of the hypoglossal nerve (arrows) caused by a

remote intubation trauma. For reference, the tongue (grey arrowhead) and region of the jugular foramen (white arrowhead) are depicted. (**e**, **f**) Patient presenting with a left recurrent laryngeal nerve palsy identified on contrast-enhanced CT. (**e**) Axial CT image shows the paramedian position of the left true vocal cord with a widened ventricle of Morgagni, in keeping with left vocal cord palsy (arrows). (**f**) Sagittal reconstruc-tion demonstrates a large diaphragmatic herniation which causes upward displacement of the pulmonary arteries (black arrowheads) and closure of the aorta-pulmonic window (arrow) with subsequent com-pression and irritation of the recurrent laryngeal nerve branch resulting in the left vocal cord palsy. Aortic arch (grey arrowheads)

mas on extracranial CNs was almost impossible before the advent of the dedicated MRN techniques like the 3D CRANI sequence (Fig. 12.6c, d).

12.4.4.6 Upper Mediastinum

The vagus nerve and its left recurrent laryngeal branch can be followed down to the upper mediastinum. The left recurrent laryngeal nerve turns superiorly after crossing the aorto-pulmonary window. Mediastinitis and inflammatory adenopathies, tumoral adenopathies and tumours of the aerodigestive tract, upper mediastinum, lymphomas, etc. can therefore damage these nerves and cause CN X or recurrent laryngeal nerve deficits. All pathologies that result in narrowing of the aorto-pulmonary window can also compress the left recurrent laryngeal nerve and cause vocal cord palsy. Examples are aortic arch aneurysms, pulmonary hypertension, and massive diaphragmatic hernias (Fig. 12.6e, f).

12.4.5 Conclusion

Cranial nerve dysfunctions warn clinicians of pathology involving the face, skull base, or brain. Guided by medical history and clinical findings, imaging should be directed to the involved CN and to the right CN segment. An enormous variety of diseases can cause CN deficits; therefore, CT and MR are used to distinguish and characterize them. Aneurysms, dissections, skull base and skull lesions, fractures, and calcifications are best demonstrated by CT and CTA. Lesions of the CN themselves are best studied on MRI with new techniques like diffusion tractography, BB imaging, and 3D CRANI MRN serving to further strengthen MRI diagnostic authority.

Take-Home Messages
- Master cranial nerve anatomy from the central nuclei to the peripheral branches.
- Adapt imaging techniques to the clinical history and clinical findings, focusing on the right CN and CN segment.
- Characterize causative lesions by using CT and/or MR, with the knowledge that different type of lesions affects the different CN segments.
- Rule out intracranial lesions, aneurysms, and dissection that require specific treatment. Employ CTA and MRA to rule out painful vascular CN disorders.
- Use the optimal adapted MR sequences such as heavy T2W, 3D FLAIR, and high-resolution T2W and T1W sequences, T1 without and with contrast and with fat saturation.
- Consider DWI and the new DWI/DTI, 3D-BB, and 3D CRANI MRN techniques in appropriate cases.

References

1. Barkhof F, Jäger R, Thurnher M, Rovira A, editors. Clinical neuroradiology: the ESNR textbook. Cham: Springer; 2019. 2272 pp.
2. Casselman J, Mermuys K, Delanote J, Ghekiere J, Coenegrachts K. MRI of the cranial nerves—more than meets the eye: technical considerations and advanced anatomy. Neuroimaging Clin N Am. 2008;18:197–231, preceding x.
3. Chapman P, Harnsberger H, Vattoth S, editors. Imaging anatomy: head and neck. Philadelphia: Elsevier; 2019. 700 pp.
4. Harnsberger H. Cranial nerves. In: Harnsberger H, Osborn A, Macdonald A, Ross J, editors. Diagnostic and surgical imaging anatomy: brain, head and neck, spine. Salt Lake City: Amirsys; 2006. p. 174–259.
5. Koch B, Hamilton B, Hudgins P, Harnsberger H, editors. Diagnostic imaging: head and neck. 3rd ed. Philadelphia: Elsevier; 2017. 1352 pp.
6. Leblanc A, editor. Encephalo-peripheral nervous system: vascularisation, anatomy, imaging. Berlin: Springer; 2004. 420 pp.
7. Osborn A, Hedlund G, Salzman K, editors. Osborn's brain. 2nd ed. Philadelphia: Elsevier; 2018. 1300 pp.
8. Romano N, Federici M, Castaldi A. Imaging of cranial nerves: a pictorial overview. Insights Imaging. 2019;10:33.
9. Jacquesson T, Cotton F, Attye A, Zaouche S, Tringali S, Bosc J, Robinson P, Jouanneau E, Frindel C. Probabilistic tractography to predict the position of cranial nerves displaced by skull base tumors: value for surgical strategy through a case series of 62 patients. Neurosurgery. 2019;85:E125–36.
10. Attye A, Jean C, Remond P, et al. Track-weighted imaging for neuroretina: evaluations in healthy volunteers and ischemic optic neuropathy. J Magn Reson Imaging. 2018;48:737.
11. Rouchy RC, Attye A, Medici M, Renard F, Kastler A, Grand S, Tropres I, Righini CA, Krainik A. Facial nerve tractography: a new tool for the detection of perineural spread in parotid cancers. Eur Radiol. 2018;28:3861–71.
12. Attye A, Karkas A, Tropres I, et al. Parotid gland tumours: MR tractography to assess contact with the facial nerve. Eur Radiol. 2016;26:2233–41.
13. Krainik A, Casselman JW. Imaging evaluation of patients with cranial nerve disorders. In: Hodler J, Kubik-Huch R, Von Schulthess G, editors. Diseases of the brain, head and neck, spine 2020–2023. Cham: IDKD Springer; 2020. p. 143–61. https://doi.org/10.1007/978-3-030-38490-6_12.
14. Klupp E, Cervantes B, Sollmann N, et al. Improved brachial plexus visualization using an adiabatic iMSDE-prepared stir 3D TSE. Clin Neuroradiol. 2019;29:631–8.
15. Van der Cruyssen F, Croonenborghs T-M, Hermans R, et al. 3D cranial nerve imaging, a novel MR neurography technique using black-blood STIR TSE with a pseudo steady-state sweep and motion-sensitized driven equilibrium pulse for the visualization of the extraforaminal cranial nerve branches. Am J Neuroradiol. 2021;42:578–80.
16. Van der Cruyssen F, Croonenborghs T-M, Renton T, et al. Magnetic resonance neurography of the head and neck: state of the art, anatomy, pathology, and future perspectives. Br J Radiol. 2021;94:20200798.
17. Casselman J, Van der Cruyssen F, Vanhove F, et al. 3D CRANI, a novel MR neurography sequence, can reliable visualise the extraforaminal cranial and occipital nerves. Eur Radiol. 2023;33:2861–70.
18. van der Zijden T, Mondelaers A, Yperzeele L, Voormolen M, Parizel P. Current concepts in imaging and endovascular treatment of acute ischemic stroke: implications for the clinician. Insights Imaging. 2019;10:64.
19. Dutra BG, da Rocha AJ, Nunes RH, Maia ACMJ. Neuromyelitis optica spectrum disorders: spectrum of MR imaging findings and their differential diagnosis. Radiographics. 2018;38:169–93.

20. Di Stefano G, Maarbjerg S, Truini A. Trigeminal neuralgia secondary to multiple sclerosis: from the clinical picture to the treatment options. J Headache Pain. 2019;20:20.
21. Bonneville F, Savatovsky J, Chiras J. Imaging of cerebellopontine angle lesions: an update. Part 1: enhancing extra-axial lesions. Eur Radiol. 2007;17:2472–82.
22. Bonneville F, Savatovsky J, Chiras J. Imaging of cerebellopontine angle lesions: an update. Part 2: intra-axial lesions, skull base lesions that may invade the CPA region, and non-enhancing extra-axial lesions. Eur Radiol. 2007;17:2908–20.
23. Radek M, Tomasik B, Wojdyn M, et al. Neurofibromatosis type 2 (NF2) or schwannomatosis? Case report study and diagnostic criteria. Neurol Neurochir Pol. 2016;50:215–9.
24. Krainik A, Cyna-Gorse F, Bouccara D, Cazals-Hatem D, Vilgrain V, Denys A, Rey A, Sterkers O, Menu Y. MRI of unusual lesions in the internal auditory canal. Neuroradiology. 2001;43:52–7.
25. Haller S, Etienne L, Kovari E, Varoquaux AD, Urbach H, Becker M. Imaging of neurovascular compression syndromes: trigeminal neuralgia, hemifacial spasm, vestibular paroxysmia, and glossopharyngeal neuralgia. AJNR Am J Neuroradiol. 2016;37:1384–92.
26. Adams ME, Linn J, Yousry I. Pathology of the ocular motor nerves III, IV, and VI. Neuroimaging Clin N Am. 2008;18:261–82, preceding x–x.
27. Kuya J, Kuya K, Shinohara Y, Kunimoto Y, Yazama H, Ogawa T, Takeuchi H. Usefulness of high-resolution 3D multi-sequences for peripheral facial palsy: differentiation between Bell's palsy and Ramsay hunt syndrome. Otol Neurotol. 2017;38:1523–7.
28. Veillon F, Taboada LR, Eid MA, Riehm S, Debry C, Schultz P, Charpiot A. Pathology of the facial nerve. Neuroimaging Clin N Am. 2008;18:309–20, x.
29. Nery B, Fernandes Costa RA, Quaggio E, et al. Jugular foramen paragangliomas. In: Morgan LR, Sarica FB, editors. Brain and spinal tumors. Rijeka: IntechOpen; 2019. https://doi.org/10.5772/intechopen.84232.
30. Zurawski J, Akhondi H. Tolosa-hunt syndrome a rare cause of headache and ophthalmoplegia. Lancet. 2013;382:912.
31. Soussan JB, Deschamps R, Sadik JC, et al. Infraorbital nerve involvement on magnetic resonance imaging in European patients with IgG4-related ophthalmic disease: a specific sign. Eur Radiol. 2017;27:1335–43.
32. Smoker WR, Reede DL. Denervation atrophy of motor cranial nerves. Neuroimaging Clin N Am. 2008;18:387–411, xi.
33. Chhabra A, Bajaj G, Wadhwa V, et al. MR neurography evaluation of facial and neck pain: normal and abnormal craniospinal nerves below the skull base. Radiographics. 2018;38:1498–513. https://doi.org/10.1148/rg.2018170194.
34. Louis D, Ohgaki H, Wiestier O, Cavenee W, editors. WHO classification of tumors of the central nervous system. 4th ed. IARC: Lyon; 2016.
35. Maroldi R, Farina D, Borghesi A, Marconi A, Gatti E. Perineural tumor spread. Neuroimaging Clin N Am. 2008;18:413–429, xi.
36. Borges A, Casselman J. Imaging the trigeminal nerve. Eur J Radiol. 2010;74:323–40.
37. Bangia M, Ahmadzai I, Casselman J, et al. Accuracy of MR neurography as a diagnostic tool in detecting injuries to the lingual- and inferior alveolar nerve in patients with iatrogenic post-traumatic trigeminal neuropathy. Eur Radiol. 2023; https://doi.org/10.1007/s00330-023-10363-2.
38. Lee JH, Cheng KL, Choi YJ, Baek JH. High-resolution imaging of neural anatomy and pathology of the neck. Korean J Radiol. 2017;18:180–93.

Part II

Brain and Spine

Demyelinating Diseases of the CNS (Brain and Spine)

13

Frederik Barkhof and Kelly K. Koeller

Abstract

Multiple sclerosis (MS) is the most important inflammatory demyelinating disorder that affects both the brain and spine. Dissemination in space and time on MRI is not limited to MS and can occur in neuromyelitis optica spectrum disorder (NMOSD) with aquaporin 4 antibodies, myelin oligodendrocyte glycoprotein-related antibody disease (MOGAD), and a series of other (inflammatory) demyelinating disorders. Spinal cord imaging is an important element of MS (differential) diagnosis and especially relevant in case of possible age-related vasculo-ischemic brain white matter lesions; a negative scan will help to rule out MS. Increasingly, MRI is used to monitor treatment and their complications such as progressive multifocal leukoencephalopathy (PML).

Keywords

Multiple sclerosis · Neuromyelitis optica · Aquaporin-4 MOG · ADEM · Progressive multifocal leukoencephalopathy · Leukoaraïosis · Wernicke · Pontine myelinolysis · CSF · Spinal cord · MRI · Gadolinium · Radiation encephalopathy · PRES

Learning Objectives
- To be familiar with the differential diagnosis of white matter diseases.
- Understand the importance of clinical setting, mode of presentation and lab results in inflammatory demyelinating disorders.
- Be able to apply MS, MOGAD, and NMOSD diagnostic criteria.
- Appreciate the value of spinal cord imaging in the work-up of MS.
- Recognize the most important variants and mimics of MS.

13.1 Introduction

Demyelinating disorders of the central nervous system (CNS) that affect the brain and spine have a variety of etiologies and can be separated into primary such as multiple sclerosis (MS) and other inflammatory-demyelinating diseases such as neuromyelitis optica spectrum disorder (NMOSD), myelin oligodendrocyte glycoprotein-related antibody disease (MOGAD) as well as secondary (e.g., infectious, ischemic, metabolic, or toxic) diseases. MRI is the imaging modality of choice to assess demyelinating disorders of the brain and the cord and, together with the clinical and laboratory findings, can accurately classify them in most cases [1–3]. This review will highlight the important imaging manifestations of some acquired demyelinating diseases that allow more specific diagnosis.

F. Barkhof (✉)
Department of Radiology and Nuclear Medicine, Amsterdam UMC, Vrije Universiteit, Amsterdam, The Netherlands

UCL Institutes of Neurology and Healthcare Engineering, London, UK
e-mail: f.barkhof@amsterdamumc.nl

K. K. Koeller
Section of Neuroradiology, Department of Radiology, Mayo Clinic, Rochester, MN, USA
e-mail: koeller.kelly@mayo.edu

© The Author(s) 2024
J. Hodler et al. (eds.), *Diseases of the Brain, Head and Neck, Spine 2024-2027*, IDKD Springer Series,
https://doi.org/10.1007/978-3-031-50675-8_13

13.2 Inflammatory-Demyelinating Diseases of the CNS

The term inflammatory demyelination encompasses a broad spectrum of CNS disorders that can be differentiated according to their severity, clinical course, and lesion distribution, as well as their imaging, laboratory, and pathological findings. The spectrum includes monophasic, multiphasic, and progressive disorders, ranging from highly localized forms to multifocal or diffuse variants [2]. Relapsing-remitting (RR) and secondary progressive (SP) MS are the two most common modes of presentation. MS can also have a progressive course from onset (primary progressive [PP]). Fulminant forms of inflammatory demyelination include a variety of disorders that have in common the severity of the clinical symptoms, an acute clinical course, and atypical findings on MRI. The classic fulminant demyelination is Marburg disease but is extremely rare. Baló concentric sclerosis and acute disseminated encephalomyelitis (ADEM) can also present with severe, acute attacks. Some inflammatory demyelinating disorders have a restricted topographic distribution, as is the case with neuromyelitis optica spectrum disorders (NMOSD), which can have a monophasic, but more often follows a relapsing course.

13.3 Multiple Sclerosis (MS)

MS is a progressive inflammatory, demyelinating and neurodegenerative autoimmune disease characterized pathologically by perivascular infiltrates of mononuclear inflammatory cells, demyelination, and axonal loss and gliosis, with the formation of focal and diffuse abnormalities in the brain and spinal cord, mainly affecting the optic nerves, brainstem, spinal cord, and cerebellar and periventricular white matter although cortical and subcortical gray matter damage is also prominent, resulting in chronic progressive disability for the majority of people with the disorder.

The high sensitivity of MRI in depicting brain and spinal cord demyelinating plaques has made this technique the most important paraclinical tool in current use, not only for the early and accurate diagnosis of MS, but also for understanding the natural history of the disease and monitoring and predicting the efficacy of disease-modifying treatments [4].

MRI is the most sensitive imaging technique for detecting MS plaques throughout the brain and spinal cord. Proton density (PD) or T2-weighted MR images (especially acquired using the fluid-attenuated inversion recovery (FLAIR) sequence) show areas of high signal intensity in the periventricular white matter in >90% of MS patients (the remainder may have cord lesions only). MS plaques are generally round

to ovoid in shape and range from a few millimeters to more than 1 cm in diameter. They are typically discrete and focal at the early stages of the disease, but become confluent as the disease progresses, particularly in the posterior hemispheric periventricular white matter. MS plaques tend to affect the periventricular and juxtacortical white matter, whereas small vessel ischemic lesions tend to involve the deep white matter without touching the cortex [4]. The total T2 lesion volume of the brain increases by approximately 5–10% each year in the relapsing forms of MS.

Both acute and chronic MS plaques appear hyperintense on T2/FLAIR sequences, reflecting their increased tissue water content. The signal increase indicates edema, inflammation, demyelination, reactive gliosis, and/or axonal loss in proportions that differ from lesion to lesion [5]. Most MS patients have at least one ovoid periventricular lesion, whose major axis is oriented perpendicular to the outer surface of the lateral ventricles. The ovoid shape and perpendicular orientation derive from the perivenular location of the demyelinating plaques noted on histopathology (Dawson's fingers).

MS lesions tend to affect specific regions of the brain, including the periventricular white matter, the inferior surface of the corpus callosum, the cortico-juxtacortical regions, the temporal lobes and the infratentorial regions (Table 13.1). Focal involvement of the periventricular white matter in the anterior temporal lobes is typical for MS and rarely seen in other white matter disorders, especially not in aging/hypertension (see Table 13.1). The lesions commonly found at the calloso-septal interface are best depicted by sagittal T2-FLAIR images—a sequence highly recommended for diagnostic MRI studies.

Histopathological studies have shown that a substantial portion of the total brain lesion load in MS is located within the cerebral cortex. Presently available MRI techniques are not optimal for detecting cortical lesions because of poor contrast resolution between normal-appearing gray matter (NAGM) and the plaques in question, and because of the partial volume effects of the subarachnoid spaces and CSF sur-

Table 13.1 Characteristic differences between small-vessel disease (SVD) and MS

Involvement	SVD	MS
Corpus callosum	Rare	Common
U-fibers	Rare	Often
Brainstem	Central pons	Peripheral
Temporal lobe	Rare[a]	Often
Gadolinium enhancement	Exceptional	Common
Black holes	Rare	Typical
Lacunes	Typical	Rare
Spinal cord	Never	Common

[a] With the exception of cerebral autosomal dominant arteriopathy with subcortical infarcts and leukoencephalopathy (CADASIL)

rounding the cortex. Cortical lesions are better visualized by 2D or 3D T2-FLAIR sequences and newer MR techniques such as 3D double inversion recovery (DIR) pulse sequences which selectively suppress the signal from white matter and cerebrospinal fluid (CSF). Juxtacortical lesions that involve the "U" fibers are seen in two-thirds of patients with MS.

Posterior fossa lesions preferentially involve the floor of the fourth ventricle, the middle cerebellar peduncles, and the brainstem. Most brainstem lesions are contiguous with the cisternal or ventricular CSF spaces, and range from large confluent patches to solitary, well-delineated paramedian lesions or discrete "linings" of the CSF border zones. Predilection for these areas is a key feature that helps to identify MS plaques and to differentiate them from focal areas of ischemic demyelination and infarction, diseases that preferentially involve the central pontine white matter.

Approximately 10–20% of T2 hyperintensities are also visible on T1-weighted images as areas of low signal intensity compared with normal-appearing gray matter. These so-called T1 black holes have a different pathological substrate that depends, in part, on the lesion age. The hypointensity is present in up to 80% of recently formed lesions and probably represents marked edema, with or without myelin destruction or axonal loss. In most cases, the acute lesions become isointense within a few months as inflammatory activity abates, edema resolves, and reparative mechanisms like remyelination, become active. Less than 40% evolve into

persisting or chronic "black holes," which correlate pathologically with the most severe demyelination and axonal loss, indicating areas of irreversible tissue damage [6]. Chronic black holes are more frequent in patients with progressive disease than in those with RRMS disease, and more frequent in the supratentorial white matter as compared with the infratentorial white matter. They are rarely found in the spinal cord and optic nerves.

MS lesions of the spinal cord resemble those in the brain. The lesions can be focal (single or multiple) or diffuse, and commonly affect the cervical cord segment (Fig. 13.1). On sagittal scans, the lesions characteristically have a cigar shape and rarely exceed two vertebral segments in length (the so-called short-segment lesions in contrast to longitudinally extensive lesions in NMOSD). On cross-section, they typically occupy the lateral and posterior white-matter columns, extend to involve the central gray matter, and rarely occupy more than one half the cross-sectional area of the spinal cord [7].

Acute spinal cord lesions can produce a mild to moderate mass effect with spinal cord swelling and may show contrast enhancement. Active lesions are rarer in the spinal cord than the brain and are more frequently associated with new clinical symptoms. The prevalence of spinal cord abnormalities is as high as 74–92% in established MS and depends on the clinical phenotype of MS. Asymptomatic spinal cord lesions are found in 30–40% of patients with a clinically isolated

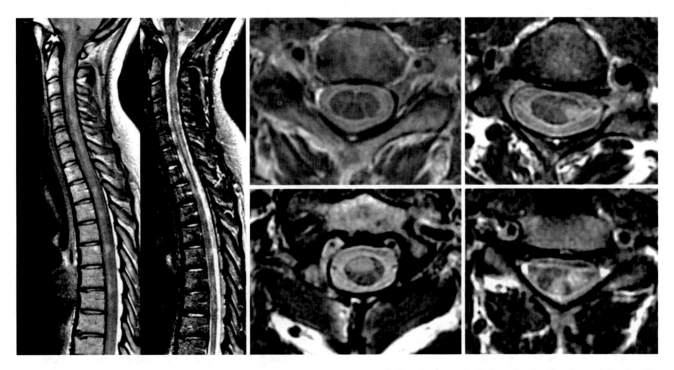

Fig. 13.1 Spinal cord lesion in MS shown on proton-density and T2-weighted sagittal and axial images. Use of at least two contrasts or planes is recommended. Typical of MS, there are multiple short-segment lesions in the sagittal plane that involve the peripheral white matter in the axial plane though lesions can also affect the central gray matter

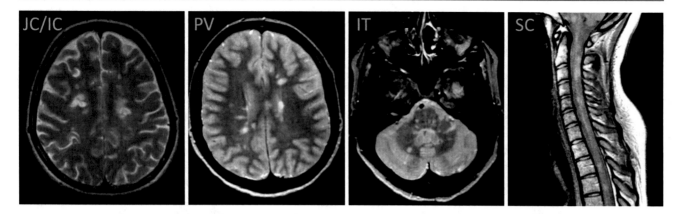

Fig. 13.2 Dissemination in space suggestive of MS is demonstrated when lesions are present in at least two of four locations regardless of whether or not they are symptomatic. *JC/IC* juxtacortical/intracortical, *PV* periventricular, *IT* infratentorial, *SC* spinal cord

syndrome (CIS), even if the presenting symptoms do not involve the spinal cord clinically. In RRMS, the spinal cord lesions are typically multifocal. In secondary progressive MS, the abnormalities are more extensive and diffuse and are commonly associated with spinal cord atrophy. In primary progressive MS, spinal cord abnormalities are quite extensive as compared with brain abnormalities. This discrepancy may help to diagnose primary progressive MS in patients with few or no brain abnormalities.

The diagnosis of MS [2] is based on a clinical symptom suggestive of MS with demonstration of dissemination in space (DIS) and time (DIT) using a combination of clinical and MRI findings. For the fulfillment of DIS based on MRI, lesions should be present in at least two typical locations (intra/juxtacortical, periventricular, infratentorial, and spinal cord) as illustrated in Fig. 13.2. For the fulfillment of DIT based on MRI, there should be either enhancing and non-enhancing lesions at one point in time, or new T2/FLAIR lesions at follow-up in typical locations. When DIT cannot be demonstrated using MRI, the presence of oligoclonal bands in CSF can be a substitute. For both clinical and MRI findings, other diagnoses should be considered and ruled out where appropriate.

Longitudinal and cross-sectional MR studies have shown that the formation of new MS plaques is often associated with contrast enhancement, mainly in the acute and relapsing stages of the disease [8, 9]. The gadolinium enhancement varies in size and shape, usually lasting a few weeks, although steroid treatment shortens this period. Incomplete ring enhancement on T1-weighted gadolinium-enhanced images, with the open border facing the gray matter of the cortex or basal ganglia is a common finding in active MS plaques and is a helpful feature for distinguishing between inflammatory-demyelinating lesions and other focal lesions such as tumors or abscesses which will have a closed ring of enhancement [10].

Contrast enhancement is a relatively good predictor of further enhancement and of subsequent accumulation of T2 lesions but shows no (or weak) correlation with progression of disability and the development of brain atrophy. In RRMS and early SPMS, enhancement is more frequent during relapses and correlates well with clinical activity. For patients with primary progressive MS, serial T2-weighted studies show few new lesions and less frequent enhancement. Contrast-enhanced T1-weighted images are used in the study of MS to provide a measure of inflammatory activity in vivo but given their potential side-effects, patient burden and costs should not routinely be used for treatment monitoring once a new post-treatment baseline is established [8].

MRI-based disease activity occurs five to ten times more frequently than clinical evaluation of relapses, suggesting that most of the enhancing lesions are clinically silent. Subclinical disease activity with contrast-enhancing lesions is four to ten times less frequent in the spinal cord than the brain, a fact that may be partially explained by the large volume of brain as compared with spinal cord. High doses of gadolinium and a long post-injection delay can increase the detection of active spinal cord lesions.

13.4 Baló Concentric Sclerosis

Baló concentric sclerosis is a rare condition, considered a variant of MS, with characteristic radiologic and pathologic features. It was formerly considered an aggressive MS variant, leading to death in weeks to months after onset, and in which the diagnosis was made on histopathologic findings at postmortem examination. However, with the widespread use of MRI, this MS variant is often identified in patients who later have a complete or almost complete clinical recovery [11]. The pathologic hallmarks include large, demyelinated lesions showing a peculiar pattern of alternating layers of preserved and destroyed myelin. One possible explanation for this pattern is that sublethal tissue injury is induced at the edge of the expanding lesion, which would then stimulate expression of neuroprotective proteins to protect the rim of peri-plaque tissue from damage, thereby resulting in alternating layers of preserved and non-preserved myelinated tissue [12]. These alternating bands are best identified with T2-weighted sequences, which typically show thick concentric hyperintense bands corresponding to areas of demyelination and gliosis, alternating with thin isointense bands corresponding to normal myelinated white matter. This pattern can also be identified on T1-weighted images as alternating isointense (preserve myelin) and hypointense (demyelinated) concentric rings. These bands, which may eventually disappear over time, can appear as multiple concentric layers (onion-skin lesion), as a mosaic, or as a "floral" configuration. The center of the lesion usually shows no layering because of massive demyelination ("storm center"). Restricted diffusion, followed by contrast enhancement are common in the outer rings (inflammatory edge) of the lesion [13].

The Baló pattern on MRI can be isolated, multiple, or combined with typical MS-like lesions, and the lesion structure can vary from one or two to several alternating bands, with a total size from one to several centimeters. Lesions occur predominantly in the cerebral white matter although brainstem, cerebellum, and spinal cord involvement has also been reported.

13.5 Neuromyelitis Optica Spectrum Disorders (NMOSD)

NMOSD is an autoimmune inflammatory disorder of the CNS with a predilection for the optic nerves and spinal cord [14]. The discovery of autoantibodies directed against aquaporin-4 (AQP4), the major water channel in the CNS, clearly identified AGP4+NMOSD as a disease separate from MS—and requiring a different treatment than MS [15, 16].

This uncommon and topographically restricted disease is characterized by severe unilateral or bilateral optic neuritis and complete transverse myelitis, which occur simultaneously or sequentially over a varying period (weeks or years). The index events of new-onset NMOSD are severe unilateral or bilateral optic neuritis, acute myelitis, or a combination of these symptoms. Myelitis attacks appear as complete transverse myelitis with severe bilateral motor deficits, sensory-level, bowel and bladder dysfunction, pain and significant residual neurologic injury. Optic neuritis attacks are generally more severe than those typically seen in MS.

Approximately 85% of patients have a relapsing course with severe acute exacerbations and poor recovery, which leads to increasing neurologic impairment and a high risk of respiratory failure and death due to cervical myelitis. Patients who experience acute optic neuritis and transverse myelitis simultaneously or within days of each other are much more likely to have a monophasic course. On the other hand, a relapsing course correlates with AQP4 seropositivity, a longer interval between attacks, older age at onset, female gender, and less severe motor impairment after the myelitic onset. Although the initial attacks are more severe in patients proven to have monophasic NMOSD, the long-term neurologic prognosis is somewhat better in this group because patients do not accumulate disability from recurrent attacks.

Clinical features alone are insufficient to diagnose NMOSD; CSF analysis and MRI are usually required to confidently exclude other disorders. CSF pleocytosis (>50 leukocytes/mm^3) is often present, while oligoclonal bands are seen less frequently (20–40%) than in MS patients (80–90%). AQP4-Ab detection is best performed using cell-based assays that have greater sensitivity. AQP4-Ab may be helpful to distinguish from MS, and it can predict relapse and conversion to NMOSD in patients presenting with a single attack of longitudinally extensive myelitis. AQP4 testing is positive in 52% of patients with relapsing transverse myelitis and in 25% of patients with recurrent idiopathic optic neuritis [17].

Wingerchuk et al. proposed a revised set of criteria for diagnosing AQP4+NMOSD [18]. These criteria remove the absolute restriction on CNS involvement beyond the optic nerves and spinal cord, allow any interval between the first events of optic neuritis and transverse myelitis, and emphasize the specificity of longitudinally extensive spinal cord lesions on MRI and AQP4-IgG seropositive status. More recently, the International Panel for NMOSD diagnosis developed new diagnostic criteria that define the unifying term NMOSD, which is stratified by serologic testing (with or without AQP4-IgG). These new criteria require, in patients with AQP4-IgG, core clinical and MRI findings related to optic nerve, spinal cord, area postrema, other brainstem, diencephalic, or cerebral presentations. However, more stringent clinical and MRI criteria are required for diagnosis of NMOSD without AQP4-IgG or when serologic testing is unavailable (Table 13.2).

MRI of the affected optic nerve demonstrates swelling and loss of blood–brain barrier integrity with gadolinium enhancement that can extend into the optic chiasm. The spinal cord lesions in NMOSD typically extend over three or more contiguous vertebral segments and occasionally the entire spinal cord (longitudinally extensive spinal cord lesions); they are centrally located (preferential central gray-matter involvement) and affect much of the cross-section on axial images. During the acute and subacute phase, the lesions are tumefactive and show contrast uptake. In some cases, the spinal cord lesions are small at the onset of symptoms, mimicking those of MS, and then progress in extent over time. The presence of very hyperintense spotty lesions on T2-weighted images ("bright spotty sign") is a specific feature that helps differentiate NMOSD from MS, particularly in patients without longitudinally extensive spinal cord

Table 13.2 Diagnostic criteria for NMOSD without or unknown AQP4-IgG status

1. At least two core clinical characteristics occurring as a result of one or more clinical attacks and meeting all of the following requirements:
    (a) At least one core clinical characteristic must be optic neuritis, acute myelitis with LETM, or area postrema syndrome
    (b) Dissemination in space (two or more different core clinical characteristics)
    (c) Fulfillment of additional MRI requirements, as applicable (see below)
2. Negative tests for AQP4-IgG using best available detection method or testing unavailable
3. Exclusion of alternative diagnoses

Additional MRI requirements

1. Acute optic neuritis: requires brain MRI showing the following:
    (a) Normal findings or only nonspecific white matter lesions
    (b) Optic nerve MRI with T2-hyperintense lesion or gadolinium-enhancing lesion extending over >1/2 optic nerve length or involving optic chiasm
2. Acute myelitis: requires associated intramedullary MRI lesion extending over ≥3 contiguous segments (LETM) or ≥3 contiguous segments of focal spinal cord atrophy in patients with history compatible with acute myelitis
3. Area postrema syndrome: requires associated dorsal medulla/area postrema lesions
4. Acute brainstem syndrome: requires associated peri-ependymal brainstem lesions

lesions and likely reflects the highly destructive component of the inflammatory lesion [7, 13, 19]. Spinal cord lesions can progress to atrophy and necrosis and may lead to syrinx-like cavities on T1-weighted images.

NMOSD was long considered a disease without brain involvement, and a negative brain MRI at disease onset was considered a major supportive criterion for the diagnosis of NMOSD. However, various studies have shown that brain MRI abnormalities exist in a significant proportion (50–85%) of patients [20]. Brain MRI lesions are often asymptomatic, but sometimes are associated with symptoms even at disease onset. The brain lesions in NMOSD are commonly nonspecific. They can be dot-like or patchy, <3 cm in diameter, and located in the deep white matter, brainstem, or cerebellum. Nonetheless, some brain MRI features appear to be quite characteristic and distinct from MS lesions. These abnormalities may parallel sites with high AQP4 expression adjacent to the ventricular system at any level, such as the hypothalamus, periependymal areas surrounding the third and lateral ventricles, cerebral aqueduct, corpus callosum, and dorsal brainstem adjacent to the fourth ventricle. The appearance of periventricular lesions in AQP4+NMOSD is quite characteristic. In contrast to MS, where periventricular lesions are discrete, oval-shaped, and perpendicular to the ependymal lining due to their perivenular distribution

(Dawson's fingers), NMOSD lesions are not oval-shaped, located immediately adjacent to the lateral ventricles following the ependymal lining in a disseminated pattern, and are often edematous and heterogeneous [20]. As opposed to what occurs in MS, NMOSD lesions do not affect the cortical gray matter.

Involvement of the corpus callosum has been described in 18% of AQP4+seropositive NMOSD patients. The lesions are multiple, large, and edematous, show heterogeneous signal intensity on T2-weighted images, and sometimes affect the entire thickness of the corpus callosum.

Lesions may also affect areas where AQP4 expression is not particularly high, such as the corticospinal tracts. These lesions, which can be unilateral or bilateral and may affect the posterior limb of the internal capsule and cerebral peduncle of the midbrain, are contiguous and often longitudinally extensive [20].

Other brain MRI findings described in AQP4+NMOSD include extensive and confluent hemispheric white-matter lesions and radial hemispheric lesions (sometimes corresponding to an extension of periventricular lesions), which are likely related to vasogenic edema involving the white-matter tracts. These lesions usually do not show mass effect or contrast enhancement, but there may be a "cloud-like" pattern of enhancement, defined as multiple patches of enhancing lesions with blurred margins [21]. In fact, the finding of large hemispheric lesions in a patient suspected of MS should trigger the option of NMOSD and testing for AQP4 antibodies.

Some of the typical brain MRI findings may be specific to clinical presentations, such as intractable vomiting and hiccup (linear dorsal medullary lesions involving the area postrema and nucleus tractus solitarius), or a syndrome of inappropriate antidiuretic hormone secretion (hypothalamic and periaqueductal lesions) [21].

Distinguishing NMOSD from MS is critical, particularly in the early stages, since the treatment and prognosis of these disorders differ. In fact, some evidence suggests that MS-modifying treatments such as interferon-ß, natalizumab, and laquinimod exacerbate AQP4+NMOSD. By contrast, several immunosuppressants (e.g., azathioprine, rituximab, mitoxantrone) seem to help in preventing NMOSD relapses.

NMOSD can be associated with systemic autoimmune diseases such as systemic lupus erythematosus and Sjögren syndrome). Whether the neurologic manifestations are solely due to NMOSD or are a manifestation of these diseases is controversial although optic neuritis and transverse myelitis are rare presentations of them, and several studies have shown that patients with systemic autoimmune diseases and AQP4-IgG antibodies always have optic neuritis, myelitis, or NMOSD.

13.6 Acute Disseminated Encephalomyelitis (ADEM)

ADEM is a severe, immune-mediated inflammatory disorder of the CNS that predominantly affects the white matter of the brain and spinal cord. In the absence of specific biologic markers, the diagnosis of ADEM is based on clinical and radiologic features [22]. This disorder affects children more commonly than adults, and, in contrast to MS, shows no gender preponderance. The estimated incidence is 0.8 per 100,000 population per year. In most cases, the clinical onset of disease is preceded by viral or bacterial infections, usually nonspecific upper-respiratory-tract infections. ADEM may also develop following a vaccination (postimmunization encephalomyelitis). Patients commonly present with nonspecific multifocal symptoms, which developed subacutely over a period of days, frequently associated with encephalopathy (relatively uncommon in MS), defined as an alteration in consciousness (e.g., stupor, lethargy) or a behavioral change unexplained by fever, systemic illness, or postictal symptoms. Although ataxia, encephalopathy, and brainstem symptoms are frequently present in both pediatric and adult cases, certain signs and symptoms appear to be age-related. In childhood ADEM, long-lasting fever and headaches occur more frequently, while in adult cases, motor and sensory deficits predominate. In general, the disease is self-limiting and the prognostic outcome favorable.

Although ADEM usually has a monophasic course, multiphasic forms have been reported, raising diagnostic difficulties in distinguishing these cases from MS. This multiphasic form, which accounts for less than 4% of ADEM cases, is defined as a new encephalopathic event consistent with ADEM, separated by 3 months after the initial illness. The second ADEM event can involve either new or re-emergent neurologic symptoms, signs, and MRI findings. Relapsing disease following ADEM that occurs beyond a second encephalopathic event is no longer consistent with multiphasic ADEM but rather indicates a chronic disorder, most often leading to the diagnosis of MS or MOGAD and should prompt testing for myelin oligodendrocyte glycoprotein (MOG) antibodies, especially in children [23, 24].

An ADEM event as the first manifestation of the classic relapsing form of MS occurs in 2–10%. According to the International Pediatric Multiple Sclerosis Study Group, the diagnosis of MS is met if, after the initial ADEM, a second clinical event meets the following three requirements: (1) it is non-encephalopathic; (2) it occurs 3 months or more after the incident neurologic illness; and (3) it is associated with new MRI findings consistent with the McDonald criteria for dissemination in space [23]. The presence of hypointense lesions and two or more periventricular lesions are MRI features that support an MS diagnosis in children

with acute CNS demyelination [23]. Unlike the lesions in MS, ADEM lesions are often large, patchy, and poorly marginated on MRI, especially when there are MOG antibodies [24]. There is usually asymmetric involvement of the subcortical and central white matter and cortical gray–white junction of the cerebral hemispheres, cerebellum, brainstem, and spinal cord. Lesions confined to the periventricular white matter and corpus callosum are less common than in MS. The gray matter of the thalamus and basal ganglia is often affected, particularly in children, and typically in a symmetric pattern. However, the frequency of thalamic involvement in adult ADEM does not differ from that of adult MS. This can be explained by the fact that involvement of this structure is less common in adult ADEM than in childhood ADEM. Four patterns of cerebral involvement have been proposed to describe the MRI findings in ADEM: (1) ADEM with small lesions (less than 5 mm); (2) ADEM with large, confluent, or tumefactive lesions, and frequent extensive perilesional edema and mass effect; (3) ADEM with additional symmetric deep gray-matter involvement; and (4) acute hemorrhagic encephalomyelitis [25]. Gadolinium enhancement of one or more lesions occurs in 14–30% of cases [23]. The pattern of enhancement varies and can be complete or incomplete ring-shaped, nodular, gyral, or spotty. Although ADEM is usually a monophasic disease, new lesions may be seen on follow-up MRI within the first month of the initial attack.

Most MRI lesions appear early in the course of the disease, supporting the clinical diagnosis of ADEM. Nonetheless, in some cases, there may be a delay of more than 1 month between the onset of symptoms and the appearance of lesions on MRI. Therefore, a normal brain MRI scan obtained within the first days after the onset of neurologic symptoms suggestive of ADEM does not exclude this diagnosis.

The spinal cord is affected in less than 30% of ADEM patients, predominantly in the thoracic region. The spinal cord lesion is typically large, causes swelling, and shows variable enhancement. In most ADEM patients, partial or complete resolution of the MRI abnormalities occurs within a few months of treatment. This course is positively associated with a final diagnosis of ADEM.

13.7 Myelin Oligodendrocyte Glycoprotein-Related Antibody Disease (MOGAD)

Beyond the setting of ADEM, the entity of MOGAD has been coined more recently [26], significantly narrowing the differential diagnosis of NMOSD without AQP4 antibodies. In older children and adults, optic neuritis is the most common mode of presentation and is bilateral in around 50% of cases, far more than in MS and even more than in AQP4-mediated disease. Transverse myelitis is the second most common mode of presentation. Infrequent modes of presentation include cerebral cortical encephalitis (with seizures), tumefactive brain lesions, brainstem, or cerebellar syndrome and even a leukodystrophy-like pattern.

Optic neuritis in MOGAD is associated with swelling and optic nerve hyperintensity on STIR or fat-saturated T2 images of the orbit, with lesions tending to involve the optic nerve over its entire length; MS lesions tend to be short (and unilateral), while AQP4-related lesions tend to be more posterior with involvement of the chiasm. MOGAD lesions show gadolinium-enhancement and peri-optic enhancement is a frequent finding.

Transverse myelitis in MOGAD tends to be longitudinally extensive (LETM) and involve the central cord more than the periphery—as in NMOSD. There can even be isolated gray matter involvement. The lower cord is frequently involved. Enhancement with gadolinium can be patchy and persistent.

Cerebral lesions in MOGAD trend to affect the gray-white matter boundaries, for example, around the cingulate cortex. Posterior fossa lesions include ill-defined ponto-mesencephalic or (sometimes bilateral) MCP lesions.

The diagnosis of MOGAD requires one of the core clinical features and clearly positive MOG-IgG test results in serum (using a fixed or live cell-based assay). In case of low-positive titers or unclear serum MOG-IgG status, one of the above-mentioned MRI findings is required to confirm the diagnosis.

13.8 Infectious Inflammatory Demyelinating Disorders

13.8.1 Progressive Multifocal Leukoencephalopathy

Progressive multifocal leukoencephalopathy (PML) is overwhelmingly a disease of the immunocompromised patient and most (55–85%) cases are related to acquired immunodeficiency syndrome (AIDS). There is a wide age range of involvement, with the peak age of presentation in the sixth decade. The disease is caused by reactivation of a papovavirus (JC virus) that selectively attacks the oligodendrocyte, leading to demyelination. Treatment with monoclonal antibody therapy (natalizumab, rituximab, efalizumab) or other immunomodulatory drugs, commonly used in patients with MS and other disorders has also been linked with PML [27]. Untreated patients with PML have an extremely poor prognosis, with death common in the

first 6 months following establishment of the diagnosis. Although there is no specific treatment, combination anti-retroviral therapy (cART) has not only resulted in a lower incidence of PML in AIDS patients, but also substantially improved survival times, now at 50% 1-year survival [27]. Unfortunately, about 20% of PML cases are linked to a robust inflammatory response to pathogens associated with recovery of the immune system after a period of immuno-suppression. This condition, known as PML-IRIS (Immune Reconstitution Inflammatory Syndrome), has been associated with intracranial masses with generous amounts of surrounding vasogenic edema on MRI. Enhancement may also occur [27].

The lesions of PML are characterized by little mass effect or enhancement. Most lesions involve the subcortical white matter and deep cortical layers of the parieto-occipital or frontal white matter although gray matter and posterior fossa lesions are also common (occurring in up to 50% of cases). PML lesions tend to be more confluent in their appearance than ADEM lesions and scalloping of the lateral margin of the lesion at the gray matter-white matter junction is common. Subtle signal intensity changes in the white matter may precede clinical suspicion of PML-IRIS. While development of mass effect and temporary enhancement in the early phase of cART has been linked to better survival, similar imaging manifestations may also be seen in monoclonal-antibody treated PML patients [27].

13.8.2 Human Immunodeficiency Virus Encephalopathy

Human immunodeficiency virus (HIV) encephalopathy results from direct infection of the brain by the virus itself. Since the advent of cART, the prevalence of the disease has markedly decreased, and the temporal progression has been slowed. Most patients are severely immunocompromised at the time of onset and exhibit psychomotor slowing, impaired mental status, and memory difficulties. Histologically, demyelination and vacuolation with axonal loss are noted, along with occasional microglial nodules. Mild cerebral atrophy is the first and sometimes only imaging feature of the disease, which is also known as AIDS dementia complex, HIV dementia, HIV-associated dementia complex, and HIV-associated neuron-cognitive disorder (HAND). Involvement of the central white matter, basal ganglia, and thalamus is characteristic. Typically, bilaterally symmetric abnormal hyperintensity in the basal ganglia and small focal areas in the periventricular regions are noted on T2-weighted MR images [28]. Regression of these findings has been seen following institution of cART.

13.9 White Matter Disease from Toxic Imbalance

13.9.1 Chronic Alcohol Ingestion and Its Consequences

Brain abnormalities in alcoholics include atrophy, Marchiafava-Bignami disease, Wernicke encephalopathy, osmotic myelinolysis, and consequences of liver cirrhosis such as hepatic encephalopathy and coagulopathy [29]. All the reported entities are not specific of alcohol and can be found in many other toxic or metabolic conditions. Ethanol direct brain toxicity is caused by up-regulation of receptors of N-methyl-D-aspartate and abnormal catabolism of homocysteine, resulting in an increased susceptibility to glutamate excitatory and toxic effects. Moreover, immune response occurs mediated by lipid peroxidation products that bind to neurons resulting in neurotoxicity. Neuroimaging studies show a characteristic distribution of loss of volume, initially with atrophy of the cerebellar vermis and hemispheres and subsequently frontal and temporal atrophy, followed by diffuse atrophy of the brain. Partial reversibility of these alterations may be observed in the early stages. In pregnancy, ethanol inhibits maturation of Bergmann's fibers of the neonatal cerebellum, with consequential marked cerebellar atrophy.

13.9.2 Hepatic Encephalopathy

The term *hepatic encephalopathy* (HE) includes a wide spectrum of neuropsychiatric abnormalities occurring in patients with liver dysfunction. Most cases are associated with cirrhosis and portal hypertension or portal-systemic shunts, but the condition can also be seen in patients with acute liver failure and, rarely, in those with portal-systemic bypass and even in the absence of associated intrinsic hepatocellular disease. Although HE is a clinical condition, several neuroimaging techniques, particularly MRI, may eventually be useful for the diagnosis because they can identify and measure the consequences of CNS increase in substances, which, under normal circumstances, are efficiently metabolized by the liver. Classical MR abnormalities in chronic HE include high signal intensity in the globus pallidus on T1-weighted images, likely a reflection of increased tissue concentrations of manganese, and an elevated glutamine/glutamate peak coupled with decreased myo-inositol and choline signals on proton MR spectroscopy, representing disturbances in cell-volume homeostasis secondary to brain hyperammonemia [30].

White matter abnormalities related to increased CNS ammonia concentration can also be detected with magnetization transfer imaging (ratio measurements show significantly low values in otherwise normal-appearing brain white matter), T2-Flair sequences (diffuse and focal high-signal intensity lesions in the hemispheric white matter), and DWI (increased white matter diffusivity). All these MR abnormalities, which return to normal with restoration of liver function, probably reflect the presence of mild diffuse interstitial brain edema, which seems to play an essential role in the pathogenesis of HE.

In acute HE, bilateral symmetric signal-intensity abnormalities on T2-weighted images, often with associated restricted diffusion involving cortical gray matter, are commonly identified. Involvement of the subcortical white matter, basal ganglia, thalami, and midbrain may also be seen. These abnormalities reflect the development of cytotoxic edema secondary to acute hyperammonemia that can lead to intracranial hypertension and severe brain injury [30].

13.9.3 Marchiafava-Bignami Disease

Marchiafava-Bignami disease is a rare complication of chronic alcoholism, characterized by demyelination and necrosis of the corpus callosum, with rare involvement of extracallosal regions. Etiology remains unknown. Initially believed to be caused by toxic agents in low-quality red wine and lack of group B vitamins, it has since been documented in those who consume other types of alcohol and even more rarely in non-alcoholics. Symptoms are mainly represented by cognitive deficits, psychosis, hypertonia, and interhemispheric disconnection, until coma and death. Typical MRI features in the acute phase are corpus callosum hyperintensity on T2-weighted sequences and FLAIR, without significant mass effect, with peripheral enhancement. Diffusion is restricted due to cytotoxic edema. In chronic forms, necrosis of the genu and splenium can be detected [31].

13.9.4 Wernicke Encephalopathy

Wernicke encephalopathy (WE) is an acute condition first described by the French ophthalmologist Gayet in 1875, and later by the German neurologist Wernicke in 1881, caused by a deficiency of 25B1 (thiamine). It develops frequently but not exclusively in alcoholics. Other potential causes include extended fasting, malabsorption, digitalis poisoning, massive infusion of glucose without 25B1 in weak patients. The autoptic incidence is reported to be 0.8–2% in random autopsies, and 20% in chronic alcoholics. The classic clinical triad of ocular dysfunctions (nystagmus, conjugate gaze palsy, ophthalmoplegia), ataxia, and confusion is observed in only 30% of cases. Treatment consists of thiamine infusion and avoids irreversible consequences including Korsakoff dementia or death. Memory impairment and dementia are related to damage of the mammillary bodies, anterior thalamic nuclei and interruption of the diencephalic-hippocampal circuits. Depletion of thiamine leads to failure of conversion of pyruvate to acetyl-CoA and α-ketoglutarate to succinate, altered pentose monophosphate shunt, and the lack of Krebs cycle, with cerebral lactic acidosis, intra- and extra-cellular edema, swelling of astrocytes, oligodendrocytes, myelin fibers, and neuronal dendrites. Neuropathological aspects include neuronal degeneration, demyelination, hemorrhagic petechiae, proliferation of capillaries and astrocytes in peri-aqueductal gray substance, mammillary bodies, thalami, pulvinar, III cranial nerves nuclei, and cerebellum. On MRI, associated bilateral and symmetrical hyperintensities on T2-weighted sequences and FLAIR are evident in these regions, most prominently in the mammillary bodies and thalami [32, 33]. Rarely, cortex of the forebrain can be involved. DWI shows areas of reduced apparent diffusion coefficient (ADC) due to cytotoxic edema although the ADC can sometimes be high due to the presence of vasogenic component. T1-weighted images may rarely show hyperintensity (related to hemorrhagic changes) in the thalami and mammillary bodies, a sign considered clinically unfavorable. In 50% of cases, contrast enhancement is present in periaqueductal regions. Marked contrast enhancement of the mammillary bodies is evident in 80% of cases, even prior to the development of visible changes in T2-weighted sequences and is considered highly specific for WE. In chronic forms, T2 signal change becomes less prominent due to diffuse brain atrophy, more pronounced at the level of mesencephalon and mammillary bodies.

13.9.5 Osmotic Demyelination Syndrome

Osmotic demyelination syndrome (ODS) usually occurs in the setting of osmotic changes, typically with the rapid correction of hyponatremia. This causes destruction of the blood-brain barrier with hypertonic fluid accumulation in extracellular space, resulting in a non-inflammatory demyelination, most conspicuously seen in the central pontine fibers [34]. ODS is mostly seen in alcoholics with nutritional deficiency, frequently in the setting of paralysis, dysphagia, dysarthria, and pseudobulbar palsy. Once regarded as nearly uniformly fatal, it is now recognized that most (~75%) afflicted patients survive and more than half show a good functional recovery. Those with prior liver transplant have higher mortality and disability rates [35]. Rarely, ODS affects other regions, especially basal ganglia, thalami, and deep white matter (extrapontine myelinolysis). MRI usually shows an area of high signal on T2-weighted sequences in the central part of the pons, sparing ventro-lateral portions and corticospinal tracts. The lesion is moderately hypointense in T1 and may show positive contrast enhance-

ment. If the patient survives, the acute phase can evolve into a cavitated pontine lesion.

13.10 White Matter Disease Associated with Radiation Therapy and Chemotherapy

Treatment strategies designed to target cancer cells are commonly associated with deleterious effects to multiple organ systems, including the CNS. As both radiation and chemotherapy alone can be associated with significant toxicity, the combination of the two modalities is particularly harmful, particularly in the CNS. With advanced treatment regimens and prolonged survival, neurological complications are likely to be observed with increasing frequency.

Neurotoxicity can result from direct toxic effects of the drug or radiation on the cells of the CNS, or indirectly through metabolic abnormalities, inflammatory processes, or vascular adverse effects. Recognition of treatment-related neurologic complications is critically important because symptoms may be confused with metastatic disease, tumor progression, paraneoplastic disorders, or opportunistic infections, and discontinuation of the offending drug may prevent irreversible CNS injury.

13.10.1 Radiation Injury and Necrosis

It is widely accepted that the white matter of the CNS is more prone to radiation-induced injury, compared with gray matter. Radiation encephalopathy has been classically divided into three stages according to its timing after radiotherapy: early, early-delayed, and late-delayed reactions [36]. Within the first several weeks of therapy, patients may experience acute declines with focal neurologic deficits. These effects are possibly related to increased edema, which has been supported by the observation that steroid treatment often results in clinical improvement. Early-delayed adverse effects usually occur within 1–6 months of treatment, and are thought to be a result of demyelination. This syndrome is characterized by somnolence, fatigue, and cognitive impairment, consistent with dysfunction of the frontal network systems. Late-delayed side-effects occur months to years after cessation of treatment, commonly associated with progressive cognitive deficits, and are largely irreversible. In more severe cases of late-delayed radiation injury, imaging and histopathological studies may demonstrate findings consistent with leukoencephalopathy and/or focal necrosis.

In all types of white matter radiation-induced damage, imaging studies, most conspicuously on MRI, may demonstrate variable degrees of white matter signal changes related to an increase in free tissue water in the involved areas. This may result from endothelial damage, causing increased capillary permeability and vasogenic edema, or from demyelination. However, the degree of these white matter changes correlates poorly with the observed functional deterioration. MRI findings in early reactions occurring during course of treatment are nonspecific. MRI may be normal or demonstrate poorly defined multifocal lesions in both hemispheres that usually disappear spontaneously. MRI in early-delayed reactions also may show signal changes involving not only the hemispheric white matter but also the basal ganglia and the cerebral peduncles, which resolve completely without treatment. These early-delayed changes have been reported in children with acute lymphocytic leukemia who have been treated with both whole brain irradiation and chemotherapy. These changes have no correlation with clinical manifestations and have no clear prognostic significance. Late-delayed reactions can be subdivided into diffuse and focal radiation necrosis injury.

Diffuse radiation injury is characterized by white matter changes that are "geographic" in nature, i.e., the areas of abnormal signal intensity or attenuation are limited to the regions of the brain that conform to the radiation portal. This can produce striking differences between the involved zones and the spared surrounding white matter. The involved territories are often symmetric and do not enhance on postcontrast studies. While originally reported in children with leukemia, diffuse necrotizing leukoencephalopathy has also been observed following treatment for many other malignancies in both children and adults. The disease may occur following chemotherapy alone, but the incidence of disease is highest when chemotherapy is combined with radiation therapy. Both the histologic findings and imaging features bear resemblance to radiation necrosis. Axonal swelling, demyelination, coagulation necrosis, and gliosis dominate the histologic picture.

Diffuse white matter changes, with hypoattenuation on CT and T1 and T2 prolongation on MRI, are common and often involve an entire hemisphere. Microbleeds can occur as a sign of vasculopathy. Radiation-induced leukoencephalopathy may be associated with progressive brain atrophy, and patients may present with cognitive decline, gait abnormalities, and urinary incontinence. However, the more common mild-to-moderate cognitive impairment is inconsistently associated with radiological findings and frequently occurs in patients with normal-appearing scans. More sensitive tools (e.g., diffusion tensor imaging) may quantify the early and progressive damage to otherwise normal-appearing white matter, consistent with radiation-induced demyelination and mild structural degradation of axonal fibers.

Focal radiation necrosis usually manifests as a ring-like or irregular enhancing mass located in the white matter, which may become hemorrhagic. The classic MRI features commonly seen in radiation necrosis include a "soap-bubble"

or larger, more diffuse, and variably sized "Swiss cheese-like" interior. This pattern reflects diffuse enhancement at the margins of the cortex and white matter with intermixed foci of necrosis [37]. The rim of enhancement is often thinner, more uniform, and more aligned to the gray matter-white matter junction than in malignant tumors. As radiation necrosis progresses, it can lead to severe shrinkage of the white matter and cortex and result in focal brain atrophy with ventriculomegaly.

Quite frequently, it is impossible to distinguish radiation necrosis from recurrent malignant brain tumor, such as glioblastoma multiforme, using conventional MRI. Metabolic imaging (e.g., positron emission tomography) may facilitate differentiating between the two diseases as radiation necrosis is iso-to-hypometabolic while recurrent high-grade tumors are typically hypermetabolic [38]. MR spectroscopy may also be useful as radiation necrosis frequently shows a characteristic lactic acid peak and near-normal peaks for N-acetyl-aspartate and choline while recurrent high-grade gliomas typically show elevated choline levels compared to NAA without or with elevated lactic acid levels. Perfusion imaging can identify the areas of increased blood flow associated with tumor recurrence whereas radiation necrosis is not expected to contain any increased blood flow [38].

13.10.2 Chemotherapy-Associated Neurotoxicity

Neurotoxicity has been observed with virtually all categories of chemotherapeutic agents [39, 40]. Neurologic complications may range from acute encephalopathy, headache, seizures, visual loss, cerebellar toxicity, and stroke to chronic side-effects, including chronic encephalopathy, cognitive decline, and dementia.

Among the most puzzling aspects of cancer therapy-related toxicity is the occurrence of delayed and progressive neurological decline, even after cessation of treatment. Anticancer agents affect brain function through both direct and indirect pathways. It is also conceivable that additional variables play important roles, including the timing of treatment, combination of different treatment modalities, patient age, integrity of the blood–brain barrier, and cognitive function prior to treatment initiation.

Imaging studies have provided evidence that structural and functional CNS changes occur in a significant number of patients treated with chemotherapy. Some agents, such as methotrexate or carmustine, are well known to cause a leukoencephalopathy syndrome, especially when administered at a high dose, intrathecally, or in combination with cranial radiotherapy. Non-enhancing, confluent, periventricular white matter lesions, necrosis, ventriculomegaly, and cortical atrophy characterize this syndrome. White matter abnormalities following high-dose chemotherapy have been detected in up to 70% of treated individuals and usually have a delayed onset of several months.

A delayed leukoencephalopathy syndrome with distinct DWI abnormalities on MRI indicative of cytotoxic edema within cerebral white matter has been previously described. This syndrome appeared to mimic a stroke-like syndrome and was seen mainly in patients receiving methotrexate, 5-fluorouracil (5-FU), carmofur, and capecitabine [41]. It has been suggested that this phenomenon may reflect the presence of intramyelinic sheath edema or myelin synthesis blockade but remains speculative.

13.11 Vascular Causes of White Matter Disease

13.11.1 Posterior Reversible Encephalopathy Syndrome

Although not a truly demyelinating condition, reversible encephalopathy syndrome is noteworthy because of its affinity for the posterior cerebral white matter territories. Under normal circumstances, cerebral perfusion pressure is maintained at a relatively constant level by autoregulation, a physiologic mechanism that compensates for wide changes in systemic blood pressure. Hypertensive encephalopathy is believed to result from loss of normal autoregulation (with competing regions of vasodilatation and vasoconstriction) and endothelial dysfunction. The vessels of the posterior cerebral circulation, lacking less sympathetic innervation compared to those of the anterior circulation, are unable to vasoconstrict in a normal manner and bear the brunt of these vascular changes. Reversible vasogenic edema is the result and is associated with visual field deficits, as well as headaches, somnolence, and an overall impaired mental status. The terms posterior reversible encephalopathy syndrome (PRES) and reversible posterior leukoencephalopathy syndrome (RPLS) have been popularized in the literature to describe this scenario that is most commonly seen in hypertensive states and/or the presence of immunosuppression (particularly cyclosporine A and tacrolimus), chemotherapy, eclampsia, and renal failure. While it commonly involves the posterior cerebral white matter, other sites may also be affected including unilateral cerebral hemispheric or isolated brainstem involvement in patients following aortic valve surgery [42, 43]. Accordingly, it has been suggested that perhaps the terminology should be changed to simply "reversible encephalopathy" [44].

On MR studies, bilaterally symmetric abnormal T2 hyperintensity, representing vasogenic edema, is most commonly seen in the distribution of the posterior circulation although other sites including the frontal lobes and corpus callosum may be noted as well. Cortical and subcortical lesions may be better detected on FLAIR sequences. DWI may be normal or show restricted water diffusion in regions of infarction that correlate with poorer prognosis [45]. Susceptibility-weighted imaging may show areas of hemorrhage within involved territories. With early treatment and limited involvement of the brain, many of these imaging abnormalities will completely resolve and most patients recover within 2 weeks [46]. However, when larger areas or regions of infarction are involved, permanent neurologic deficits or even death are possible. Vascular narrowing has been observed on angiographic studies. Perfusion studies reported in the literature indicate normal to increased perfusion in these zones. When biopsies of these regions have been performed, white matter edema is seen histologically.

13.12 Aging and Ischemic Demyelinating Disorders

Small focal lesions on T2-weighted images are quite common in the white matter of adult subjects [47]. They are not associated with mass effect, do not enhance, and are typically isointense compared to normal white matter on T1-weighted images. When these lesions have been biopsied, histologic examination reveals a spectrum of findings including gliosis, partial loss of myelination, and vasculopathy. They tend to be located in the deep white matter of the centrum semiovale. In contrast to MS, they do not involve the corpus callosum or the juxtacortical U-fibers, important distinguishing features [3]. Since the lesions are so ubiquitous and appear to be a part of "normal" aging, various terms have been proposed: senescent white matter changes or disease, deep white matter ischemia, leukoaraiosis, etc. In general, the more lesions present, the more likely it is that the patient will have cognitive problems or difficulties with neuropsychologic testing. However, it is not possible to predict a particular patient's status simply based on the imaging appearance alone.

In adult patients between 30 and 50 years of age, the presence of periventricular and subcortical lesions in a patient with a family history of similarly affected relatives should raise the possibility of cerebral autosomal dominant arteriopathy with subcortical infarcts and leukoencephalopathy (CADASIL). A defect in the notch3 gene on the long arm of chromosome 19 has been identified and apparently evokes an angiopathy affecting small and medium-sized vessels. Most lesions occur in the frontal and temporal lobes and less commonly in the thalamus, basal ganglia, internal and external capsules, and brainstem [48].

13.13 Conclusion

MRI of the brain and spinal cord is of vital importance in the diagnosis of MS, the most important idiopathic inflammatory CNS disorder. Dissemination in space and time on MRI is not limited to MS and can occur in NMOSD, and spinal cord imaging is important in the differential diagnosis. Increasingly, MRI is used to monitor MS treatment and their complications such as PML. Numerous other diseases may also involve the white matter of the brain and spinal cord but can be differentiated from demyelinating disease by clinical, imaging, and laboratory features.

> **Key Points**
> - Age-related white matter changes are extremely prevalent and affect the deep white matter with sparing of the U-fibers and spinal cord.
> - The McDonald criteria for MS include cortico/juxtacortical, periventricular, infratentorial and spinal cord lesions.
> - Longitudinally extensive spinal cord lesions and large/atypical brain lesions should prompt antibody testing to rule out NMOSD and MOGAD.
> - The differential diagnosis of symmetric white lesions includes toxic and metabolic disorders.

References

1. Solomon AJ, Arrambide G, Brownlee WJ, et al. Differential diagnosis of suspected multiple sclerosis: an updated consensus approach. Lancet Neurol. 2023;22(8):750–68.
2. Thompson AJ, Banwell BL, Barkhof F, et al. Diagnosis of multiple sclerosis: 2017 revisions of the McDonald criteria. Lancet Neurol. 2018;17(2):162–17.
3. Aliaga ES, Barkhof F. MRI mimics of multiple sclerosis. Handb Clin Neurol. 2014;122:291–316.
4. Rovira À, Barkhof F. Multiple sclerosis and variants. In: Barkhof F, Jager R, Thurnher M, Rovira Cañellas A, editors. Clinical neuroradiology. Cham: Springer; 2018.
5. Filippi M, Rocca MA. MR imaging of multiple sclerosis. Radiology. 2011;259:659–81.
6. Bagnato F, Jeffries N, Richert ND, et al. Evolution of T1 black holes in patients with multiple sclerosis imaged monthly for 4 years. Brain. 2003;126:1782–9.
7. Ciccarelli O, Cohen JA, Reingold SC, Weinshenker BG. Spinal cord involvement in multiple sclerosis and neuromyelitis optica spectrum disorders. Lancet Neurol. 2019;18(2):185–97.
8. Wattjes MP, Ciccarelli O, Reich DS, et al. 2021 MAGNIMS-CMSC-NAIMS consensus recommendations on the use of MRI in patients with multiple sclerosis. Lancet Neurol. 2021;20(8):653–70.
9. Cotton F, Weiner HL, Jolesz FA, et al. MRI contrast uptake in new lesions in relapsing-remitting MS followed at weekly intervals. Neurology. 2003;60:640–6.
10. Masdeu JC, Quinto C, Olivera C, et al. Open-ring imaging sign: highly specific for atypical brain demyelination. Neurology. 2000;54:1427–33.
11. Popescu BF, Lucchinetti CF. Pathology of demyelinating diseases. Annu Rev Pathol. 2012;7:185–217.
12. Stadelmann C, Ludwin S, Tabira T, et al. Tissue preconditioning may explain concentric lesions in Baló's type of multiple sclerosis. Brain. 2005;128:979–87.
13. Wuerfel J, Rovira A, Paul F, Barkhof F. Neuromyelitis optica spectrum disorders (NMOSD). In: Barkhof F, Jager R, Thurnher M, Rovira Cañellas A, editors. Clinical neuroradiology. Cham: Springer; 2019.
14. Hardy TA, Miller DH. Baló's concentric sclerosis. Lancet Neurol. 2014;13:740–6.
15. Trebst C, Jarius S, Berthele A, et al. Update on the diagnosis and treatment of neuromyelitis optica: recommendations of the Neuromyelitis Optica Study Group (NEMOS). J Neurol. 2014;261:1–16.
16. Lennon VA, Wingerchuk DM, Kryzer TJ, et al. A serum autoantibody marker of neuromyelitis optica: distinction from multiple sclerosis. Lancet. 2004;364:2106–12.
17. Wingerchuk DM, Lennon VA, Pittock SJ, et al. Revised diagnostic criteria for neuromyelitis optica. Neurology. 2006;66:1485–9.
18. Wingerchuk DM, Banwell B, Bennett JL, et al. International consensus diagnostic criteria for neuromyelitis optica spectrum disorders. Neurology. 2015;85:177–89.
19. Yonezu T, Ito S, Mori M, et al. "Bright spotty lesions" on spinal magnetic resonance imaging differentiate neuromyelitis optica from multiple sclerosis. Mult Scler. 2014;20:331–7.
20. Kim HJ, Paul F, Lana-Peixoto MA, et al. MRI characteristics of neuromyelitis optica spectrum disorder: an international update. Neurology. 2015;84:1165–73.
21. Misu T, Fujihara K, Nakashima I, et al. Intractable hiccup and nausea with periaqueductal lesions in neuromyelitis optica. Neurology. 2005;65:1479–82.
22. Auger C, Rovira A. Acute disseminated encephalomyelitis and other acute parainfectious syndromes. In: Barkhof F, Jager R, Thurnher M, Rovira Cañellas A, editors. Clinical neuroradiology. Cham: Springer; 2018.
23. Verhey LH, Branson HM, Shroff MM, et al. MRI parameters for prediction of multiple sclerosis diagnosis in children with acute CNS demyelination: a prospective national cohort study. Lancet Neurol. 2011;10:1065–73.
24. Hacohen Y, Mankad K, Chong WK, et al. Diagnostic algorithm for relapsing acquired demyelinating syndromes in children. Neurology. 2017;89:269–78.
25. Tenembaum SN. Chapter 132: Acute disseminated encephalomyelitis. In: Dulac O, Lassonde M, Sarnat HB, editors. Handbook of clinical neurology, pediatric neurology part II, vol. 112 (series 3). Elsevier; 2013. p. 1253–62.
26. Banwell B, Bennett JL, Marignier R, et al. Diagnosis of myelin oligodendrocyte glycoprotein antibody-associated disease: international MOGAD panel proposed criteria. Lancet Neurol. 2023;22(3):268–82.
27. Wattjes MP, Barkhof F. Diagnosis of natalizumab-associated progressive multifocal leukoencephalopathy using MRI. Curr Opin Neurol. 2014;27:260–70.
28. Gottumukkala RV, Romero JM, Riascos RF, et al. Imaging of the brain in patients with human immunodeficiency virus infection. Top Magn Reson Imaging. 2014;23:275–91.
29. Geibprasert S, Gallucci M, Krings T. Alcohol-induced changes in the brain as assessed by MRI and CT. Eur Radiol. 2010;20:1492–501.
30. Rovira A, Alonso J, Cordoba J. MR imaging findings in hepatic encephalopathy. AJNR Am J Neuroradiol. 2008;29:1612–21.

31. Arbelaez A, Pajon A, Castillo M. Acute Marchiafava-Bignami disease: MR findings in two patients. AJNR Am J Neuroradiol. 2003;24:1955–7.

32. Gallucci M, Bozzao A, Splendiani A, et al. Wernicke encephalopathy: MR findings in five patients. AJR Am J Roentgenol. 1990;155:1309–14.

33. Zuccoli G, Santa Cruz D, Bertolini M, et al. MR imaging findings in 56 patients with Wernicke encephalopathy: nonalcoholics may differ from alcoholics. AJNR Am J Neuroradiol. 2009;30:171–6.

34. Ruzek KA, Campeau NG, Miller GM. Early diagnosis of central pontine myelinolysis with diffusion-weighted imaging. AJNR Am J Neuroradiol. 2004;25:210–3.

35. Singh AJ, Fugate JE, Rabinstein AA. Central pontine and extrapontine myelinolysis: a systematic review. Eur J Neurol. 2014;21:1443–50.

36. Soussain C, Ricard D, Fike JR, et al. CNS complications of radiotherapy and chemotherapy. Lancet. 2009;374:1639–51.

37. Kumar AJ, Leeds NE, Fuller GN, et al. Malignant gliomas: MR imaging spectrum of radiation therapy- and chemotherapy-induced necrosis of the brain after treatment. Radiology. 2000;217:377–84.

38. Mayo ZS, Halima A, Broughman JR, Smile TD, Tom MS, Murphy ES, Suh JH, Lo SS, Barnett GH, Wu G, Johnson S, Chao ST. Radiation necrosis or tumor progression? A review of the radiographic modalities used in the diagnosis of cerebral radiation necrosis. J Neuro-Oncol. 2023;161:23–31.

39. de Medeiros Rimkus C, Andrade CS, da Costa Leite C, et al. Toxic leukoencephalopathies, including drug, medication, environmental, and radiation-induced encephalopathic syndromes. Semin Ultrasound CT MR. 2014;35:97–117.

40. Godi C, Falini A. Radiological findings of drug-induced neurotoxic disorders. In: Barkhof F, Jager R, Thurnher M, Rovira Cañellas A, editors. Clinical neuroradiology. Cham: Springer; 2019.

41. Baehring JM, Fulbright RK. Delayed leukoencephalopathy with stroke-like presentation in chemotherapy recipients. J Neurol Neurosurg Psychiatry. 2008;79:535–9.

42. Wijdicks EF, Campeau N, Sundt T. Reversible unilateral brain edema presenting with major neurologic deficit after valve repair. Ann Thorac Surg. 2008;86:634–7.

43. McKinney AM, Short J, Truwit CL, et al. Posterior reversible encephalopathy syndrome: incidence of atypical regions of involvement and imaging findings. AJR Am J Roentgenol. 2007;189:904–12.

44. Casey SO, Sampaio RC, Michel E, Truwit CL. Posterior reversible encephalopathy syndrome: utility of fluid-attenuated inversion recovery MR imaging in the detection of cortical and subcortical lesions. AJNR Am J Neurodiol. 2000;21:1199–206.

45. Covarrubias D, Luetmer P, Campeau N. Posterior reversible encephalopathy syndrome: prognostic utility of quantitative diffusion-weighted MR images. AJNR Am J Neuroradiol. 2002;23:1038–48.

46. Geocadin RG. Posterior reversible encephalopathy syndrome. N Engl J Med. 2023;388:2171–8.

47. Kloppenborg RP, Nederkoorn PJ, Geerlings MI, van den Berg E. Presence and progression of white matter hyperintensities and cognition: a meta-analysis. Neurology. 2014;82:2127–38.

48. van dem Boom R, Lesnick Oberstein S, et al. Cerebral autosomal dominant arteriopathy with subcortical infarcts and leukoencephalopathy: MR imaging changes and apolipoportein E genotype. AJNR Am J Neuroradiol. 2006;27:359–62.

Child with Acute Neurological Emergency

14

Livja Mertiri, Andrea Rossi, Laura M. Huisman, and Thierry A. G. M. Huisman

Abstract

Children with acute neurological emergencies present to the ER with a wide spectrum of symptoms and signs. Neuroimaging plays an important role because of limitations such as gathering an accurate patient history and difficulties in performing a detailed neurological examination in the ER, particularly in young patients. The goal of this chapter is to discuss the neuroimaging findings of the most frequent causes of acute emergencies in children, as well as of some less frequently encountered entities.

Keywords

Neurological emergencies · Stroke · Hemorrhages Infections · Trauma · Seizures

Learning Objectives
- To understand the common acute neurological disorders in children encountered in the emergency room.
- To learn basic neuroimaging findings of acute pediatric neurological emergencies.

L. Mertiri (✉) · Thierry A. G. M. Huisman
Edward B. Singleton Department of Radiology, Texas Children's Hospital and Baylor College of Medicine, Houston, TX, USA
e-mail: lxmertir@texaschildrens.org; huisman@texaschildrens.org

A. Rossi
Neuroradiology Unit, IRCCS Istituto Giannina Gaslini, Genoa, Italy

Department of Health Sciences (DISSAL), University of Genoa, Genoa, Italy
e-mail: andrearossi@gaslini.org

L. M. Huisman
Tufts University, Boston, MA, USA
e-mail: Laura.Huisman@tufts.edu

14.1 Introduction

Neurological emergencies account for about one-third of the highest severity codes encountered in the pediatric emergency department [1]. Children present to the emergency room (ER) with a wide range of symptoms, including headache, fever, nausea, vomiting, altered mental status, coma, and physical signs of trauma. Neuroimaging plays an important role because of limitations such as gathering an accurate patient history and difficulties in performing a detailed neurological examination in the ER, particularly in young patients. When faced with a child with an acute neurological emergency, radiologists have to (1) decide whether neuroimaging is required emergently, (2) choose the most appropriate imaging modality based on the institutional availability and the clinical status of the patient, and (3) consider specific issues related to the pediatric age (e.g., higher sensitivity to radiation compared to adults, need for sedation or general anesthesia, different appearance of the pediatric brain related to the age of maturation and development) [2].

Computed tomography (CT) is most often the initial neuroimaging modality of choice in acutely ill children. This method is widely available and fast, and with modern multidetector CT scanners, it is possible to acquire submillimeter-thin cross-sectional images that can be used to render multiplanar reformats and three-dimensional (3D) images. This allows rapid detection of skull and facial fractures. However, the primary disadvantage of CT is that it requires ionizing radiation [2].

Magnetic resonance imaging (MRI) overcomes CT's ionizing radiation limitation and also allows superior anatomic details and various tissue contrast (especially for the evaluation of the posterior fossa). It may also give more accurate information about the timing and quality of injury. Furthermore, MRI can provide multiple advanced and functional sequences progressively incorporated into acute pediatric neuroimaging protocols [2]. These advantages make MRI the preferred diagnostic modality in children with acute

J. Hodler et al. (eds.), *Diseases of the Brain, Head and Neck, Spine 2024-2027*, IDKD Springer Series,
https://doi.org/10.1007/978-3-031-50675-8_14

neurological emergencies. Advanced MRI techniques include susceptibility-weighted imaging (SWI), diffusion-weighted imaging (DWI), diffusion-tensor imaging (DTI), magnetic resonance spectroscopy (MRS), and perfusion-weighted imaging (PWI) including arterial spin labeling (ASL). MRI's main disadvantage is that it generally requires longer scan times, but ultrafast MRI protocols may be considered instead of CT in a time-sensitive setting [3].

Lastly, among the challenges radiologists face is the consideration that children are not small adults and pediatric neuroimaging differs from adults [4]. When evaluating brain MRIs of children, radiologists should be familiar with normal variants, congenital or developmental disorders, and age-dependent changes to provide reliable differential diagnosis and reduce morbidity and mortality.

This chapter aims to discuss the neuroimaging findings of the most frequent causes of acute emergencies in children as well as of some less frequently encountered entities.

14.2 Stroke

Arterial ischemic stroke (AIS) is considered a rare entity in the pediatric population. However, a lack of familiarity often results in delayed diagnosis and high morbidity and mortality rates. Compared to adults, stroke in children has different risk factors and clinical presentations that affect the diagnostic approach, management, and outcome. The most relevant risk factors include (1) cardiac causes (e.g., congenital heart defects, endocarditis, cardiomyopathies, valvulopathies), (2) hematological diseases (e.g., sickle cell disease, coagulopathies), (3) vascular causes (e.g., arteriovenous malformations (AVM), arteriopathies), and (4) genetic/hereditary conditions (e.g., neurofibromatosis type I, Fabry disease) [5]. Acute ischemic strokes presenting in the perinatal period are a specific subset of vascular injury in term newborns and, while they are characterized by different etiologies than in older age groups (i.e., placental emboli, coagulopathies), are often eventually labeled as idiopathic [6].

Acute infarctions may not be visible on ultrasound (US) and CT within the first 24 h of the event. In contrast, MRI provides high sensitivity in detecting acute stroke in children and is considered the preferred imaging modality. DWI and ADC mapping sequences are pivotal. Arterial infarcts appear hyperintense on DWI and hypointense on ADC maps within minutes of occurrence (Fig. 14.1a, b). T2*gradient echo

(GRE) and SWI are the most sensitive in detecting intracranial blood and should also be included. Other recommended MRI sequences include T1- and T2-weighted images (WI) to assess myelination, intra- or extra-axial products, and edema [7].

Furthermore, combined analysis of DWI/PWI findings can identify potentially salvageable brain tissue, i.e., "ischemic penumbra." The ischemic penumbra appears hypoperfused but does not reveal a matching diffusion restriction (DWI/PWI mismatch), unlike the ischemic core which shows matching areas of hypoperfusion and restricted diffusion (Fig. 14.1c) [8].

In addition, MRA of the brain should be performed to assess vascular supply, stenosis, or occlusion (Fig. 14.1d).

Hemorrhagic venous stroke (VS) in the neonatal period may occur as a cerebral venous sinus thrombosis (CVST) complication. Multiple risk factors include maternal and fetal causes (e.g., gestational diabetes, preeclampsia, neonatal sepsis, dehydration, prothrombotic state) [8]. Imaging findings may be misleading and include (1) intraventricular hemorrhage in a term neonate, (2) thalamic, caudate, or parietal hemorrhage, and (3) ischemia not respecting an arterial distribution [7]. MRI remains the preferred modality to diagnose CVST. The appearance of venous thrombus on T1- and T2-WI depends on the age of the clot. T2*GRE and SWI are both indicated to detect venous stasis. Along with MRI, magnetic resonance venography (MRV) should be considered in the setting of an "unexplained" spontaneous hemorrhage (Fig. 14.2) [9].

Numerous other neurologic conditions may clinically mimic pediatric stroke (e.g., hypoglycemia, hemiplegic migraine, seizure, postictal paresis, infection) in up to 20% of children with the initial suspicion of acute stroke [9, 10]. The high frequency underlines the value of MRI in evaluating suspected acute stroke.

> **Key Points**
> - Neuroimaging is extremely time sensitive in children with suspected ischemic or hemorrhagic stroke.
> - MRI with DWI/DTI and ADC sequences is the established modality of choice for accurate diagnosis.

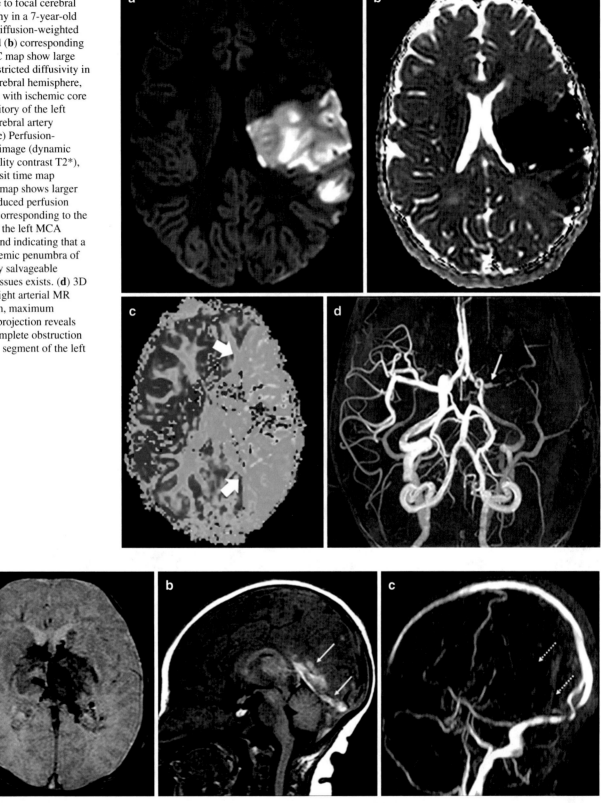

Fig. 14.1 Acute ischemic stroke due to focal cerebral arteriopathy in a 7-year-old girl. (**a**) Diffusion-weighted image and (**b**) corresponding axial ADC map show large area of restricted diffusivity in the left cerebral hemisphere, consistent with ischemic core in the territory of the left middle cerebral artery (MCA). (**c**) Perfusion-weighted image (dynamic susceptibility contrast T2*), mean transit time map colorized map shows larger area of reduced perfusion (arrows) corresponding to the totality of the left MCA territory and indicating that a large ischemic penumbra of potentially salvageable nervous tissues exists. (**d**) 3D time-of-flight arterial MR angiogram, maximum intensity projection reveals almost complete obstruction of the M1 segment of the left MCA

Fig. 14.2 Straight sinus thrombosis in a 6-year-old boy. (**a**) Gradient-echo T2*-weighted image shows venous infarction involving both thalami with a focal hemorrhage on the left side. (**b**) Sagittal T1-weighted image shows subacute thrombus in straight sinus (arrows). (**c**) MR venogram confirms absent flow in straight sinus (dashed arrows)

14.3 Intracranial Hemorrhages

Excluding head trauma, an important cause of intracranial hemorrhages (ICH), spontaneous ICH is a rare, but potentially fatal event in childhood [11]. The most common causes of ICH include vascular malformations (e.g., AVM, cavernous angiomas, and aneurysms), hematological diseases (e.g., coagulopathies and thrombocytopenias), brain tumors, and rare entities (e.g., Moyamoya disease). In addition, ICH may be observed as a complication of AIS and VS. Higher morbidity and mortality are seen particularly in infratentorial hemorrhages, aneurysms, children younger than 3 years, and children with underlying hematological disorders [11]. The presenting symptoms are non-specific, especially in children younger than 3 years of age, including headache, vomiting, impaired consciousness, convulsions, and focal neurological defects. Subacute courses are frequent and result in delayed diagnosis.

US, CT, and MRI may be used depending on the child's age, clinical presentation, location, and availability. ICH follows a well-defined evolution, and neuroimaging appearance varies with the stage of hematoma: hyperacute (<12 h), acute (12 h to 2 days), early subacute (2–7 days), late subacute (8 days to a month), and chronic (more than 1 month) [12] (Table 14.1).

Table 14.1 Evolution of intra-parenchymal hematoma characteristics on CT and MRI

Hematoma age/phase	CT	T1-weighted MRI	T2-weighted MRI
Hyperacute (<12 h)	Isodense	Iso/hypointense	Hyperintense
Acute (12 h–2d)	Increasing density	Iso/hypointense	Hypointense
Early subacute (2–7 days)	Increased density	Hypointense	Hypointense
Late subacute (8d–1m)	Decreasing density	Hyperintense	Hyperintense
Chronic (>1m)	Hypodense	Hypointense	Hyperintense (hypointense rim)

h hours, *d* days, *m* months

On US, exact differentiation between each phase of the hematoma is limited. Acute hematomas typically appear as iso- or hyperechogenic focal mass lesions. Progressively they become centrally hypoechogenic with decreased mass effect, and in the chronic stage, hematomas may dissolve, leaving a hypoechoic CSF-filled brain defect.

On CT, early hyperacute hematomas are isodense compared to normal brain tissue, and consequently it can be difficult to identify hyperacute hematomas. However, intravenous contrast injection may increase the sensitivity of CT in detecting these lesions. Progressive blood clot retraction increases the density of hematomas in the early subacute phases (Fig. 14.3a), while late subacute hematomas show decreasing density due to progressive red blood cell lysis. In the chronic phase, progressive hematoma resorption results in a hypodense, CSF-filled brain lesion.

Similar temporal signal changes are observed on MRI (Fig. 14.3b–d) depending on (1) magnetic susceptibility effects of the evolving blood products and the different oxidation states of the iron within the hemoglobin, (2) magnetic field strength, and (3) applied MRI sequence. T2*GRE and SWI should be included due to the paramagnetic susceptibility effects of hemosiderin. DWI also shows a well-defined temporal evolution of hematomas [12]. Contrast-enhanced sequences and MRA and MRV sequences may be used to exclude vascular malformations or neoplasms as underlying causes of ICH.

Key Points
- ICH is a frequent cause of high morbidity and mortality in children.
- Depending on the etiology and evolutionary phase of the ICH, CT, and MRI imaging characteristics change over time.

Fig. 14.3 Ruptured AVM in a 13-year-old boy. (**a**) Axial CT scan shows hyperdense hematoma in right frontal lobe. (**b**) Axial T1-weighted image and (**c**) Axial T2-weighted image shows hematoma is mainly T1-hyperintense and T2-hypointense, consistent with an early subacute phase (intracellular methemoglobin) and elicits vasogenic edema. Notice intraventricular penetration, with dependent layering in the right occipital horn (thin arrow, **b** and **c**) suggesting more recent bleeding (isointense in T1 and T2—oxyhemoglobin). Also notice prominent vascularity consisting of hypertrophied anterior and middle cerebral artery branches (thick arrows, **c**). (**d**) 3D TOF MR angiogram confirms hypertrophied arterial afferent converging on to a nidus (arrow)

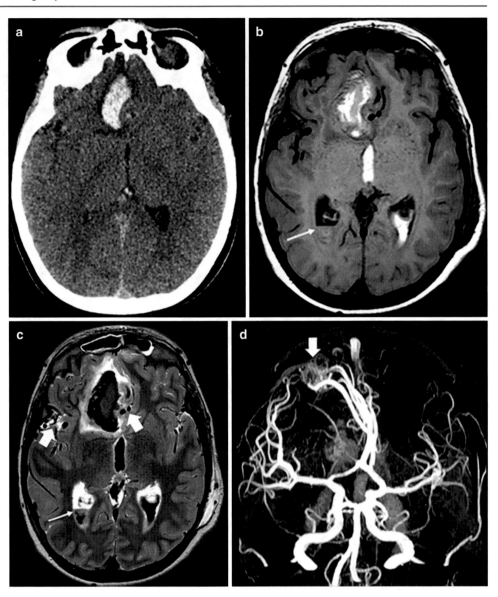

14.4 Seizures

Acute seizures are the most common neurologic emergencies in neonates [13]. Seizures are sudden, uncontrolled bursts of electrical activity in the brain that cause changes in behavior, movements, and levels of consciousness. The increased susceptibility of the neonatal brain is related to age-dependent physiologic features of the developing brain that lead to increased neuronal excitation and decreased inhibition. Seizures are most commonly caused by acute brain injuries. Hypoxic/ischemic encephalopathy is responsible for seizures in up to 90% of full-term newborns [2], followed by intracranial hemorrhages, stroke, infections, acute hydrocephalus, electrolyte and metabolic disturbances, leukodystrophies, and congenital CNS malformations [13]. In a minority of children, seizures may be unprovoked and secondary to epilepsy.

Timely and accurate diagnosis is critical for optimizing management and determining prognosis.

Initial assessment includes general physical and neurological examination, laboratory tests, and EEG monitoring. Neuroimaging is required depending on testing results, and MRI without contrast (Fig. 14.4) is the preferred imaging modality because it has a superior anatomic resolution and is more detailed than CT in assessing potential causative entities. Functional MRI provides further information and helps localize the epileptogenic foci even in cases where structural MRI is normal [14]. In neonates, US may be performed as an initial imaging investigation. Neuroimaging is not indicated in children with febrile seizures but should be considered for

Fig. 14.4 Peri-ictal changes in a 15-year-old girl with ongoing complex partial seizures. (**a**) Coronal FLAIR image shows right hippocampal sclerosis. (**b**) Colorized arterial spin labeling (ASL) image shows markedly increased perfusion signal in the anterior temporal lobe, which normalized at 7-day follow-up (not shown)

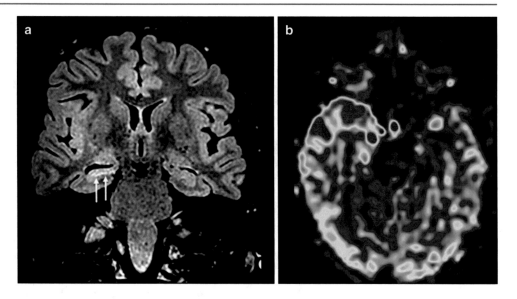

complex seizures or new-onset seizures without a febrile illness [3]. The aim is to detect focal disorders that need immediate intervention.

Key Points
- Seizures are the most common neurologic emergencies of children presenting to the ER and EEG is mandatory.
- Neuroimaging should be saved for cases with history of long-time seizures with focal onset and focal neurological deficits, and in neonates.

14.5 Trauma

Traumatic brain injury (TBI) is a leading cause of disability and mortality in children. Birth trauma resulting from instrumental delivery is responsible for almost all cases of neonatal traumas. In contrast, non-accidental trauma is the most common cause of traumatic death in the first 2 years of life. In toddlers and adolescents, falls and motor vehicle accidents represent the main cause of TBJ [15]. Clinical assessment is often challenging, and the emergency work-up requires a multidisciplinary approach. Pediatric TBJ may occur because of the initial trauma (primary injury) or as a complication of it (secondary injury). Secondary injuries are largely preventable and treatable and imaging plays a key role in limiting their extension [15].

Primary injuries can be extra-cranial (epidural, subdural hemorrhage, subarachnoid, and intraventricular hemor-

rhage), intra-axial (cortical contusion, intracerebral hematoma, and diffuse axonal injury), or vascular (carotid cavernous fistula, arteriovenous dural fistula, vascular dissection, and pseudoaneurysm) (Fig. 14.5). Secondary injuries may be acute (diffuse cerebral edema, brain herniation, and infection) or chronic (hydrocephalus, encephalomalacia, cerebrospinal fluid leak, and leptomeningeal cyst). Multiple imaging modalities are currently available depending on the type, quality, degree, and time of injury. The minimal standard MRI protocol includes (1) sagittal 3D T1WI, which allows multiplanar reconstruction, (2) axial T2WI, (3) axial DWI or DTI sequence, and (4) axial SWI sequence from the skull base to the vertex [16].

In an emergency setting, the presence of hemorrhages of different ages, retinal hemorrhages, change or inconsistency in the reported trauma history, delay in seeking medical care by the caregivers, overall poor care, or when the encountered imaging findings are inconsistent with the trauma history, non-accidental head trauma should be suspected. The most common mechanisms of injury in abusive head trauma include blunt impact, acceleration/deceleration injuries, neck strangulation, and chest compression that may lead to reduced blood flow and consequent brain ischemia (Fig. 14.6). In the setting of accidental and non-accidental trauma, elevated lactate, reduced N-acetyl aspartate, and elevated choline/related compounds on MRS have been demonstrated to indicate poor outcomes by some authors [17].

Further diagnostic workup should include spinal cord injuries, but this topic will be covered in a separate paragraph dedicated to spinal emergencies.

Fig. 14.5 Accidental head trauma. (**a**) Axial gradient-echo T2*-weighted image in a 3-year-old girl shows epidural hematoma; notice typical biconvex shape of the blood collection (arrows). (**b**) Axial susceptibility-weighted image in a 3-year-old boy who was in a motor vehicle accident shows large hemorrhagic (thick arrows) and punctate (thin arrow) areas of traumatic axonal damage

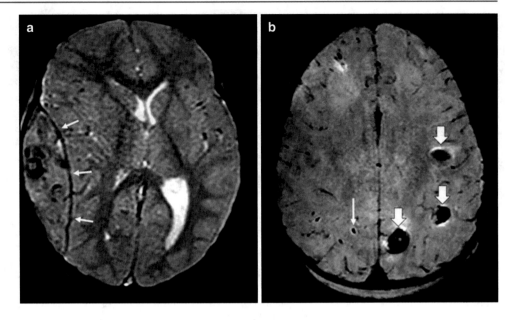

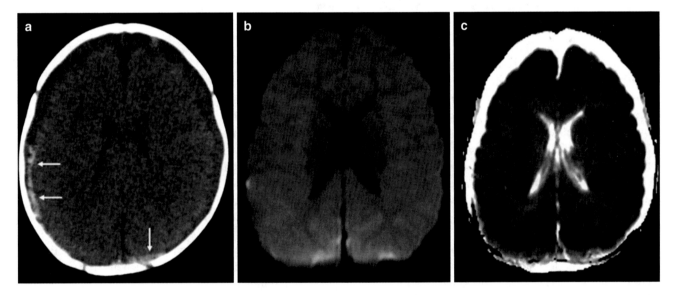

Fig. 14.6 Abusive head trauma in a 2-month-old boy who was found unresponsive. (**a**) Axial CT scan shows diffuse cerebral edema with loss of demarcation between gray and white matter; mixed density subdural hematoma with hyperdense components (arrows) are seen bilaterally. (**b**) Diffusion-weighted image and (**c**) corresponding ADC map confirm diffuse cytotoxic edema with profoundly restricted diffusion

Key Points
- Trauma is a leading cause of disability and mortality in children and depending on the etiology of TBJ and age of the child, CT and MRI are the primary modality of choice.
- It is important to keep in mind child abuse when dealing with trauma in children in an emergency setting. Particularly, in presence of delay in medical care, overall poor care, or when the encountered imaging findings are inconsistent with the trauma history.

14.6 Infections

Infections of the central nervous system (CNS) can be life-threatening if not promptly diagnosed and treated. When a child presents to the ER with non-specific signs and symptoms, including headache, fever, altered mental status, and behavioral changes, CNS infections should be suspected and considered in the differential diagnoses [18]. In an emergency setting, in conjunction with medical history and clinical and laboratory findings, neuroimaging accurately determines brain involvement and suggests the diagnosis in cases where this has yet to be established [19].

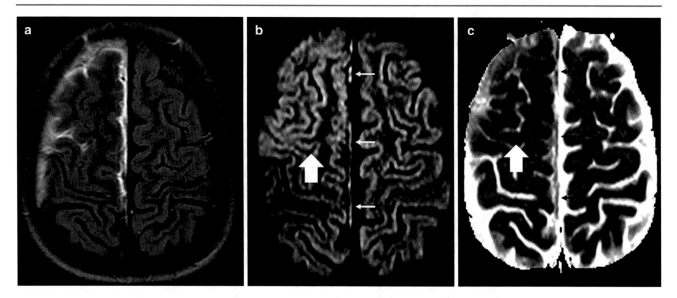

Fig. 14.7 Bacterial meningoencephalitis in a 7-year-old girl. (**a**) Axial post-contrast FLAIR image shows enhancement of the right frontal subarachnoid spaces, consistent with arachnoiditis. (**b**) Axial diffusion-weighted image and (**c**) corresponding ADC map reveal restricted diffusion affecting the right frontal lobe (thick arrow), suggesting cerebritis. Also notice restricted diffusion of the dura along the falx (thin arrows)

Meningitis is the most common form of CNS infection, and bacterial meningitis is usually associated with a higher morbidity and mortality than viral meningitis [18, 19]. Group B streptococcus and *Neisseria meningitidis* are the most common causative bacteria in the neonatal period and in children older than 2 years, respectively [19]. In most cases, meningitis occurs by hematogenous spread from bacterial infection outside the CNS. However, it may also develop from an adjacent infective focus (e.g., sinusitis, mastoiditis), or direct invasion after a skull fracture.

The diagnosis of meningitis is clinical and based on laboratory analysis. A lumbar puncture demonstrating increased white blood cells in the CSF confirms the diagnosis. Neuroimaging is generally used to evaluate complications, including hydrocephalus, subdural effusion, empyema, cerebritis, brain abscess, and infarctions (including strokes secondary to vasculitis). MRI is the modality of choice and T1- and T2WI, fluid-attenuated inversion recovery (FLAIR), SWI, and DWI are especially helpful in evaluating the full extension of CNS affection [2] (Fig. 14.7).

Cerebritis and brain abscesses typically present with focal neurological deficits, seizures, visual defects, personality changes, and more generic symptoms (e.g., fever, headache, nausea/vomiting). Classic MR imaging findings of an abscess include a contrast-enhanced rim surrounding a necrotic core. They appear hyperintense on T1WI, hypointense on T2 WI, and show true restricted diffusion on DWI (Fig. 14.8).

Pyogenic ventriculitis is a life-threatening form of infection. Contrast-enhanced MRIs typically show ependymal enhancement (Fig. 14.9) and restricted diffusion on DWI with reduced ADC values, especially if pus is collecting within the ventricles [20].

Subdural empyema is an infected fluid collection between the dura and arachnoidea. It is a neurologic emergency that can progress rapidly, increasing intracranial pressure and leading to coma and death within 24–48 h. They appear hyperintense on T2WI, isointense on T1WI and show peripheral enhancement [3] (Fig. 14.10).

Acute viral encephalitis is the most common type of encephalitis and often occurs with meningeal involvement [21]. It is caused by direct cytotoxic neurotropic action of viruses that reach the CNS by hematogenous spread or retrograde axonal transport.

Herpes simplex virus (HSV) type 1 is the most common causative agent [3]. Infection predominately affects the limbic system, particularly the medial temporal and inferior frontal lobes [22]. MRI is superior to CT in detecting the often-subtle edema involving the limbic system in the initial stages (Fig. 14.11). In later stages, progressing edema and hemorrhagic necrosis are seen in the hippocampus, cingulate gyrus, and insular and frontobasal regions [19]. Gyral swelling and edema appear hypointense on TWI, hyperintense on T2W- and FLAIR images, and show restricted diffusion on DWI. It is important to note that the enhancement on DWI may disappear within 2 weeks, whereas the hyperintense signal on T2W/FLAIR images may last longer [19].

HSV type 2 encephalitis occurs more often in neonates and immunocompromised patients. Imaging findings of HSV-2 encephalitis are much less uniform, and lesions can

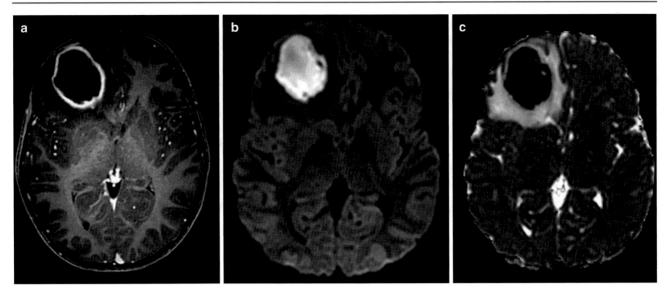

Fig. 14.8 Pyogenic abscess in an 8-year-old boy. (a) Axial post-contrast T1-weighted image shows ring-enhancing mass in the right frontal lobe. (b) Axial diffusion-weighted image and (c) corresponding ADC map show profoundly restricted diffusion consistent with a pyogenic core. Notice marked vasogenic edema surrounding the abscess, characterized by increased diffusion

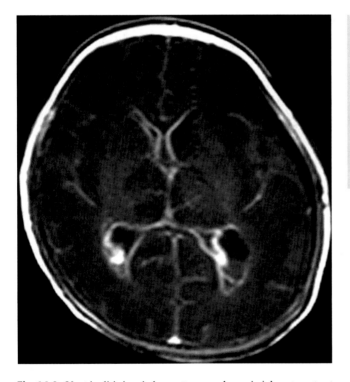

Fig. 14.9 Ventriculitis in a 1-day preterm newborn. Axial post-contrast enhancement shows diffuse ependymal enhancement. Also notice enhancing subarachnoid spaces due to concurrent meningitis

Key Points
- The diagnosis of uncomplicated meningitis is based on laboratory testing and neuroimaging is limited to evaluate threating complications including empyema or parenchymal infections. MRI is the diagnostic modality of choice.
- Acute viral encephalitis is most commonly caused by HSV type 1 and neuroimaging shows typical lesions involving the limbic system on initial stages.

be either multifocal or limited to the temporal lobes, cerebellum, or brainstem [23]. Watershed distribution ischemic injury may be described in areas remote from the primary herpetic lesions (Fig. 14.12). Hemorrhage is less often compared with HSV-1 encephalitis [24].

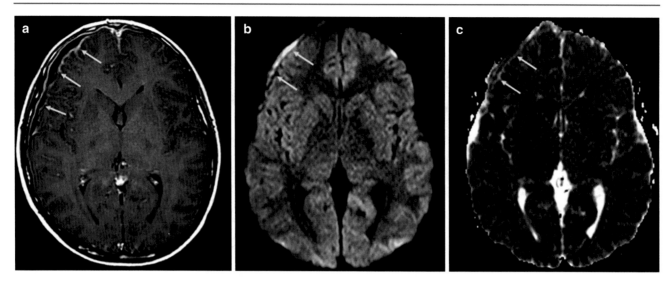

Fig. 14.10 Subdural empyema in a 9-year-old boy presenting with fever and convulsions. (**a**) Axial post-contrast T1-weighted image shows enhancing arachnoid (arrows) underlying a subdural collection along the surface of the right frontal lobe. (**b**) Axial diffusion-weighted image and (**c**) corresponding ADC map shows the subdural collection gives restricted diffusion consistent with a pyogenic collection

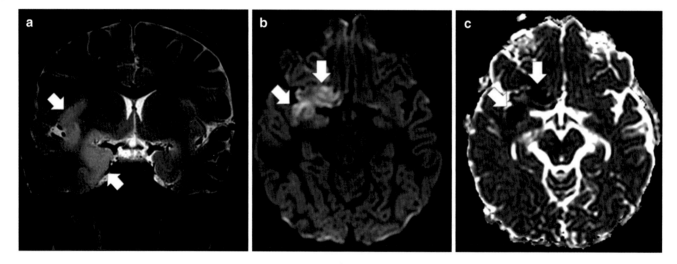

Fig. 14.11 Encephalitis due to herpes simplex virus-1 in a 3-year-old boy presenting with seizures, hemiparesis, and impairment of consciousness. (**a**) Coronal T2-weighted image shows swollen, hyperintense cortex in the right mesial temporal lobe and insula. (**b**) Axial diffusion-weighted image and (**c**) corresponding ADC map show restricted diffusion in the involved cortex

Fig. 14.12 Encephalitis due to herpes simplex virus-2 in a 15-day newborn presenting with seizures. (**a**) Axial diffusion-weighted image and (**b**) corresponding ADC map show multifocal areas of restricted diffusion involving the cortical gray matter of both cerebral hemispheres. (**c**) Coronal T2-weighted image is unrevealing; however, (**d**) coronal T2-weighted image obtained after 1 month reveals severe brain damage with extensive cortico-subcortical liquefaction

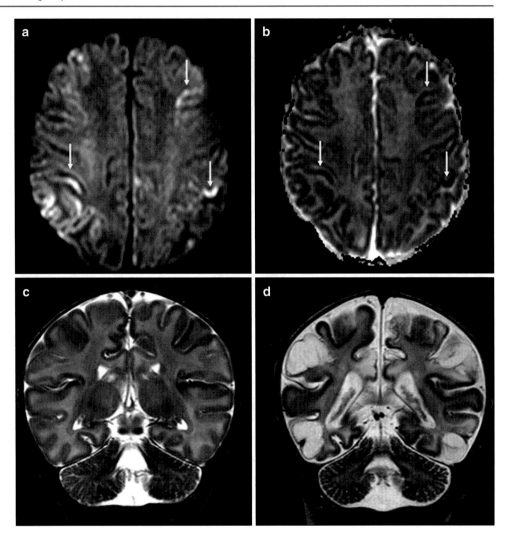

14.7 Metabolic and Toxic Imbalances

Neurometabolic imbalances are characterized by acute onset in a previously healthy child, and manifest with progressive and rapid worsening of the symptoms. Laboratory testing is fundamental and neuroimaging may provide further information to diagnose or evaluate the degree of brain injury and estimate the prognosis.

Diabetic ketoacidosis (DKA) is a serious complication in children with type 1 diabetes that may lead to significant long-term neurological morbidity or mortality. Neuroimaging typically shows brain edema and, in severe cases, may cause focal stroke and subfalcine or transtentorial brain herniation. Focal infarctions typically occur in the mesial basal ganglia, thalamus, periaqueductal gray matter, and dorsal pontine nuclei [25] (Fig. 14.13).

Methotrexate (MTX)-induced leukoencephalopathy is an adverse neurologic effect that may occur in children with leukemia after receiving MTX both intravenously and intra-

thecally [26]. Children may present with stroke-like symptoms, including headache, confusion, lethargy, seizures, transient paresis, aphasia, and dysarthria. MRI shows diffuse T2/FLAIR hyperintensities in the deep white matter of the centrum semiovale and initial sparing of the subcortical U-fibers (Fig. 14.14). DWI will often demonstrate cytotoxic edema as areas of restricted diffusion across multiple vascular territories in the involved regions. These lesions typically resolve once MTX is withdrawn [27].

Osmotic demyelination syndrome (ODS) is an acute demyelination process associated with electrolyte imbalance. Most frequently, it occurs after too rapid medical correction of hyponatremia and is rare in children. It may present with central pontine myelinolysis (CPM) or extrapontine myelinolysis (EPM). On MRI, CPM shows T2-hyperintensity in the central pons, with sparing of the ventrolateral pons, tegmentum, and corticospinal tracts. This produces a characteristic trident-shaped, bat-winged, or piglet appearance. The lesion is hypointense on T1 with no mass

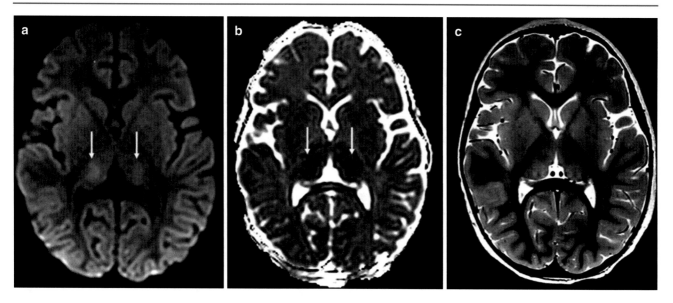

Fig. 14.13 Diabetic ketoacidosis in a 1-year-old boy presenting with impaired consciousness. (**a**) Axial diffusion-weighted image and (**b**) corresponding ADC map reveal reduced diffusivity in both thalami (arrows). (**c**) Axial T2-weighted image shows corresponding mild, ill-defined hyperintensity

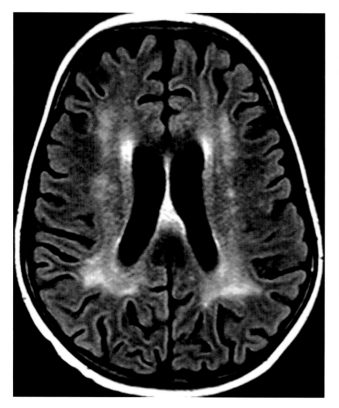

Fig. 14.14 Acute toxic leucoencephalopathy in a 9-year-old girl with relapse of acute myeloid leukemia treated with methotrexate and intrathecal steroids. Axial FLAIR image shows ill-defined, partially confluent, mostly symmetric hyperintense areas involving the deep white matter of the bilateral centrum semiovale

effect. In EPM, lesions are usually bilateral and noted over cerebellar peduncles, globus pallidus, thalamus, lateral geniculate body, putamen, external and extreme capsule, splenium of corpus callosum, and supratentorial white matter [27] (Fig. 14.15).

> **Key Points**
> - In children with toxic/metabolic imbalances, along with laboratory testing, neuroimaging may provide further information to make the diagnosis and to evaluate the degree of brain injury and estimate the prognosis.
> - Localization of the lesions depends on the etiology and MRI is typically the diagnostic modality of choice.

Fig. 14.15 Extrapontine myelinolysis in a 2.5-year-old patient with recent hypothalamic surgery and presenting with diabetes insipidus and hyponatremia. (**a**) Axial diffusion-weighted image and (**b**) corresponding ADC map shows extensive areas of restricted diffusion at level of the subcortical white matter bilaterally. Complete resolution was noted at 6-month follow-up (not shown)

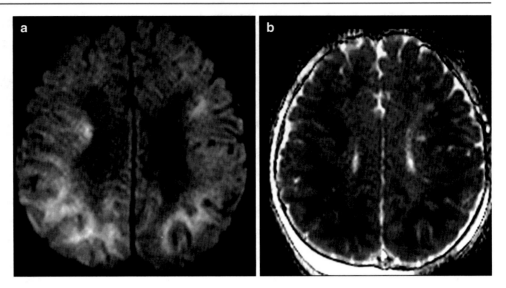

14.8 Autoimmune Pathologies

Acute disseminated encephalomyelitis (ADEM) is an immune-mediated inflammatory disease characterized by perivenular lymphocytic inflammation with acute demyelination in the CNS that occurs 1–3 weeks following an upper respiratory infection or vaccination. It is a monophasic disease with sudden onset, causing rapidly progressive impairment of consciousness and multifocal neurologic symptoms. Brain MRI shows focal or multifocal, patchy, and bilateral T2W and FLAIR hyperintense areas, mainly affecting the basal nuclei and white matter [3, 19] (Fig. 14.16). The cerebellum and spinal cord may also be involved, but these rarely present as isolated lesions without an accompanying lesion in the brain [28]. Acute hemorrhagic encephalomyelitis (AHEM) is a hyperacute variant of ADEM that rapidly progresses to coma and may be fatal. Similarly to ADEM, AHEM occurs in response to a preceding infection or immunization and presents with symmetric multifocal neurologic deficits, headache, and seizures [29].

ADEM is typically a diagnosis of exclusion; therefore, demyelinating disorders, particularly multiple sclerosis (MS), and myelin oligodendrocyte glycoprotein-associated disease (MOGAD) should be considered in the differential diagnosis.

MS most commonly affects adults, whereas ADEM presents at an early age. Furthermore, follow-up MRIs in MS usually demonstrate new and often asymptomatic demyelinating lesions [30].

Neuromyelitis optica spectrum disorder (NMOSD) is an inflammatory disorder of the CNS characterized by severe, immune-mediated demyelination, and axonal damage predominantly targeting optic nerves and the spinal cord. Serum titer of anti-aquaporin-4 antibodies is an important biomarker for the diagnosis. However, MRI also plays an important role in the differential diagnosis of NMOSD, particularly with MS. Longitudinally extending myelitis (>3 vertebral segments) appears hyperintense on T2WI and hypointense on T1W sequences. In most cases, it involves the cervical and upper thoracic spinal cord segments with a central gray matter predominance [31] (Fig. 14.17a, b). Optic nerve sheath thickening, with T2-hyperintensity and gadolinium enhancement on T1-weighted sequences (Fig. 14.17c) has been described in both NMOSD and MS. In contrast to MS, in NMSOD, the optic nerve involvement is typically bilateral and lesions are seen in the optic chiasm as well. Brain lesions include periependymal T2- and FLAIR hyperintense diencephalic lesions surrounding the third ventricles and cerebral aqueduct, dorsal brainstem lesions adjacent to the fourth ventricle, periependymal lesions surrounding the lateral ventricles as well as hemispheric white matter and corticospinal tracts involving lesions [31].

Key Points

- Children with autoimmune CNS diseases may present to the ER with acute signs and symptoms.
- In addition to CSF and serum laboratory findings, brain and spinal cord MRI is helpful to differentiate MS from ADEM and NMSOD.

Fig. 14.16 Acute disseminated encephalomyelitis (ADEM) in a 2-year-old girl presenting with reduced consciousness 2 weeks after an upper airway infection. (**a**) Axial FLAIR image and (**b**) coronal T2-weighted image show hyperintense signal involving the striatum bilaterally

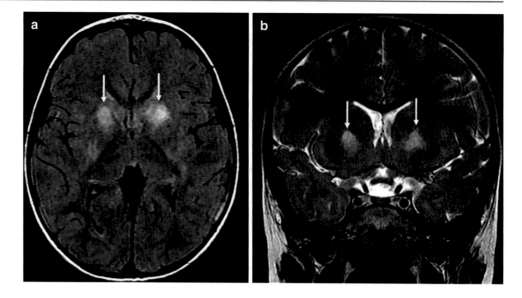

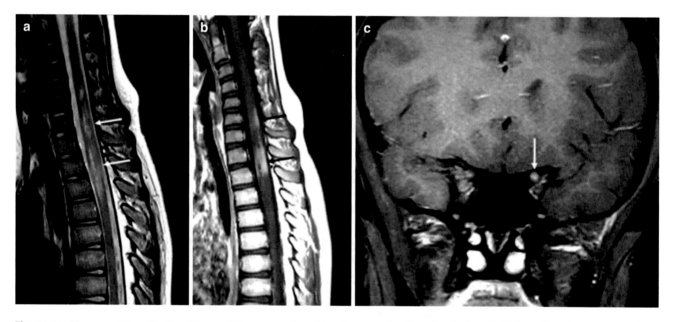

Fig. 14.17 Neuromyelitis optica in a 10-year-old boy presenting with tetraparesis and visual impairment. (**a**) Sagittal T2-weighted image and (**b**) post-contrast sagittal T1-weighted image shows swollen, hyperin-tense cervico-thoracic spinal cord with irregular enhancement. (**c**) Post-contrast, fat-suppressed coronal T1-weighted image shows enhancing intraforaminal segment of the left optic nerve

14.9 Acute Facial Nerve Palsy

Facial nerve palsy (FNP) is frequently presented in pediatric emergency departments. Bell's palsy is an idiopathic or potentially post-viral peripheral form of FNP and constitutes the most common cause of FNP in the pediatric population [32]. Other causes include (1) infectious diseases (e.g., otitis media, mastoiditis, Herpes Zoster, Lyme disease); (2) neoplasms/malignancies (e.g., posterior fossa tumors, parotid gland tumors, leukemia, lymphoma); (3) trauma/nerve compression (perinatal trauma, temporal bone fractures, otic

barotrauma); (4) congenital (facial nerve malformation, cardiofacial syndrome), (5) inflammatory; and (6) metabolic disorders [33]. FNP results from a peripheral lesion of the facial nerve or a central lesion involving the upper motor neuron due to damage above the facial nucleus. Clinical symptoms include immobility of the brow, incomplete lid closure, drooping of the corner of the mouth, impaired closure of the lips, dry eye, hyperacusis, impaired taste, and pain around the ear [34].

Bell's palsy is an exclusion diagnosis, and imaging is not typically required to confirm the diagnosis. Imaging is indi-

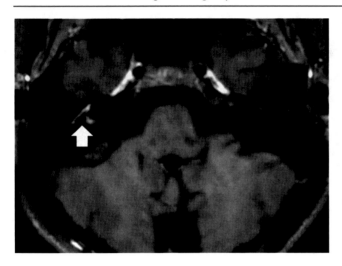

Fig. 14.18 Facial neuritis in a 9-year-old girl presenting with peripheral facial paralysis. Post-contrast axial T1-weighted image shows enhancement of geniculate and tympanic segments of right facial nerve

cated only in the presence of symptoms inconsistent with Bell's palsy, such as progressive onset or paralyses, multiple cranial nerve involvement, no signs of recovery after 3/6 months from the onset, recurrent paralysis, suspected malignancy, or in traumatic cases [33, 35]. Contrast-enhanced CT and MRI are beneficial in these cases, allowing evaluation of all portions of the facial nerve [33, 36] (Fig. 14.18).

> **Key Points**
> - FNP is a frequent presentation in pediatric emergency department and, idiopathic FNP (Bell's palsy) constitutes the most common cause of FNP in children.
> - Bell's palsy is an exclusion diagnosis and neuroimaging is indicated only in the presence of recurrent paralysis, suspected malignancy, progressive onset, and multiple cranial nerve involvement.

14.10 Hydrocephalus

Hydrocephalus in children can occur due to CSF overproduction, obstruction of the CSF flow (communicating and non-communicating type), or decreased CSF absorption due to dysfunctional Pachionic granulations. Pediatric patients may present to the emergency department with symptoms related to acute hydrocephalus or secondary to the complications of shunted hydrocephalus. Clinical presentation varies with age and includes irritability, vomiting, and bulging of the fontanelle in infants. In older children, headache, vomiting, diplopia, or papilledema can be seen [37]. Neuroimaging is necessary to identify the underlying causes, and MRI is the diagnostic modality of choice. Recommended sequences include axial thin-section T2WI, followed by coronal and sagittal reconstruction [3]. The most common imaging findings (Fig. 14.19) include (1) ventriculomegaly, (2) enlargement of the third ventricular recesses and lateral ventricular and/or temporal horns, (3) decreased mamillopontine distance and frontal horn angle, (4) thinning and elevation of the corpus callosum, (5) normal or narrowed cortical sulci, (6) periventricular white matter interstitial edema, and (7) aqueductal flow void phenomenon on T2W images (a sign of communicating hydrocephalus) [38].

Complications of shunted hydrocephalus include infections and shunt malfunctions. CT is often the primary imaging modality because it is readily available and can assess the length of the shunt catheter, the causes of the obstruction and the site of tubing disconnections or migration [3]. Scout views can be useful for detecting possible shunt disconnections below or outside the scanned region that may be missed on axial or reconstructed cross/sectional CT images [39].

CSF cultures are usually sufficient for the diagnosis in children with infections due to a shunted hydrocephalus. Imaging may be indicated in children that along with fever, altered mental status, nausea, and vomiting, present with abdominal symptoms from a peritoneal CSF pseudo-cyst. Abdominal US or CT are helpful in these cases [2].

> **Key Points**
> - Children may present to the ER with acute finding of hydrocephalus or complications of shunted hydrocephalus including shunt malfunction and infection.
> - MRI and CT are useful to differentiate the etiology.

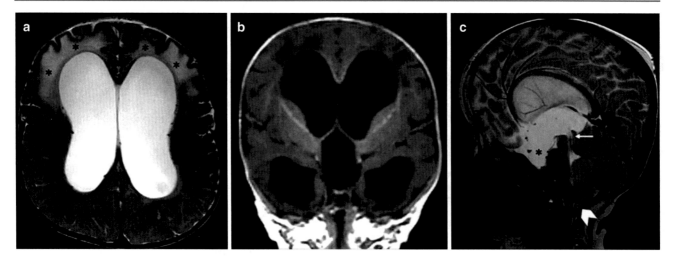

Fig. 14.19 Obstructive hydrocephalus in a 1-year-old girl with Chiari I deformity presenting with severe headache and a large head. (**a**) Axial T2-weighted image shows marked ventriculomegaly with periventricular edema (asterisks) suggesting an unbalanced condition which may herald rapid clinical deterioration. (**b**) Coronal T1-weighted image shows commensurate dilatation of the temporal and frontal horns, an important element in the differentiation from ex-vacuo ventriculomegaly. (**c**) Sagittal T2-weighted image shows marked ectasia of the third ventricle, prominently including the anterior recesses (asterisk); the aqueduct is patent as shown by flow artifact (arrow), while the cerebellar tonsils are protruded into the foramen magnum (arrowhead)

14.11 Drowning/Near Drowning

Anoxic brain injury is a well-known consequence of drowning and may cause severe lifelong neurologic disabilities or, in severe cases, death. Irreversible injury of the hippocampi, basal ganglia, and cerebral cortex have been demonstrated within 4–10 min following the anoxic event. Therefore, early imaging is important for prompt detection of injuries and treatment. CT is useful to detect head and neck trauma, cerebral edema, and loss of white matter differentiation; however, a normal appearing brain parenchyma on early CT does not exclude brain injury. DWI/DTI with ADC mapping on MRI imaging improves the ability to detect brain injuries within minutes of the incident and predict the outcome.

Cortical and deep brain DWI abnormalities, and lower ADC values are associated with poor outcomes (Fig. 14.20). MRS best predicts outcome 3–4 days after drowning [40].

> **Key Points**
> - Pediatric brain is extremely sensitive to hypoxia and irreversible brain injury develops within 4–10 min after drowning.
> - DWI/DTI and ADC mapping on MRI are the most useful sequences to detect brain injuries in children after drowning.

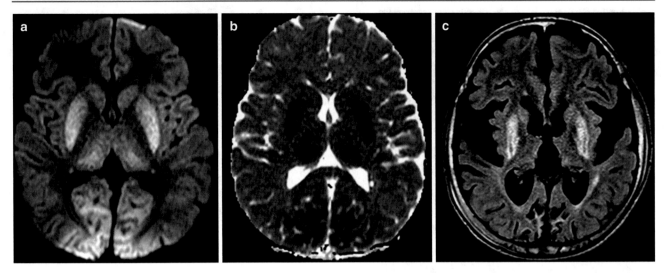

Fig. 14.20 Near drowning in an 8-year-old boy. (**a**) Axial diffusion-weighted image and (**b**) corresponding ADC map show restricted diffusion in the bilateral caudate nucleus, putamen, thalamus, and occipital cortex. (**c**) Axial FLAIR image after 3 months shows profound cerebral atrophy and residual signal changes in the putamen, optic radiations, and calcarine cortex bilaterally

14.12 Spinal Cord Emergencies

Spinal cord emergencies manifest with acute onset of upper and/or lower extremity symptoms (paresis/paralysis), sphincter dysfunction, difficulty walking, and paresthesias in the extremities. Trauma is the most common etiology for pediatric spinal emergencies; other causes include infectious and inflammatory diseases and, more rarely, neoplasms and vascular emergencies [41].

Pediatric spinal trauma is often secondary to motor vehicle accidents, sports-related injuries, falls, and child abuse [42]. Injury location depends on the age of the patients (more often cervical spine due to anatomic differences in the developing spine) [41] and on the injury mechanism (L2–L4 levels in seat-belt flexion-distraction injury) (Fig. 14.21). CT is typically the first imaging study to be performed, and multiplanar reconstructions of the spine show fractures and dislocations with high sensitivity. MRI is necessary to detect spinal cord injuries, epidural hematomas, and intramedullary hemorrhages and allows a better depiction of the adjacent soft tissue [16].

Apart from ADEM, NMOSD, or MS that may involve the spine (previously described), acute spine inflammatory diseases include Guillain-Barre syndromé. It is a demyelinating polyradiculopathy, typically preceded by Campylobacter and Cytomegalovirus infection. MRI demonstrates non-nodular enhancement of the spinal nerve roots, particularly of the cauda equine (Fig. 14.22). Similar lesions and T2-hyperintensities in the anterior spinal cord gray matter are found in acute infection from West Nile virus, too. It results in extremity weakness due to viral tropism for the anterior horn cells of the spinal cord [41].

> **Key Points**
> - Trauma is the leading cause of spinal acute emergencies in pediatric population followed by infectious and inflammatory diseases.
> - CT is typically the first imaging study to be performed showing fractures and dislocations with high sensitivity. MRI is necessary to detect spinal cord injuries, epidural hematomas, intramedullary hemorrhages, and allows a better depiction of the adjacent soft tissue.

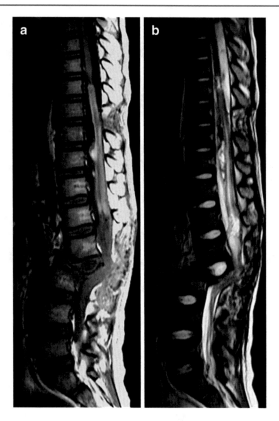

Fig. 14.21 Chance fracture due to seat-belt injury in a 7-year-old boy. (**a**) Sagittal T1-weighted image and (**b**) sagittal T2-weighted image show posteriorly dislocated L2 vertebral body and underlying L2–3 disc with resulting kyphosis and extensive intraspinal hemorrhage, involving both the spinal cord and thecal sac

Fig. 14.22 Guillain-Barré syndrome in an 8-year-old boy presenting with lower limb hypotonia and hyporeflexia. (**a**) Sagittal and (**b**) axial post-contrast fat-suppressed T1-weighted images show enhancing cauda equina nerve roots

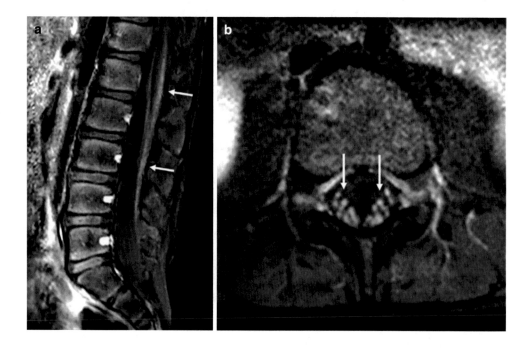

14.13 Conclusion

Children with acute neurological emergencies present to the ER with a wide spectrum of symptoms and signs. Several challenges are faced by radiologists. Firstly, they should decide if neuroimaging is required emergently. Typically, neuroimaging is necessary in cases where it is difficult to gather good and reliable patient history or adequate physical/neurological examination. Secondly, radiologists must be able to choose the most appropriate imaging modality. CT and MRI are used most often in the emergency setting. Lastly, radiologists should be familiar with the age-specific anatomy and maturational changes related to the pediatric age in order to provide reliable differential diagnosis and prompt patient management.

Take-Home Messages
- Children with acute neurological emergencies may present to the ER with non-specific symptoms or subtle findings.
- Radiology is an integral part of the ER and the choice of the appropriate imaging modality depends on the symptoms, age of the patient, and institution availability.
- Radiologists should be familiar with the CNS biologic and morphologic changes related to the pediatric age in order to provide reliable differential diagnosis and prompt patient management.

References

1. Mastrangelo M, Baglioni V. Management of neurological emergencies in children: an updated overview. Neuropediatrics. 2021;52(4):242–51.
2. Prabhu SP, Young-Poussaint T. Pediatric central nervous system emergencies. Neuroimaging Clin N Am. 2010;20(4):663–83.
3. Saigal G, Ezuddin NS, Vega G. Neurologic emergencies in pediatric patients including accidental and nonaccidental trauma. Neuroimaging Clin N Am. 2018;28(3):453–70.
4. Baheti AD, et al. "Children are not small adults": avoiding common pitfalls of normal developmental variants in pediatric imaging. Clin Imaging. 2016;40(6):1182–90.
5. Hollist M, et al. Pediatric stroke: overview and recent updates. Aging Dis. 2021;12(4):1043–55.
6. Stence NV, Mirsky DM, Neuberger I. Perinatal ischemic stroke: etiology and imaging. Clin Perinatol. 2022;49(3):675–92.
7. Lee S, et al. Pathways for neuroimaging of neonatal stroke. Pediatr Neurol. 2017;69:37–48.
8. Chen F, Ni YC. Magnetic resonance diffusion-perfusion mismatch in acute ischemic stroke: an update. World J Radiol. 2012;4(3):63–74.
9. Lall NU, Stence NV, Mirsky DM. Magnetic resonance imaging of pediatric neurologic emergencies. Top Magn Reson Imaging. 2015;24(6):291–307.
10. Shellhaas RA, et al. Mimics of childhood stroke: characteristics of a prospective cohort. Pediatrics. 2006;118(2):704–9.
11. Meyer-Heim AD, Boltshauser E. Spontaneous intracranial haemorrhage in children: aetiology, presentation and outcome. Brain Dev. 2003;25(6):416–21.
12. Huisman TA, Singhi S, Pinto PS. Non-invasive imaging of intracranial pediatric vascular lesions. Childs Nerv Syst. 2010;26(10):1275–95.
13. Shellhaas RA. Chapter 17: Seizure classification, etiology, and management. In: de Vries LS, Glass HC, editors. Handbook of clinical neurology. Elsevier; 2019. p. 347–61.
14. Shaikh Z, Torres A, Takeoka M. Neuroimaging in pediatric epilepsy. Brain Sci. 2019;9(8):190.
15. Pinto PS, et al. The unique features of traumatic brain injury in children. Review of the characteristics of the pediatric skull and brain, mechanisms of trauma, patterns of injury, complications and their imaging findings—part 1. J Neuroimaging. 2012;22(2):e1–e17.
16. Pinto PS, et al. The unique features of traumatic brain injury in children. review of the characteristics of the pediatric skull and brain, mechanisms of trauma, patterns of injury, complications, and their imaging findings—part 2. J Neuroimaging. 2012;22(2):e18–41.
17. Makoroff KL, et al. Elevated lactate as an early marker of brain injury in inflicted traumatic brain injury. Pediatr Radiol. 2005;35(7):668–76.
18. Dorsett M, Liang SY. Diagnosis and treatment of central nervous system infections in the emergency department. Emerg Med Clin North Am. 2016;34(4):917–42.
19. Triulzi F. Paediatric neuroimaging. Neurol Sci. 2008;29(Suppl 3):342–5.
20. Nickerson JP, et al. Neuroimaging of pediatric intracranial infection—part 2: TORCH, viral, fungal, and parasitic infections. J Neuroimaging. 2012;22(2):e52–63.
21. Said S, Kang M. Viral Encephalitis. [Updated 2023 Aug 8]. In: StatPearls [Internet]. Treasure Island (FL): StatPearls Publishing; 2023 Jan-. Available from: https://www.ncbi.nlm.nih.gov/books/NBK470162/
22. Bello-Morales R, Andreu S, López-Guerrero JA. The role of herpes simplex virus type 1 infection in demyelination of the central nervous system. Int J Mol Sci. 2020;21(14):5026.
23. Liu F-Y, et al. A case of herpes simplex 2 encephalitis with an unusual radiographic manifestation. IDCases. 2020;21:e00884.
24. Vossough A, et al. Imaging findings of neonatal herpes simplex virus type 2 encephalitis. Neuroradiology. 2008;50(4):355–66.
25. Barrot A, Huisman TA, Poretti A. Neuroimaging findings in acute pediatric diabetic ketoacidosis. Neuroradiol J. 2016;29(5):317–22.
26. Cruz-Carreras MT, et al. Methotrexate-induced leukoencephalopathy presenting as stroke in the emergency department. Clin Case Rep. 2017;5(10):1644–8.
27. Inaba H, et al. Clinical and radiological characteristics of methotrexate-induced acute encephalopathy in pediatric patients with cancer. Ann Oncol. 2008;19(1):178–84.
28. Stoian A, et al. The occurrence of acute disseminated encephalomyelitis in SARS-CoV-2 infection/vaccination: our experience and a systematic review of the literature. Vaccine. 2023;11(7):1225.
29. Kits A, et al. Fatal acute hemorrhagic encephalomyelitis and antiphospholipid antibodies following SARS-CoV-2 vaccination: a case report. Vaccines (Basel). 2022;10(12):2046.
30. Tenembaum SN. Pediatric multiple sclerosis: distinguishing clinical and MR imaging features. Neuroimaging Clin N Am. 2017;27(2):229–50.
31. Kim HJ, et al. MRI characteristics of neuromyelitis optica spectrum disorder: an international update. Neurology. 2015;84(11):1165–73.
32. Yılmaz U, et al. Peripheral facial palsy in children. J Child Neurol. 2014;29(11):1473–8.
33. Wohrer D, et al. Acute facial nerve palsy in children: gold standard management. Children. 2022;9(2):273.

34. Stew B, Williams H. Modern management of facial palsy: a review of current literature. Br J Gen Pract. 2013;63(607):109–10.

35. Su BM, Kuan EC, St John MA. What is the role of imaging in the evaluation of the patient presenting with unilateral facial paralysis? Laryngoscope. 2018;128(2):297–8.

36. Bilge S, et al. Peripheral facial nerve palsy in children: clinical manifestations, treatment and prognosis. Egypt J Neurol Psychiatr Neurosurg. 2022;58(1):152.

37. Kahle KT, et al. Hydrocephalus in children. Lancet. 2016;387(10020):788–99.

38. Kartal MG, Algin O. Evaluation of hydrocephalus and other cerebrospinal fluid disorders with MRI: an update. Insights Imaging. 2014;5(4):531–41.

39. Orman G, et al. Scout view in pediatric CT neuroradiological evaluation: do not underestimate! Childs Nerv Syst. 2014;30(2):307–11.

40. Topjian AA, et al. Brain resuscitation in the drowning victim. Neurocrit Care. 2012;17(3):441–67.

41. Traylor KS, Kralik SF, Radhakrishnan R. Pediatric spine emergencies. Semin Ultrasound CT MR. 2018;39(6):605–17.

42. Basu S. Spinal injuries in children. Front Neurol. 2012;3:96.

Part IV

Head and Neck

Evaluation of Tinnitus and Hearing Loss in the Adult

15

Graham C. Keir, Jenny K. Hoang, and C. Douglas Phillips

Abstract

Tinnitus and hearing loss in the adult can have profound effects on quality of life. The imaging workup for tinnitus and hearing loss in adults follows otoscopic exam and audiometry testing. CT and MR imaging have different and often complimentary roles in the evaluation of tinnitus and hearing loss, depending on the clinical scenario and the suspected underlying etiology. Imaging can often identify the cause and evaluate the extent of disease for surgical planning. This article discusses anatomy, imaging techniques, and pathologies that cause tinnitus and hearing loss with a mass and without a mass.

Keywords

Temporal bone · Hearing loss · Tinnitus · Otospongiosis
Labyrinthitis ossificans · Superior semicircular canal
dehiscence · Enlarged vestibular aqueduct syndrome
Vestibular schwannoma

Learning Objectives
- Identify key anatomical structures in the temporal bone.
- Describe the role of CT and MRI for temporal bone imaging.
- Differentiate between diseases of the temporal bone on imaging and describe their clinical presentation.

Key Points
- Imaging can identify the cause and evaluate the extent of disease for surgical planning.
- The common causes of tinnitus and hearing loss without a mass include otospongiosis, labyrinthitis ossificans, superior semicircular canal dehiscence, and enlarged vestibular aqueduct syndrome.
- Otospongiosis affects the bony labyrinth while labyrinthitis ossificans affects the membranous labyrinth.
- Vestibular schwannomas often present with non-pulsatile tinnitus and high frequency sensorineural hearing loss.

15.1 Introduction

Tinnitus and hearing loss in the adult can have profound effects on quality of life. Tinnitus is relatively common, with an estimated prevalence of 10–15%, severely impairing approximately 1–2% of all people [1]. Tinnitus is the perception of sound when no external sound is present and may be described as ringing, buzzing, swishing, or clicking sensations. Hearing loss is also common, causing disability in approximately 5% of the world population is indeed "common" and it is indeed referred to as one of the most common disabilities [2]. Hearing loss has several diverse causes and ranges from a partial to total inability to hear sounds. Hearing loss and tinnitus can occur concurrently or in isolation. The role of imaging is to help identify the etiology of these symptoms and evaluate the extent of disease.

G. C. Keir · C. D. Phillips (✉)
Weill Cornell Medical College, New York-Presbyterian Hospital,
New York, NY, USA
e-mail: qgk9003@nyp.org; cdp2001@med.cornell.edu

J. K. Hoang
Johns Hopkins School of Medicine, Baltimore, MD, USA

© The Author(s) 2024
J. Hodler et al. (eds.), *Diseases of the Brain, Head and Neck, Spine 2024-2027*, IDKD Springer Series,
https://doi.org/10.1007/978-3-031-50675-8_15

15.2 Causes of Tinnitus and Hearing Loss

15.2.1 Tinnitus

Tinnitus may be categorized as (1) pulsatile or non-pulsatile, (2) primary (idiopathic) or secondary (due to another condition), and (3) subjective or objective. Evaluation of tinnitus begins with otoscopic examination to evaluate for a vascular retro-tympanic mass, audiometric examination, and a review of the patient's medical history and medications. This evaluation helps to determine if imaging is necessary and if so, what study or studies are indicated.

15.2.1.1 Pulsatile Tinnitus

Causes include vascular masses (glomus tympanicum), aberrant arterial or venous anatomy, vascular malformations, and intracranial hypertension. Objective tinnitus (auscultation of a bruit on physical examination) is uncommon and has been attributed to turbulent flow in the setting of dural fistulas, atherosclerotic carotid artery disease, jugular bulb abnormalities, and large condylar or mastoid emissary veins.

15.2.1.2 Non-pulsatile Tinnitus

Causes include cerumen impaction, middle ear infection, mass, medications, noise-induced hearing loss, presbycusis or chronic bilateral hearing loss, hemorrhage, neurodegeneration, and spontaneous intracranial hypotension.

15.2.2 Hearing Loss

Clinical assessment and audiometric testing can determine the type of hearing loss as conductive, sensorineural, or mixed and guide subsequent diagnostic imaging. Conductive hearing loss results from diseases affecting the conduction of mechanical sound wave energy to the cochlea. Sensorineural hearing loss is caused by diseases that impair the cochlear function or the transmission of electrical signal along the auditory pathway.

15.2.2.1 Conductive Hearing Loss

Causes include otospongiosis (commonly a mixed conductive/sensorineural loss), ossicular erosion or fusion, round window occlusion, dehiscence of the superior semicircular canal, and cholesteatoma or neoplasm with suspected intracranial or inner ear extension.

15.2.2.2 Sensorineural Hearing Loss

Causes include labyrinthine ossificans, vestibular schwannoma, and fractures extending across the otic capsule.

15.3 Anatomy

The temporal bone is comprised of five parts: the petrous, tympanic, mastoid, styloid, and squamous segments. The petrous, tympanic, and mastoid segments form the external auditory canal, middle ear, inner ear, and internal auditory canal. These are the most relevant areas to review for hearing loss and tinnitus.

15.3.1 External Auditory Canal

The external auditory canal (EAC) extends from the auricle to the tympanic membrane. The lateral one third of the EAC is fibrocartilaginous, while the medial two-thirds are surrounded by the tympanic portion of the temporal bone.

15.3.2 Middle Ear

The middle ear cavity contains the ossicular chain which conducts sound from the tympanic membrane laterally, to the oval window and inner ear structures medially. The roof of the middle ear is the tegmen tympani and the jugular wall is the floor. The middle ear can be subdivided into the epitympanum (attic) superior to the level of the tympanic membrane, mesotympanum at the level of tympanic membrane, and hypotympanum inferior to the level of tympanic membrane. The epitympanum communicates with the mastoid via the aditus ad antrum.

The mesotympanum contains the majority of the ossicular chain. The ossicular chain is composed of three bones: the malleus, incus, and stapes. Since the stapes is anchored to the oval window, a mnemonic for the order of the ossicles is "MISO" representing *M*alleus, *I*ncus, *S*tapes, and *O*val window. The manubrium of the malleus is attached to the tympanic membrane, and the head of the malleus articulates with the body of the incus in the epitympanum forming the incudomalleolar joint, which has a characteristic "ice cream cone" configuration on axial sections. The lenticular process of the incus extends at approximately a right angle from the long process of the incus to articulate with the capitulum (head) of the stapes, forming the incudostapedial joint.

An important middle ear structure is the scutum, an angular bony projection to which the tympanic membrane attaches superiorly. Prussak space or the lateral epitympanic space, the location for pars flaccida cholesteatomas, is bounded by the scutum laterally and the neck of the malleus medially. The posterior wall of the middle ear is irregular and includes the sinus tympani, pyramidal eminence, and facial recess.

15.3.3 Inner Ear

The inner ear consists of the osseous labyrinth, which includes the cochlea, vestibule, and semicircular canals. The cochlea contains the end organ for hearing while the vestibule and semicircular canals are responsible for balance and equilibrium. The otic capsule surrounds the osseous labyrinth and is considered the densest bone in the human skeleton [3]. The osseous labyrinth encapsulates the membranous labyrinth, which contains endolymph and is separated from the bony walls by perilymph. The endolymph and perilymph do not usually communicate, and there are contrast-enhanced MRI techniques that allow their separate visualization [4].

The cochlea is a spiral-shaped structure with 2½ to 2¾ turns, including the basal, middle, and apical turns, which are separated by interscalar septae. The lateral aspect of the basal turn of the cochlea bulges into the middle ear cavity, forming the cochlear promontory. The nerve of Jacobson (a branch of cranial nerve IX) courses over the cochlear promontory. The cochlear nerve passes from the internal auditory canal through the bony canal for the cochlear nerve (also referred to as the cochlear fossette or cochlear aperture) into the modiolus, a crown-shaped structure centered within the cochlea that transmits branches of the cochlear nerve to the organ of Corti. The organ of Corti is the end organ for hearing and is not visible on CT images.

The bony vestibule is an ovoid space located superior and posterior to the cochlea, which connects to the semicircular canals. There are three semicircular canals—superior, posterior, and lateral, oriented orthogonally to one another. The endolymphatic duct extends from the posterior aspect of the vestibule toward the posterior cranial fossa, ending in a blind pouch, the endolymphatic sac, at the posterior margin of the petrous ridge. The osseous vestibular aqueduct surrounds the endolymphatic duct and normally measures up to 1 mm at the midpoint and 2 mm at the operculum, according to the Cincinnati criteria [5].

The cochlear aqueduct should not be mistaken for a fracture. It is a narrow bony channel that surrounds the perilymphatic duct and extends from the basal turn of the cochlea to the subarachnoid space adjacent to the pars nervosa of the jugular foramen.

15.3.4 Internal Auditory Canal

The internal auditory canal (IAC) is a channel in the petrous bone extending from the fundus, which abuts the labyrinth, to the porus acusticus. At the fundus, a horizontal crest (crista falciformis) divides the IAC into superior and inferior compartments. A vertical crest ("Bill's bar") divides the superior compartment into anterior and posterior components. The facial nerve is in the anterosuperior compartment, the cochlear nerve in the anteroinferior compartment, and the superior and inferior vestibular nerves in the superoposterior and inferoposterior compartments, respectively. A mnemonic for the location of the nerves in the anterior compartment is "Seven (cranial nerve VII) Up, Coke (cochlear nerve) down."

15.4 Imaging Modalities and Techniques

While CT is often the first modality utilized to assess suspected pathology involving the inner ear structures (cochlea and labyrinth), certain lesions such as a cochlear schwannoma and labyrinthine hemorrhage are better detected with MRI. In the workup of subjective pulsatile tinnitus, CT is frequently the preferred modality. However, MR imaging with MRA and MRV may be more appropriate in the workup of objective pulsatile tinnitus (audible bruit on auscultation by the clinician). Conventional catheter angiography may then follow to further characterize the vascular abnormality as well as to provide therapeutic management (embolization) of lesions such as dural fistulas. MR imaging is the primary modality for evaluating the non-osseous components of the temporal bone, suspected retrocochlear pathology, and sensorineural hearing loss. Magnetic resonance imaging is required when temporal bone pathology is suspected to involve the intracranial compartment.

15.4.1 Computed Tomography

15.4.1.1 Temporal Bone CT Technique

Dual acquisition temporal bone CT (separately acquired direct axial and direct coronal images) has been replaced with multi-detector row CT (MDCT) in which a single set/volume of axial images are acquired and reformatted in multiple planes. Thoughtfully performed MDCT reduces radiation dose, and its rapid acquisition minimizes artifact from patient motion. Intravenous contrast is typically not used with temporal bone CT. When contrast is necessary (tumors, vascular pathology such as dural fistulas), higher resolution MRI, MRI with MRA, or CTA are more commonly.

To acquire temporal bone CT, the patient lies supine in the gantry with the head angled superiorly and posteriorly. The neck is hyperextended so that the orbits are canted out of the pathway of the X-ray beam, minimizing exposure to the lens. Gantry tilt may need to be avoided to facilitate image reconstruction and reformats. The scan coverage is from the roof of the temporal bone (the arcuate eminence) through the mastoid tip. A collimation of 0.5–1.0 mm provides appropriate resolution. The raw data from each ear is most often reconstructed into 0.6–0.75 mm thin axial images using an edge-enhancing (bone) algorithm at a DFOV of 70–100 mm that effectively magnifies the images. Technologists provide reconstructed images including 0.6–1.0 mm reformats in the axial plane parallel to the lateral semicircular canal created from a sagittal plane, and 0.6–1.0 mm reformats in the coronal plane. Axial images with 2–3 mm section thickness of the entire scan volume are also provided in soft tissue algorithm.

Reformats may be obtained in sagittal or oblique planes to improve the detection of pathology in specific clinical settings such as superior semicircular canal dehiscence.

Stenvers reformat: On the console, the technologist scrolls through the sagittal plane until a view of the lateral semicircular canal is obtained. A reformatted axial plane parallel to the lateral semicircular canal is made. The technologist then scrolls through this axial data set and Stenvers reformats are made by tracing a line perpendicular to the long axis of the summit of the superior semicircular canal at submillimetric intervals. This plane is perpendicular to the roof of the superior semicircular canal displaying it in cross section.

Pöschl reformat: On the console, the technologist scrolls through the sagittal plane until a view of the lateral semicircular canal is obtained. A reformatted axial plane parallel to the lateral semicircular canal is made. The technologist then scrolls through this axial data set and Poschl reformats are made by tracing a line parallel to the long axis of the summit of the superior semicircular canal at submillimetric intervals.

15.4.2 Magnetic Resonance Imaging

MRI of the temporal bones is performed in a head coil and should include thin section unenhanced and enhanced axial T1-weighted images, and enhanced coronal T1-weighted images. Fat suppression in at least one enhanced plane may be performed to distinguish fat from enhancement, particularly in the region of the petrous apex. A maximum section thickness of 3 mm with no interslice gap and a small FOV are required to provide images able to depict the fine detail of the anatomy and pathology in the temporal bone. 3D T1-weighted techniques may allow submillimetric scanning on many platforms. 3D T2-weighted techniques are commonly available and valuable in temporal bone imaging to evaluate the relationship of pathologic processes such as a vestibular schwannoma with the surrounding nerves, the patency of labyrinthine structures, the size of the endolymphatic duct and sac, and the extent of cochlear dysplasia in congenital or developmental hearing loss. Reformatted oblique sagittal images perpendicular to the long axis of the

internal auditory canal are helpful in identifying cranial nerve hypoplasia or aplasia. Diffusion-weighted imaging (DWI) can help in distinguishing cholesteatoma (restricted diffusion) from inflammatory middle ear cavity opacification (facilitated diffusion). For this purpose, non-echo planar diffusion-weighted imaging outperforms echo-planar imaging as it is less prone to susceptibility artifact and is capable of thin-slice imaging [4, 6].

Axial T2-weighted, T2 FLAIR, and enhanced T1-weighted images of the brain should be performed to assess for intracranial extension of temporal bone pathology. These brain sequences may also exclude central nervous system pathology such as demyelinating disease, stroke, or inflammation/infection that might produce tinnitus, vertigo, hearing loss, or cranial nerve symptoms.

15.5 Tinnitus and Hearing Loss Without a Mass

When no mass is seen on imaging, the radiologist should closely review the inner ear structures. The common causes of tinnitus and hearing loss without a mass include otospongiosis, labyrinthitis ossificans, superior semicircular canal dehiscence, and enlarged vestibular aqueduct syndrome.

15.5.1 Otospongiosis

Otospongiosis (also referred to as otosclerosis) is an idiopathic progressive disease of pathological bone remodeling that causes conductive, sensorineural, or mixed hearing loss. It results in spongiosis or sclerosis of portions of the petrous bone. Conductive hearing loss is usually secondary to abnormal bone encroaching on stapes with impingement on the stapes footplate. Therefore, stapes surgery is the traditional initial treatment for otosclerosis, but is being augmented or replaced by innovations in hearing aid technology and cochlear implants.

Symptoms typically start in the second or third decade of life and presentation is with progressive conductive hearing loss (approximately 80% bilateral [7]) with a normal tympanic membrane, and no evidence of middle ear inflammation. On otoscopic examination, the promontory may have a faint pink tinge reflecting the vascularity of the lesion, referred to as the Schwartze sign.

On imaging, the disease is seen as lucency in the otic capsule. The most common location of involvement of otosclerosis is the bone just anterior to the oval window at a small cleft known as the fissula ante fenestram (*fenestral otosclerosis*) (Fig. 15.1). Involvement of the otic capsule separable from the oval window is referred to as "retrofe-

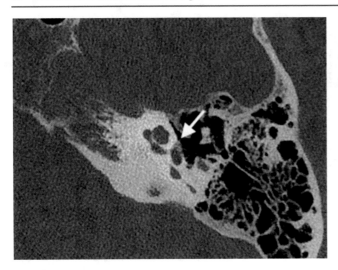

Fig. 15.1 Fenestral otospongiosis on the left with signs of lucency in the fissula ante fenestram (arrow)

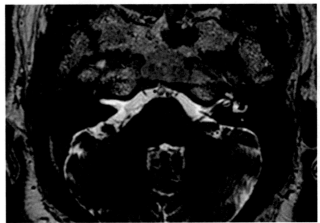

Fig. 15.2 Labyrinthitis ossificans on the right with loss of fluid signal intensity on heavily T2-weighted sequence images

nestral otosclerosis" or "cochlear otosclerosis" and can give a sensorineural component to the hearing loss. The Symons and Fanning grading system for otospongiosis has shown to have excellent inter- and intra-observer agreement [7, 8].

A later presumably less active phase can occur where the bone becomes denser and more sclerotic. The bone still appears to encroach on the footplate but has a density closer to that of the otic capsule making it more difficult to identify.

15.5.2 Labyrinthitis Ossificans

Labyrinthitis ossificans is the late stage of labyrinthitis, in which there is pathologic ossification of spaces within the membranous labyrinth. Profound bilateral hearing loss from labyrinthitis ossificans is most commonly due to bacterial meningitis with onset of symptoms 3–4 months after the episode [9]. Other causes include trauma, hemorrhage, autoimmune disease, vascular obstruction of labyrinthine artery, and surgical insult.

Imaging can detect the evolution of labyrinthitis in three stages: acute, fibrous, and ossification. In the acute stage, enhancement of the inner ear is noted on MR images, while the CT images may appear normal. In the intermediate fibrous stage of labyrinthitis, there is loss of fluid signal intensity on heavily T2-weighted sequence images (Fig. 15.2), while the CT scan may still appear normal. In the late ossific stage, there is replacement of the normal cochlea, vestibule, and/or semicircular canals by bone attenuation, now evident on CT [10].

15.5.3 Superior Semicircular Canal Dehiscence

Superior semicircular canal dehiscence is the most common type of third window abnormalities. The labyrinth is normally in a closed hydraulic system with the oval and round windows. Defects in the integrity of the bony structure of the inner ear can decompress/dampen the energy of the sound wave resulting in conductive hearing loss.

In addition to conductive hearing loss, superior semicircular canal dehiscence can present with characteristic symptoms of vertigo when exposed to loud sounds (Tullio phenomenon). This is because of movement of fluid in the superior canal without movement in other canals. Other symptoms include autophony and pulsatile tinnitus. At audiometry, there is a characteristic low-frequency air-bone gap due to decreased air conduction and increased bone conduction.

On imaging, there is a defect in the superior semicircular canal, best seen in the coronal plane, and on reformatted oblique images in the Stenvers plane (perpendicular to the canal). The Pöschl plane shows the superior canal as a ring and helps to determine the length of a dehiscence (Fig. 15.3). The defect is typically along the superior arc of the superior canal along the floor of the middle cranial fossa. However, a defect can also occur along the posterior limb of the canal facing the posterior fossa.

Other third windows abnormalities present with similar symptoms and include enlargement of the opening of the vestibular aqueduct, dehiscence of the scala vestibuli side of the cochlea, erosion of the lateral semicircular canal by cholesteatoma, and abnormal bony thinning between the cochlea and vascular channels. The presence of a defect does not mean that the patient will necessarily have symptoms or will benefit from surgery. Asymptomatic defects are rare (2% of

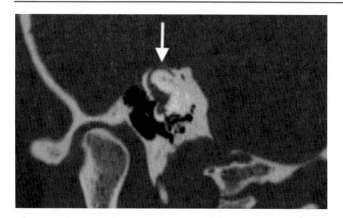

Fig. 15.3 Superior semicircular canal dehiscence on the left. There is a bone defect (arrow) in the superior semicircular canal. Pöschl plane shows the superior canal as a ring and helps to determine the length of a dehiscence

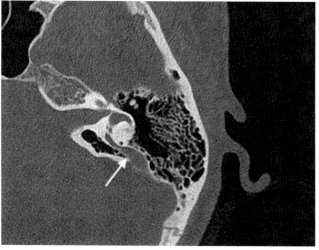

Fig. 15.4 Enlarged vestibular aqueduct. The vestibular aqueduct extends from the posterior aspect of the vestibule toward the posterior cranial fossa (arrow)

the population) so further audiometric evaluation is recommended for all patients with imaging findings [11].

15.5.4 Enlarged Vestibular Aqueduct Syndrome

Most congenital hearing malformations are detected after birth on newborn hearing screening. The exception is enlarged vestibular aqueduct syndrome (EVA) which can progress in childhood or less commonly early adulthood [12]. Stable hearing is observed in 67% of ears with EVA of which 34% will demonstrate fluctuations in hearing. Progression of hearing loss is seen in 33% of ears of which half will demonstrate fluctuations [13].

During fetal development, the vestibular aqueduct starts out as a wide tube. By the fifth week it narrows, and by midterm it approaches adult dimension and shape. However, the vestibular aqueduct continues to grow and change until a child is 3–4 years old. Yet incompletely understood genetic and/or environmental conditions cause EVA.

It is unclear whether EVA actually causes hearing loss, or if instead EVA and hearing loss are caused by the same underlying defect (gene mutation). Supporting this latter theory is the observation that there is an association of EVA with modiolar deficiency [14] as well as the discovery of a specific gene mutation, SLC26A4, which is found in approximately ¼ of patients with EVA [15] and seen in many patients with Pendrad syndrome. Other syndromic causes of EVA include branchio-oto-renal syndrome and CHARGE syndrome.

On clinical exam, hearing loss can be conductive, mixed or sensorineural, and the loss may be stable or fluctuating. Imaging is both diagnostic and prognostic (Fig. 15.4). There are several definitions of an enlarged vestibular aqueduct. The most sensitive criteria are the Cincinnati criteria which

defines abnormal as greater than 0.9 mm at the midpoint or greater than 1.9 mm at the operculum in the axial view [5]. Another frequently used criterion is comparison with the semicircular canals—the vestibular aqueduct is considered enlarged if the width of the proximal intraosseous portion exceeds that of the adjacent posterior semicircular canal. A retrospective study has found the severity of hearing loss in patients with an EVA is influenced by degree of widening of the vestibular aqueduct midpoint width [16].

15.6 Tinnitus and Hearing Loss with a Mass

15.6.1 Vestibular Schwannoma

Vestibular schwannomas typically arise from perineural Schwann cells of the superior or inferior vestibular nerve in the internal auditory canal, near the porus acusticus. They may extend into the cerebello-pontine angle. Vestibular schwannomas often present with non-pulsatile tinnitus and high frequency sensorineural hearing loss. Less often, they may present with symptoms related to mass effect upon the middle cerebellar peduncle, lateral pons, and/or the cisternal trigeminal nerve. The presence of bilateral vestibular schwannomas is diagnostic of neurofibromatosis type II.

Vestibular schwannomas are typically difficult to identify on CT unless quite large. Expansion of the internal auditory canal may be present. On MR imaging, they are heterogeneous on T1- and T2-weighted images and enhance following contrast administration. When large (greater than 2 cm), they often show cystic degeneration. Approximately 5–10% of vestibular schwannomas may have a co-existent arachnoid cyst. Hemorrhage and calcification are rare, unless previously treated [17]. Foci of micro-hemorrhage, identified as susceptibility-related signal loss, is a highly specific finding in schwannomas as compared with meningiomas [18]. When evaluating a patient with a vestibular schwannoma, it is important to identify the full extent of the neoplasm including extension to the cochlear aperture and/or cerebello-pontine angle, and to describe the presence of mass effect on the middle cerebellar peduncle and brainstem. Approximately 60–75% of vestibular schwannomas involve the internal auditory canal and the cerebello-pontine angle.

The goal of management of vestibular schwannomas over the last decade has shifted from "complete resection" to hearing preservation. Treatment may include surgical resection or stereotactic radiosurgery. Clinical and radiologic observation is now common for small, stable tumors [19].

15.6.2 Cholesteatoma

Cholesteatoma is an expansile erosive mass lined by keratinizing stratified squamous epithelium. It may result from a congenital inclusion of squamous epithelium in the middle ear cavity (congenital cholesteatoma), or more commonly from abnormal migration of squamous epithelium into the middle ear cavity through a perforated tympanic membrane because of chronic infection/inflammation. Otoscopic examination typically reveals a pearly white mass behind the tympanic membrane. Erosive enzymes and osteoclast-stimulating agents within the epithelial debris cause bone destruction, the radiologic hallmark of this pathology. Acquired cholesteatomas most often occur in the setting of an under-pneumatized mastoid, a perforation of the pars flaccida (Shrapnell's membrane), involve Prussak space, and erode the adjacent bone including the scutum and ossicles (the mallear head and incus body). The ossicles may be displaced medially. Cholesteatomas related to pars tensa perforations are less common. In these lesions, the sinus tympani, pyramidal eminence, and facial nerve recess may be involved, as well as the long process of the incus and the stapes suprastructure.

In the imaging evaluation of patients with a cholesteatoma, it is important to comment on the extent of middle ear cavity opacification. Specifically, it is important to note if there is involvement of the anterior epitympanic recess, round window niche, sinus tympani, and/or facial recess. The radiologist should comment on the integrity of adjacent bone including the roof of the epitympanum (the tegmen tympani), the lateral semicircular canal, and the facial nerve canal. It is also important to address relevant surgical anatomy, such as the presence of a high or dehiscent jugular bulb, or an anteriorly positioned sigmoid sinus plate. Non-echo planar diffusion-weighted MR imaging is valuable in distinguishing cholesteatomas (which typically have restricted dif-

fusion) from inflammatory opacification in the middle ear cavity (which typically have facilitated diffusion). Frequently both are present, and DWI can distinguish the cholesteatoma from areas of inflammation [20, 21]. Inflammatory disease also typically enhances, contributing to the distinction of these entities.

15.6.3 Glomus Tumor

Glomus tympanicum is a paraganglioma that arises from glomus bodies along the course of Jacobson's nerve (the tympanic branch of CN IX) along the lateral aspect of the cochlea in the middle ear cavity. Glomus tympanicum is the most common primary tumor of the middle ear in adults and presents in middle age with a slight female predominance. The typical clinical presentation is pulsatile tinnitus. Patients may also have conductive hearing loss. On otoscopic examination, a fleshy vascular mass behind the tympanic membrane in the middle ear cavity is most often identified.

When imaging a patient with a suspected glomus tympanicum, the radiologist should first evaluate for and exclude other causes of pulsatile tinnitus. These include vascular anomalies such as an aberrant internal carotid artery, high riding dehiscent jugular bulb, jugular vein or sigmoid diverticulum (outpouching of the jugular bulb or sigmoid sinus, respectively, into adjacent pneumatized temporal bone), and large condylar or mastoid emissary veins that traverse air cells.

The classic imaging appearance is a demarcated mass along the cochlear promontory (Fig. 15.5). These tumors are soft tissue in density on CT, and on MR imaging they are iso- to mildly hyperintense to CSF on T1-weighted imaging, mildly hyperintense on T2-weighted imaging, and enhance

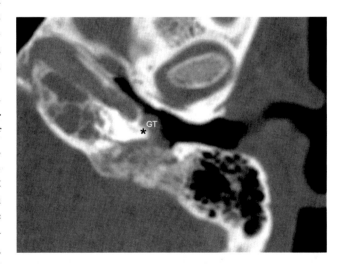

Fig. 15.5 Glomus tympanicum. Axial multi-detector CT image of the left temporal bone shows a soft tissue mass (GT) at the cochlear promontory (asterisk)

intensely following contrast administration [22]. DOTATATE Positron Emission Tomography (PET) has recently emerged as a valuable adjunct to CT and MR imaging for the evaluation of these lesions [23]. While these tumors are very vascular, the typical "salt and pepper" appearance seen in other glomus tumors/paragangliomas is frequently not seen in glomus tympanicum tumors due to their relatively small size. Once establishing the presence of a glomus tympanicum it is important to determine the extent of disease. These tumors are classified based on their spread from the cochlear promontory to the middle ear cavity/ossicles, inner ear structures, external auditory canal, carotid canal, and the mastoid air cells. The radiologist should specify if the tumor is confined to the middle ear cavity (glomus tumors tend to engulf rather than erode the ossicles), identify if there is fistulization to the inner ears structures due to bone erosion, and identify extension of tumor into adjacent structures.

When there is tumor in the jugular foramen, it is important to establish if the middle ear tumor is a projection of a larger glomus tumor arising in the jugular fossa—a glomus jugulare-tympanicum. Glomus jugulare paragangliomas arise from glomus bodies in the jugular foramen, either in the adventitia of the jugular bulb, the superior ganglion of cranial nerve CN X, or along Arnold or Jacobsen nerves (auricular branch of CN X and tympanic branch of CN IX, respectively). They frequently grow directly into the jugular vein (Fig. 15.6a, b).

15.6.4 Cholesterol Granuloma

Lucent, expansile lesions of the petrous apex (cholesterol granuloma, mucocele, epidermoid, meningocele) are com- mon. They are frequently incidental lesions detected on head CTs performed for unrelated reasons. These lesions may be symptomatic when they produce mass effect on adjacent structures. The management of each petrous apex lesion is different, and the clinical history is often of limited use. Biopsy is often difficult to perform, and in certain instances are contraindicated as they may potentially harm the patient. Fortunately, a specific diagnosis can usually be made using a combination of CT and MR imaging [24, 25]. On CT, the pattern of bone expansion, remodeling, and/or erosion are important. On MR imaging, the signal intensity on T1, T2, T2 FLAIR, DWI, and enhanced T1 weighting are often diagnostic-cholesterol granulomas are typically hyperintense on unenhanced T1-weighted imaging and epidermoids classically have restricted diffusion [24, 25]. It is important to describe the size, the location of the lesion, and its relationship to adjacent critical structures, including the petrous internal carotid artery and the internal auditory canal.

Cholesterol granulomas typically arise in a pneumatized space, most often the petrous apex of the temporal bone. It is thought that these develop due to recurrent microhemorrhages at the capillary level, which may result from negative pressures in petrous air cells. The blood incites a mucosal reaction, giant cells, and cholesterol crystal deposition leading to recurrent hemorrhage. This cycle results in petrous apex expansion which can cause cranial nerve symptoms (CNs V and VIII) and tinnitus. The resulting appearance is an expansile, lytic, circumscribed mass centered in the petrous apex, that is often unilocular (Fig. 15.7a). On MR imaging, cholesterol granulomas are characteristically hyperintense on T1-weighted images related to methemoglobin (Fig. 15.7b) though they may be heterogeneous on all pulse sequences due to blood products of varying ages.

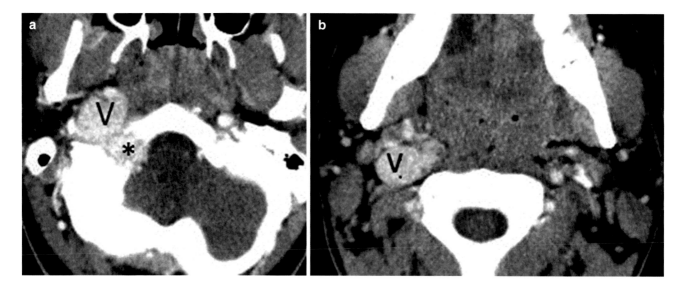

Fig. 15.6 (a, b) Glomus jugulare. Axial enhanced CT images show a vascular avidly enhancing mass in the jugular foramen (*), with direct inferior growth into the internal jugular vein (V)

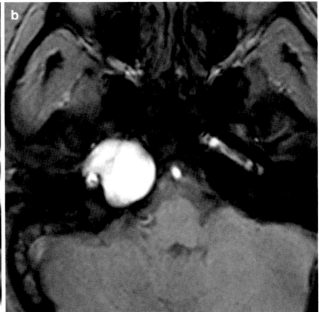

Fig. 15.7 (**a, b**) Cholesterol granuloma. (**a**) Axial CT image in bone window shows a unilocular, expansile mass of the right petrous apex. (**b**) Axial unenhanced T1-weighted gradient image shows the character- istic hyperintensity of these lesions related to blood products. The right mastoid air cells are opacified

15.7 Conclusion

The imaging workup for tinnitus and hearing loss in adults follows otoscopic exam and audiometry testing. Computed tomography and MR imaging have different and often complimentary roles in the evaluation of tinnitus and hearing loss depending on the clinical scenario and the suspected underlying cause. Imaging can often identify the cause and evaluate the extent of disease for surgical planning.

Take-Home Messages
- The radiologist should be familiar with a few key temporal bone anatomical structures and levels on axial and coronal imaging.
- The imaging approach and differential for hearing loss and tinnitus can be based on whether a mass is present or absent.
- MR and CT are complementary modalities. The choice of imaging modality depends on the most likely clinical diagnosis following history and otoscopic examination.

References

1. Langguth B, Kreuzer PM, Kleinjung T, De Ridder D. Tinnitus: causes and clinical management. Lancet Neurol. 2013;12(9):920–30.
2. Deafness and hearing loss fact sheet. World Health Organization. 27 Feb 2023. Retrieved 25 Aug 2023.
3. Little SC, Kesser BW. Radiographic classification of temporal bone fractures: clinical predictability using a new system. Arch Otolaryngol Head Neck Surg. 2006;132(12):1300–4.
4. Benson JC, Carlson ML, Lane JI. MRI of the internal auditory canal, labyrinth, and middle ear: how we do it. Radiology. 2020;297(2):252–65.
5. El-Badry MM, Osman NM, Mohamed HM, Rafaat FM. Evaluation of the radiological criteria to diagnose large vestibular aqueduct syndrome. Int J Pediatr Otorhinolaryngol. 2016;81:84–91.
6. van Egmond SL, Stegeman I, Grolman W, Aarts MCJ. A systematic review of non-echo planar diffusion-weighted magnetic resonance imaging for detection of primary and postoperative cholesteatoma. Otolaryngol Head Neck Surg. 2016;154(2):233–40.
7. Lee TC, Aviv RI, Chen JM, Nedzelski JM, Fox AJ, Symons SP. CT grading of otosclerosis. AJNR Am J Neuroradiol. 2009;30(7):1435–9.
8. Marshall AH, Fanning N, Symons S, et al. Cochlear implantation in cochlear otosclerosis. Laryngoscope. 2005;115:1728–33.
9. Hartnick CJ, Kim HY, Chute PM, Parisier SC. Preventing labyrinthitis ossificans. Arch Otolaryngol Neck Surg. 2001;127(2):180.
10. Juliano AF, Ginat DT, Moonis G. Imaging review of the temporal bone: part I. Anatomy and inflammatory and neoplastic processes. Radiology. 2013;269(1):17–33.

11. Berning AW, Arani K, Branstetter BF. Prevalence of superior semicircular canal dehiscence on high-resolution CT imaging in patients without vestibular or auditory abnormalities. AJNR Am J Neuroradiol. 2019;40(4):709–12.

12. Wieczorek SS, Anderson ME, Harris DA, Mikulec AA. Enlarged vestibular aqueduct syndrome mimicking otosclerosis in adults. Am J Otolaryngol. 2013;34(6):619–25.

13. Mori T, Westerberg BD, Atashband S, Kozak FK. Natural history of hearing loss in children with enlarged vestibular aqueduct syndrome. J Otolaryngol Head Neck Surg. 2008;37(1):112–8.

14. Naganawa S, Ito T, Iwayama E, et al. MR imaging of the cochlear modiolus: area measurement in healthy subjects and in patients with a large endolymphatic duct and sac. Radiology. 1999;213(3):819–23.

15. Madden C, Halsted M, Meinzen-Derr J, et al. The influence of mutations in the SLC26A4 gene on the temporal bone in a population with enlarged vestibular aqueduct [published correction appears in Arch Otolaryngol Head Neck Surg. 2007 Jun;133(6):607]. Arch Otolaryngol Head Neck Surg. 2007;133(2):162–8.

16. Saliba I, Gingras-Charland M-E, St-Cyr K, Décarie J-C. Coronal CT scan measurements and hearing evolution in enlarged vestibular aqueduct syndrome. Int J Pediatr Otorhinolaryngol. 2012;76(4):492–9.

17. Shahbazi T, Sabahi M, Arjipour M, Adada B, Borghei-Razavi H. Hemorrhagic vestibular schwannoma: case report and literature review of incidence and risk factors. Cureus. 2020;12(9):e10183.

18. Thamburaj K, Radhakrishnan VV, Thomas B, Nair S, Menon G. Intratumoral microhemorrhages on T2*-weighted gradient-echo imaging helps differentiate vestibular schwannoma from meningioma. AJNR Am J Neuroradiol. 2008;29(3):552–7.

19. Lin EP, Crane BT. The management and imaging of vestibular schwannomas. Am J Neuroradiol. 2017;38(11):2034–43.

20. Schwartz KM, Lane JI, Bolster BD, Neff BA. The utility of diffusion-weighted imaging for cholesteatoma evaluation. Am J Neuroradiol. 2011;32(3):430–6.

21. Dremmen MH, Hofman PA, Hof JR, Stokroos RJ, Postma AA. The diagnostic accuracy of non-echo-planar diffusion-weighted imaging in the detection of residual and/or recurrent cholesteatoma of the temporal bone. AJNR Am J Neuroradiol. 2012;33(3):439–44.

22. Alaani A, Chavda SV, Irving RM. The crucial role of imaging in determining the approach to glomus tympanicum tumours. Eur Arch Otorhinolaryngol. 2009;266(6):827–31.

23. Rini JN, Keir G, Caravella C, Goenka A, Franceschi AM. Somatostatin receptor-PET/CT/MRI of head and neck neuroendocrine tumors. AJNR Am J Neuroradiol. 2023;44(8):959–66.

24. Schmalfuss IM. Petrous apex. Neuroimaging Clin N Am. 2009;19(3):367–91.

25. Chapman PR, Shah R, Cure JK, Bag AK. Petrous apex lesions: pictorial review. Am J Roentgenol. 2011;196(3):WS26–37.

Approach to Masses in Head and Neck Spaces

16

Brianna E. Damadian, Patricia A. Rhyner, and Deborah R. Shatzkes

Abstract

The neck is anatomically complex and exhibits a wide range of pathologies, making the imaging diagnosis of masses in this region challenging. Organizing the neck into specific "spaces" based on fascial planes and individual contents is a helpful approach to generating a differential diagnosis. Once a mass is localized within a neck space, then specific imaging features and clinical context can be applied to narrow these different considerations. In this chapter, we will review the normal anatomy and contents of each space in the suprahyoid and infrahyoid neck and discuss the specific pathologies typically found in each space.

Keywords

Head and neck spaces · Head and neck masses Suprahyoid neck · Infrahyoid neck · Neck anatomy Cervical fascia

Learning Objectives
- To understand how the layers of the deep cervical fascia, along with muscles and bones, help define "spaces" or compartments in the neck.
- To understand the normal anatomy and contents of each of the spaces in the suprahyoid and infrahyoid neck.
- To accurately localize neck pathology into a specific space in order to generate the most appropriate differential diagnosis.

B. E. Damadian · D. R. Shatzkes (✉)
Department of Radiology, Zucker School of Medicine at Hofstra/Northwell Health, New York, NY, USA
e-mail: bdamadian@northwell.edu

P. A. Rhyner
Department of Radiology, Mayo Clinic, Jacksonville, FL, USA

16.1 Introduction to Head and Neck Spaces

While the neck is anatomically complex, it can be organized into specific "spaces" or compartments based on fascial planes and individual contents [1, 2]. Some authors argue that the term "space" may be an oversimplification and lead to confusion. These authors propose naming fascial layers in functional terms and using the term "compartment," which can be bound by bone, muscle, and/or fascia. For consistency with radiologic literature, this review will use the term "space" but will attempt to point out any potentially confusing terms and propose newer terminology to promote interdisciplinary communication. The ability to place pathology within a neck space is the first step to generating a differential diagnosis; then, specific imaging features and clinical context can be applied to narrow these different considerations.

The neck can be divided into suprahyoid and infrahyoid spaces by the hyoid bone. Some head and neck spaces traverse both the suprahyoid and infrahyoid neck. Two layers of fascia, superficial and deep, are commonly used to define the spaces of the neck. The superficial cervical fascia (SCF) is a thin layer, investing loose connective and adipose tissue, the platysma muscle, superficial lymph nodes, and muscles of facial expression. Some surgeons refer to SCF simply as "subcutaneous tissue" [3] to prevent confusion with the superficial layer of the deep cervical fascia (SLDCF), which is described below.

The deep cervical fascia is further subdivided into three layers: superficial, middle, and deep. The superficial layer of deep cervical fascia (SLDCF) lies between the SCF (or subcutaneous tissue) and the muscles of the neck; it attaches anteriorly to the hyoid, superiorly to the mandible, and to the mastoid process and external occipital protuberance. The "rule of twos" is a helpful way to remember that the SLDCF encloses two glands (submandibular and parotid) and two muscles (sternocleidomastoid and trapezius).

J. Hodler et al. (eds.), *Diseases of the Brain, Head and Neck, Spine 2024-2027*, IDKD Springer Series,
https://doi.org/10.1007/978-3-031-50675-8_16

Some surgeons refer to the subdivisions of the SLDCF as the masticator fascia, submandibular fascia, and sternocleidomastoid/trapezius fascia, choosing to define fascia by function.

The middle layer of deep cervical fascia (MLDCF) extends from the skull base to the mediastinum and is divided into a muscular layer and a visceral layer. The muscular layer invests the strap muscles, while the visceral layer (also called buccopharyngeal in the suprahyoid neck) invests the larynx, pharynx, trachea, esophagus, and thyroid. The deep layer of deep cervical fascia (DLDCF) surrounds the vertebral column and paravertebral muscles with two distinct components: the alar and prevertebral fascia. The alar layer forms the posterior and lateral walls of the retropharyngeal space and bridges the transverse processes of the vertebrae. The prevertebral layer encloses the paraspinal muscles: the longus colli and longus capitis muscles; the anterior, middle, and posterior scalene muscles; and the levator scapulae. The carotid sheath is generally thought to be composed of all three layers of DCF though the thickness of the carotid sheath varies among individuals and at different levels in the neck.

The suprahyoid neck spaces comprise the area from the base of skull to the hyoid bone, excluding the orbits, paranasal sinuses, and oral cavity. The spaces of the suprahyoid neck include the pharyngeal mucosal space (PMS), the sublingual space (SLS), the submandibular space (SMS), the parapharyngeal space (PPS), the parotid space (PS), and the masticator space (MS). Those spaces traversing the entire neck (suprahyoid and infrahyoid) include the carotid space (CS), the retropharyngeal and danger space (RPS), and the perivertebral space (PVS). In addition to the entire neck spaces (listed above), the infrahyoid neck also contains the visceral space (VS), which includes the thyroid and parathyroid glands and the larynx, hypopharynx, trachea, and cervical esophagus.

16.2 Suprahyoid Neck: Pharyngeal Mucosal Space (PMS)

16.2.1 Anatomy and Contents

The contents of the pharyngeal mucosal space include the mucosa of the nasopharynx and oropharynx, as well as submucosal structures such as Waldeyer's ring, minor salivary glands (MSGs), the pharyngeal constrictor and levator veli palatine muscles, and the torus tubarius bordering the Eustachian tube orifice [4]. Waldeyer's ring comprises the adenoids and the palatine and lingual tonsils; the ring-like configuration of lymphoid tissue can be thought of as a mechanism to protect the body from inhaled and ingested antigens. Deep mucosa-lined tonsillar crypts result in a char-

acteristic striped appearance on contrast-enhanced imaging and may hide small primary tumors.

> **Key Point**
> • While squamous cell carcinoma is the most common tumor of the PMS, the presence of Waldeyer's ring lymphoid tissue and submucosal minor salivary glands may result in lymphoproliferative and salivary neoplasms, respectively.

16.2.2 Pathology

The most common malignant neoplasm in this space is squamous cell carcinoma arising from the mucosa, which is covered in a separate chapter. Tumors arising from Waldeyer's ring lymphoid tissue and MSGs are considerably less common. Inflammatory disease of the oropharynx represents a spectrum ranging from non-focal tonsillitis to tonsillar or peritonsillar abscess (Fig. 16.1). Congenital lesions of the PMS include the central nasopharyngeal Tornwaldt cyst and those related to the embryologic thyroglossal duct, including cysts and the lingual thyroid (Fig. 16.2).

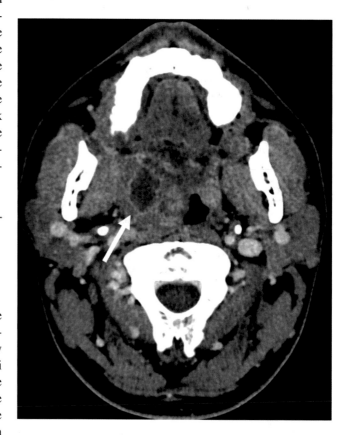

Fig. 16.1 Axial CECT shows a discrete rim-enhancing fluid collection (arrow) lateral to an enlarged and inflamed tonsil in a patient with tonsillitis and peritonsillar abscess

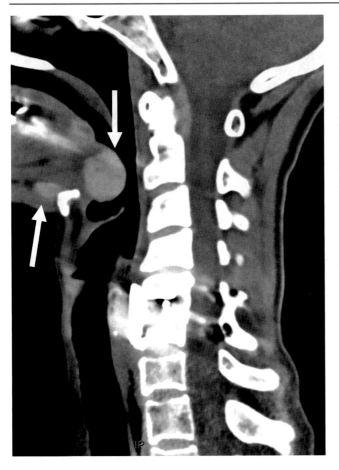

Fig. 16.2 Sagittal CECT shows two sites of ectopic lingual thyroid tissue, one in the pharyngeal mucosal space at the base of tongue and the other anterior to the hyoid bone. Additional images confirmed absence of normal thyroid tissue in the thyroid bed

16.3   Suprahyoid Neck: Parapharyngeal Space (PPS)

16.3.1 Anatomy and Contents

The PPS is a triangular fat-containing space lateral to the PMS. It is bound laterally by the masticator and parotid spaces, posteriorly by the retropharyngeal and carotid spaces, and superiorly by the skull base, with inferior extension into the submandibular space. The PPS contents are simple: fat, minor salivary glands, and, rarely, lymph nodes.

16.3.2 Pathology

Primary pathology of the PPS is rare, with the majority of lesions originating from minor salivary glands and representing benign mixed tumors (BMTs) [5]. The PPS is most often affected by pathology of neighboring spaces, and the pattern of deviation or deformity of the PPS fat may be helpful in identifying the space of origin. For example, while a well-defined markedly T2-hyperintense mass bounded entirely by fat is likely a primary PPS BMT, a similar lesion contiguous with the deep lobe of the parotid and displacing the PPS fat anteromedially more likely originates in the parotid space (Fig. 16.3). Similarly, masticator space lesions displace the PPS fat posteromedially, PMS lesions laterally, and carotid space lesions anteriorly.

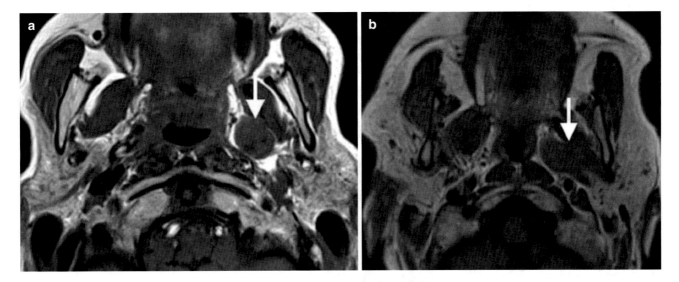

Fig. 16.3 (**a**) Primary BMT of the left PPS (arrow) is surrounded entirely by fat on axial T1-weighted image. (**b**) Axial T1-weighted image shows a primary BMT of the left parotid space (arrow) inseparable from the deep lobe and displacing PPS fat medially

16.4 Suprahyoid Neck: Masticator Space (MS)

16.4.1 Anatomy and Contents

Located lateral to the PPS, the MS contains the muscles of mastication (masseter, temporalis, and medial and lateral pterygoids), the posterior body and ramus of the mandible, and the mandibular nerve (a branch of the trigeminal nerve).

16.4.2 Pathology

As with the PPS, most pathology of the MS originates in the neighboring spaces, the most common being odontogenic infection arising from molar teeth within the neighboring oral cavity [6]. Dental abscesses may extend to the medial pterygoid or masseter muscles and may also result in osteomyelitis of the posterior mandibular body and condyle (Fig. 16.4). Another common non-neoplastic lesion affecting the MS is the venous malformation (VM), which has a predilection for the muscles of mastication and is a frequent incidental finding on imaging studies performed for unrelated indications (Fig. 16.5). The presence of phleboliths within a

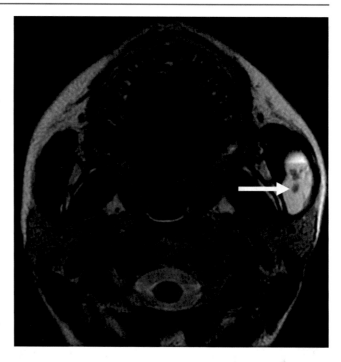

Fig. 16.5 Axial T2-weighted image shows a markedly hyperintense mass in the left masseter muscle with fluid-fluid level and internal rounded areas of signal void (arrow). These represent phleboliths, which are virtually pathognomonic for a venous malformation

markedly T2-hyperintense and heterogeneously enhancing mass is virtually pathognomonic for VM. Neoplastic entities of the MS include perineural spread of tumor to cranial nerve V3 or, much less commonly, primary nerve sheath tumors of cranial nerve V3 such as schwannomas. Primary neoplasms of the muscles of mastication, such as sarcomas and lymphoproliferative malignancies, are exceedingly rare. More often, malignant MS disease results from spread of tumors arising in the pharynx, oral cavity, or parotid space.

16.5 Suprahyoid Neck: Parotid Space (PS)

16.5.1 Anatomy and Contents

The PS contains the parotid gland, facial nerve, retromandibular vein, and branches of the external carotid artery. The plane of the facial nerve bisects the parotid gland into superficial and deep lobes; localization of lesions into one of these lobes is key to prevent inadvertent facial nerve injury during resection. The plane may be approximated on cross-sectional imaging by identifying the stylomandibular tunnel, located between the styloid process and the posterior cortex of the mandibular condyle, as well as by the position of the retromandibular vein.

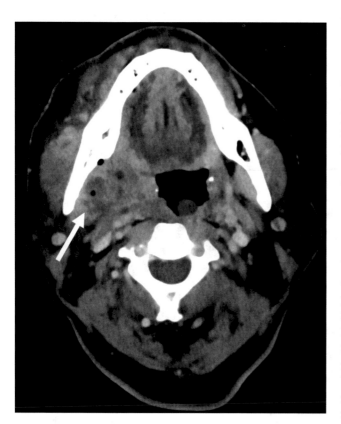

Fig. 16.4 Axial CECT image shows a fluid and gas collection centered in the right medial pterygoid muscle (arrow), representing odontogenic abscess arising from the right mandibular third molar

16.5.2 Pathology

The parotid gland is the only salivary gland to contain lymph nodes, with the important consequence that the differential diagnosis for lymphadenopathy, including neoplastic and inflammatory etiologies, must be considered for any PS mass [7]. The parotid lymph nodes also represent first echelon drainage for cancers of the external auditory canal as well skin cancers of portions of the scalp and facial skin. Fortunately, most primary salivary epithelial neoplasms represent benign mixed tumors; these typically demonstrate very high signal on T2-weighted and ADC scans (Fig. 16.6). This is one of the few parotid neoplasms that demonstrates characteristic imaging features. In general, given the very diverse neoplastic histology of this region, a specific diagnosis cannot be reliably predicted based on CT or MR imaging.

Infectious/inflammatory diagnoses in the PS include both acute and chronic parotitis. Acute parotitis may occur secondary to obstruction by calculi, retrograde migration of oral flora due to poor salivary flow, or hematogenic viral infection. Chronic parotitis is typically bilateral and reflects underlying systemic disease such as Sjogren syndrome or sarcoidosis.

> **Key Point**
> - The parotid gland is the only salivary gland to contain lymph nodes; the differential diagnosis for lymphadenopathy must be considered for any PS mass.

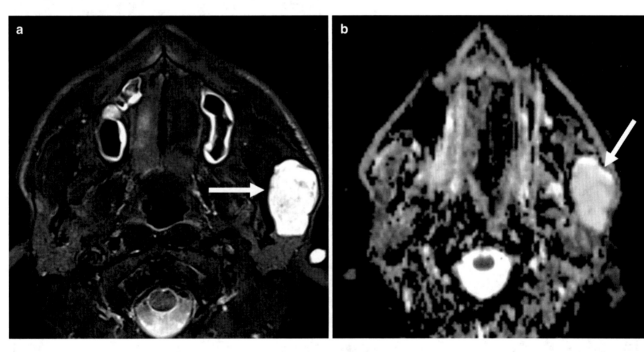

Fig. 16.6 (**a**) Axial STIR image demonstrates a well-circumscribed markedly T2 hyperintense mass in the superficial lobe of the right parotid, a pathologically proven benign mixed tumor (arrow). (**b**) The corresponding ADC map demonstrates high signal, indicating relatively free diffusivity of water in these gelatinous tumors

16.6 Suprahyoid Neck: Sublingual (SLS) and Submandibular Space (SMS)

16.6.1 Anatomy and Contents

The oral cavity (OC) is anatomically complex with an extensive, convoluted mucosal surface covering its constituent structures: the tongue, floor of mouth, hard palate, cheeks, and gingiva. The SLS is the portion of the floor of mouth below the tongue and above the mylohyoid muscle, a sling-like structure that separates the OC above from the SMS below (Fig. 16.7) [8]. The SLS contains the sublingual glands (SLGs), the deep lobes of the submandibular glands (SMGs) and submandibular ducts, the "neurovascular bundles" (lingual nerves, arteries, and veins), and cranial nerves 9 and 12. The SMS is relatively simple in composition, containing only the SMG superficial lobe, fat, lymph nodes, and the facial artery and vein.

16.6.2 Pathology

Much like in the MS, inflammatory disease is a common entity in the SLS and SMS, with the teeth and salivary glands as the principal sources. It is important to recognize that symptoms localized to the SMS could be caused by pathology in the SLS. For example, sialoliths frequently impact distally at the punctum of the submandibular duct, which is

part of the SLS. An obstructing sialolith in the SLS may cause upstream inflammatory disease of the SMG, part of which is located in the SMS. Dental artifact frequently obscures calculi at the anterior floor of mouth, making a high index of suspicion and careful search imperative to diagnosis (Fig. 16.8). Obstruction of the SLG or a submucosal MSG

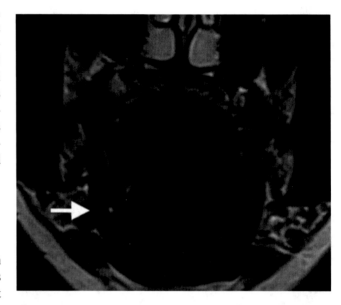

Fig. 16.7 Coronal T2-weighted image shows the mylohyoid (arrow), the sling-like muscle that separates the oral cavity above from the SMS below

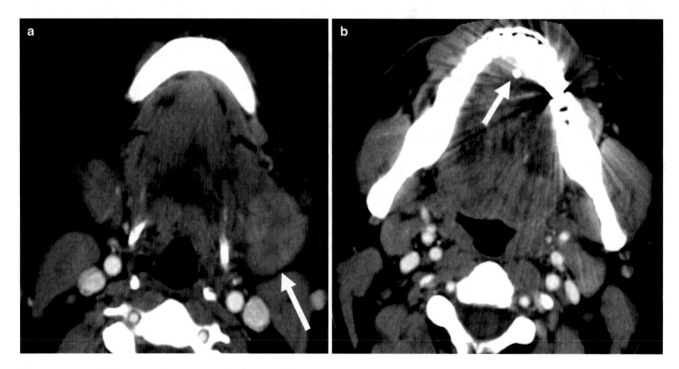

Fig. 16.8 (**a**) Axial CECT depicts an enlarged, edematous SMG (arrow) in the SMS, representing acute sialadenitis. (**b**) Axial CECT identifies the causative obstructing calculus (arrow), located in the submandibular duct at anterior floor of mouth in the SLS

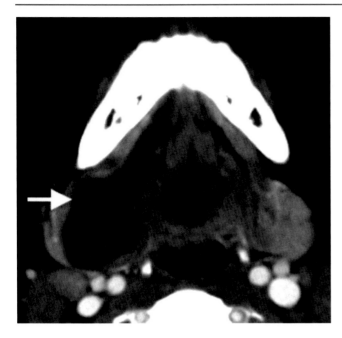

Fig. 16.9 Axial CECT depicts a "diving" or "plunging" ranula (arrow) extending from the SLS to the SMS behind the posterior free edge of the mylohyoid muscle

duct may result in formation of a ranula, an epithelial-lined cyst within the SLS. When these rupture, they may form pseudocysts that may "dive" or "plunge" behind the posterior free edge of the mylohyoid muscle into the SMS (Fig. 16.9). The vast majority of neoplasms in this region are squamous cell carcinomas originating from the OC mucosa. Salivary epithelial tumors may arise from the major salivary glands (SLG, SMG) or from minor salivary glands (MSGs) lying within the SLS submucosal space.

16.7 Infrahyoid Neck: Visceral Space (VS)

16.7.1 Anatomy and Contents

The VS is a central tubular space extending from the hyoid to the mediastinum. Enclosed by the middle layer of deep cervical fascia, the VS is the only space confined entirely to the infrahyoid neck. Its contents include: the thyroid and parathyroid glands, the recurrent laryngeal nerve, the larynx, hypopharynx, trachea, and cervical esophagus. The thyroid gland is located anterior to the prevertebral musculature and posterior to the infrahyoid strap musculature, in close proximity to other vital structures of the VS such as the larynx, trachea, and esophagus. The tracheoesophageal groove lies posteromedial to the thyroid lobe and contains several important structures including the recurrent laryngeal nerve, paratracheal nodes, and parathyroid glands.

16.7.2 Thyroid and Parathyroid Pathology

Abnormalities of the thyroid gland are a major indication for imaging the VS. In general, ultrasound is the workhorse imaging modality for inflammatory (i.e., Hashimoto's) or infectious thyroiditis and for evaluation of the intrathyroidal nodule. Intrathyroidal nodules may represent colloid cysts, adenomas, differentiated thyroid cancer, or rarely, metastases. Many ultrasound classification systems exist to risk stratify these nodules and determine whether biopsy is indicated, including ones by the American Thyroid Association (ATA) and the Society of Radiologists in Ultrasound (SRU). Newer systems such as European Thyroid Imaging and Reporting Data System (EU-TIRADS) and the American College of Radiology Thyroid Imaging and Reporting Data System (ACR TIRADS) are gaining acceptance for their point-based approach [9, 10], particularly ACR TIRADS, with emerging studies demonstrating its high diagnostic performance and reduction of unnecessary biopsies [11, 12].

Thyroid cancer is a heterogeneous group of malignancies, including differentiated thyroid carcinomas (papillary and follicular), medullary and anaplastic carcinomas, and non-Hodgkin lymphoma. Cross-sectional imaging is most appropriate when there is a concern for extrathyroidal extension of tumor [13, 14] into surrounding structures such as the trachea or esophagus (Fig. 16.10). For rapidly enlarging thyroid masses, both anaplastic carcinoma and lymphoma should be considered. For multinodular goiters (MNG), ultrasound is used for surveillance of individual nodules, but non-contrast CT (NCCT) is often the choice for presurgical evaluation if airway compression necessitates removal. NCCT is helpful to evaluate the extent of airway compression and substernal

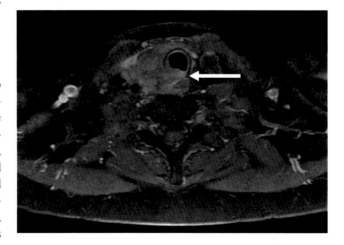

Fig. 16.10 Post-contrast axial T1-weighted image with fat saturation demonstrates a papillary thyroid cancer with extra-thyroidal extension and invasion of the trachea and esophagus (arrow)

extension for surgical planning and to exclude overt signs of malignancy. Local extension into trachea, tracheoesophageal (TE) groove, or infrahyoid strap muscles, vocal cord paralysis from involvement of the recurrent laryngeal nerve in TE groove, and pathologic cervical adenopathy are imaging findings that suggest thyroid malignancy.

Key Point
- US is the primary imaging modality for both inflammatory disease and work-up of thyroid nodules, with cross-sectional imaging used when there is concern for extrathyroidal extension of tumor, or to evaluate potential airway compression or substernal extension of goiter.

Congenital lesions in the VS include infrahyoid thyroglossal duct cysts or ectopic thyroid tissue along the course of the thyroglossal duct. Thyroglossal duct cysts are the most common congenital neck masses (Fig. 16.11); most present before age 10 as a painless, movable mass that may fluctuate in size after upper respiratory tract infection. When suprahyoid they are characteristically midline while infrahyoid lesions are often paramidline. Nodules in the tracheoesopha-

geal groove may represent parathyroid adenomas (or rare carcinomas), lymph nodes, or unusual schwannomas of the recurrent laryngeal nerve. Parathyroid adenomas are characteristically hypervascular, demonstrating rapid wash-in on early arterial phase and relatively rapid wash-out on venous phase multiphase contrast-enhanced CT [15].

16.7.3 Larynx, Hypopharynx, Trachea, and Esophagus Pathology

The most common indication for imaging of larynx and hypopharynx is staging of squamous cell carcinoma (a primary mucosal space abnormality), which will be discussed in a separate chapter. Much less common, submucosal tumors are usually well circumscribed on imaging and will not have an overlying mucosal abnormality on endoscopy. The differential diagnosis for submucosal masses includes minor salivary gland tumors, sarcomas such as laryngeal chondrosarcoma, and lymphoma. Benign lesions of the larynx, including papillomas and hemangiomas, are also uncommon. Laryngoceles, also called saccular cysts, are seen as dilated laryngeal ventricular saccules extending cranially within the paraglottic fat (Fig. 16.12). These are almost always unilateral and may be confined to the paralaryngeal space ("internal") or may extend laterally into the cervical soft tissues through the thyrohyoid membrane ("external").

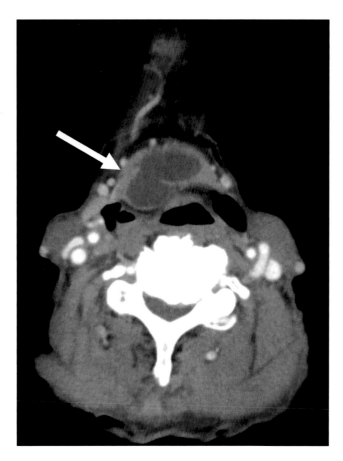

Fig. 16.11 Axial CECT demonstrates a paramidline infrahyoid cystic lesion (arrow) consistent with thyroglossal duct cyst

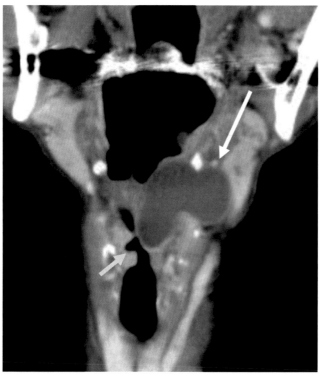

Fig. 16.12 Coronal CECT demonstrates a dilated, fluid-filled left ventricular saccule, consistent with laryngocele. There is lateral extension through the thyrohyoid membrane indicative of an external component (white arrow). A normal right laryngeal ventricle is seen (yellow arrow)

Laryngoceles that contain both an internal and external component are classified as mixed type. While this benign entity is usually functional and related to chronic increased glottic pressure, a small number (5–20%) may herald obstructing squamous cell carcinoma [16].

In the inflammatory category, epiglottitis should be suspected in a child with difficulty breathing and swallowing and may initially be evaluated with plain film. When there is a classic "thumb" sign reflecting the swollen epiglottis, treatment may be initiated and CECT may not even be required. Adults may have supraglottitis with CECT showing thickened, edematous epiglottis and aryepiglottic folds.

16.8 Entire Neck: Carotid Space (CS)

16.8.1 Anatomy and Contents

The carotid space spans the suprahyoid and infrahyoid neck, extending from the skull base to the aortic arch, with all three layers of the deep cervical fascia contributing to the carotid sheath [17]. It is located posterior to the styloid process (and is therefore termed the post-styloid PPS by some authors), anterior to the prevertebral muscles, and lateral to the retropharyngeal space. The CS can be further subdivided into nasopharyngeal, oropharyngeal, cervical and mediastinal components. The suprahyoid CS contains the carotid artery, internal jugular vein (IJV), cranial nerves 9–12, and the sympathetic chain. The infrahyoid CS differs in that all cranial nerves have exited except the vagus nerve. Lymph nodes are closely associated with the carotid space, along its lateral

border. The carotid artery is located medially, IJV laterally, vagus nerve posteriorly along the vessels, and the sympathetic chain posteriorly within the sheath.

> **Key Point**
> • The CS spans the suprahyoid and infrahyoid neck, with all three layers of the DCF contributing to the carotid sheath.

16.8.2 Pathology

Masses in the suprahyoid CS classically displace the parapharyngeal fat anteriorly and splay the carotid and jugular vein, often displacing the ICA anteriorly and IJV posterolaterally. Vascular pathology, primarily dissection or pseudoaneurysm of the carotid artery or thrombosis/thrombophlebitis of the IJV, may easily be overlooked on routine neck CT or MRI. Special attention should be paid to the CS to exclude dissection in any patient presenting with Horner's syndrome. An IJV thrombophlebitis caused by extension of oropharyngeal or odontogenic infection is referred to as Lemierre syndrome (Fig. 16.13). CT and MR angiography or venography are studies of choice if there is high clinical suspicion for a vascular lesion.

The most common masses in the high nasopharyngeal CS often dumbbell inferiorly from the jugular foramen and include glomus jugular paraganglioma, schwannoma, and meningioma. Close attention to the skull base is important in

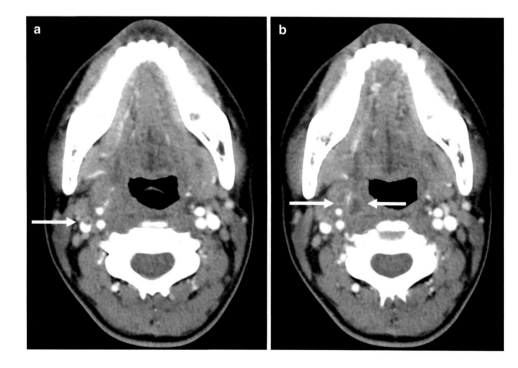

Fig. 16.13 (**a**) Axial CECT demonstrates a filling defect in the right IJV (arrow), consistent with thrombophlebitis. (**b**) In close proximity to the IJV thrombus, axial CECT identifies a right peritonsillar abscess in the PMS (arrows). The combination of these findings is consistent with Lemierre syndrome

Fig. 16.14 (a) Axial CECT demonstrates an avidly enhancing mass (arrow) at the right carotid bifurcation splaying the internal and external carotid arteries. (b) Axial T2w with fat saturation image demonstrates characteristic flow voids (the "pepper" of the "salt and pepper" appearance) within the mass (arrow). These findings are consistent with carotid body paraganglioma

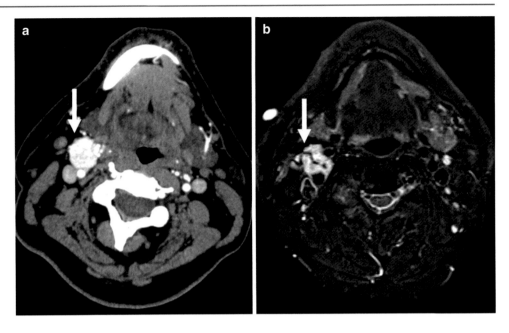

any patient presenting with hoarseness/vocal cord palsy or other cranial neuropathy involving CNs 9–12. Bony changes on CT are an important clue to the correct diagnosis of a jugular foramen/CS mass at the skull base. Permeative destruction favors paraganglioma, smooth remodeling is characteristic of schwannoma, and hyperostosis suggests a CS mass is a meningioma. On MRI, paragangliomas are intensely enhancing and can have the classic "salt and pepper" appearance with the "salt" representing microhemorrhages on T1-weighted (T1W) images and the "pepper" representing flow voids on T2-weighted (T2W) images. Carotid body and glomus vagale paragangliomas are also found in the CS. Carotid body tumors are located at the carotid bifurcation in the infrahyoid neck and splay the internal and external carotid arteries (Fig. 16.14). CS nerve sheath tumors include schwannomas and neurofibromas. Schwannomas are typically fusiform enhancing tumors, sometimes with cystic change, whereas neurofibromas are classically hypodense and hypoenhancing on CT and have a characteristic target sign on MRI.

16.9   Entire Neck: Retropharyngeal, Danger, and Prevertebral Spaces (RPS)

16.9.1 Anatomy and Contents

As mentioned in the introduction, the DLDCF has two components, the alar and prevertebral fascia. This results in the formation of three posterior neck spaces: (1) retropharyngeal space (RPS), between the visceral and alar fascia, (2) danger space, between the alar and prevertebral fascia, and (3) prevertebral space, between the prevertebral fascia and the vertebral periosteum (part of the perivertebral space, discussed below). The importance of recognizing the division into these spaces

primarily relates to their inferior extent. While the RPS terminates at the level of the T3 vertebra, the danger space extends more inferiorly to a point just above the diaphragm, and the prevertebral space continues to the coccyx. Though we typically cannot distinguish these spaces on imaging, we must remember to follow a posterior neck space collection to its inferior extent and be cognizant of the fact that this may lie within the chest or below. Contents of the suprahyoid RPS are simple: fat and lymph nodes. The RPS in the infrahyoid neck is a potential space, collapsed in the normal setting.

> **Key Point**
> • Retropharyngeal collections that have entered the danger or prevertebral spaces can descend to the mediastinum and as far inferiorly as the coccyx.

16.9.2 Pathology

Disease processes in the RPS can be categorized as related to the presence of fluid and/or nodal pathology. Fluid within the RPS may be encapsulated and represent an abscess or, much less commonly, a pseudomeningocele as a complication of spinal surgery. More frequent is unencapsulated edema or effusion of the RPS, and this may occur as a reaction to a wide variety of disease processes such as pharyngitis, lymphatic or venous obstruction, angioedema (Fig. 16.15), or radiation therapy [18]. Cervical osteomyelitis/discitis can secondarily result in fluid in the RPS. Nodal enlargement may occur in the setting of inflammatory or neoplastic processes. When there is pharyngitis, lymphadenopathy may be reactive and homogenous, or, particularly in children, an intranodal abscess may develop and rupture into the

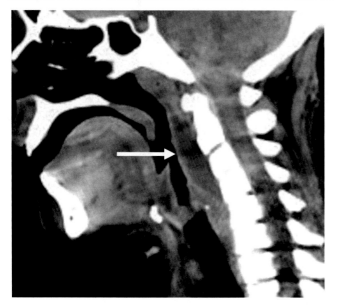

Fig. 16.15 Sagittal CECT demonstrating unencapsulated fluid in the retropharyngeal space in a patient presenting with angioedema

RPS. RPS lymph nodes may be involved in hematologic malignancy, such as lymphoma, or may represent sites of metastatic disease from local malignancies, particularly those of the pharynx, paranasal sinuses, and thyroid gland.

16.10 Entire Neck: Perivertebral Space (PVS)

16.10.1 Anatomy and Contents

The perivertebral space (PVS) is a cylindrical space around the vertebral column, invested in the DLDCF from the skull base to the mediastinum. The PVS can be subdivided into the prevertebral space and the paraspinal space [19]. The contents of the PVS include the vertebral bodies, disc spaces, musculature, and the vertebral arteries in the foramen transversarium. The RPS lies directly anterior to the PVS, and the paired carotid spaces lie anterolateral. The prevertebral muscles are invested in the anterior DLDCF, known as the "carpet" by surgeons. It is tenacious and serves as a barrier to infection and neoplasm. Lesions in the PVS tend to lift or displace the prevertebral muscles anteriorly, whereas RPS lesions displace these muscles posteriorly.

16.10.2 Pathology

The vast majority of pathologic lesions in the perivertebral space involve the vertebral bodies and disc spaces, and the minority of lesions are centered in the paraspinal musculature. Therefore, pyogenic discitis/osteomyelitis and bone metastasis are the most common pathologies found in this space. Atypical infections such as tuberculosis are less common but have characteristic imaging features such as sparing of the disc spaces. Primary bone tumors are also uncommon but have characteristic locations and appearance. For example, chordomas can be suggested when a lesion is found in the upper cervical spine with characteristic bright T2 signal and enhancement. An important differential diagnosis to consider in a patient with acute onset neck pain and dysphagia is calcific tendinitis of the longus colli muscle (Fig. 16.16), also referred to as prevertebral calcific tendinitis. Imaging features include prevertebral edema and calcification anterior to C2.

Fig. 16.16 (**a**) Sagittal CECT soft tissue window demonstrates prevertebral edema (arrow) in a patient with 3 days of acute onset neck pain. (**b**) Sagittal bone windows show calcification anterior to C2 (arrow), diagnostic of longus colli calcific tendinitis (prevertebral calcific tendinitis)

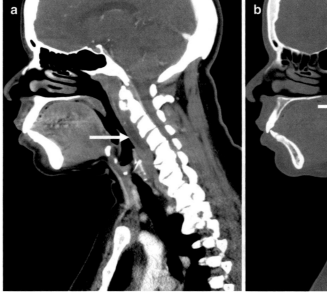
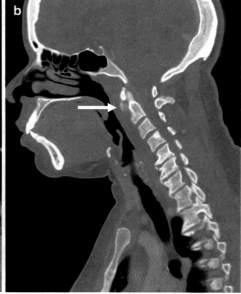

16.11 Concluding Remarks

The neck is anatomically complex but can be organized into compartments or "spaces" to help organize the approach to neck masses. A thorough understanding of fascial planes, the various spaces and their normal contents will help the radiologist generate the best differential diagnoses to appropriately guide management. The parapharyngeal space (PPS) fat is especially important in the analysis of most suprahyoid neck masses, as the mass effect on this triangular fat pad often helps to localize the space of origin. Pathology will displace the PPS in a predictable pattern. For example, masses arising in the deep lobe of the parotid tend to displace the PPS anteromedially, carotid space masses displace the PPS anteriorly, masticator space masses push the PPS posteriorly, and pharyngeal mucosal space masses often push the PPS laterally. Each compartment has common and uncommon pathology, typically based on the normal contents. Therefore, once a lesion is localized to the correct space, the radiologist can utilize imaging features and clinical information to provide a tailored list of differential considerations, or in some cases, a specific most likely diagnosis.

H&N Space Contents

Space	Boundaries	Major contents	Common pathology
Pharyngeal mucosal (PMS)	Mucosa to pharyngeal constrictors of nasopharynx and oropharynx (some include hypopharynx and oral cavity)	Mucosa, Waldeyer's ring, minor salivary glands, constrictor and levator palatine muscles, cartilaginous Eustachian tube	Malignant tumors (mucosal = SCC or NPC and submucosal = minor salivary tumors or lymphoma) Pharyngitis, tonsillitis
Parapharyngeal (PPS)	Skull base to mandibular angle, borders PPS, CS, PS, MS	Fat, minor salivary glands	Benign salivary tumors, rare branchial cleft cyst or vascular malformation
Masticator (MS)	Skull base to mandibular angle, lateral to PPS	Muscles of mastication, posterior body and ramus of mandible, CNV3	Odontogenic infections, venous malformations, sarcomas
Parotid (PS)	Enclosed within the parotid fascia, lateral to PPS, MS	Parotid gland, CN7, lymph nodes, retromandibular vein, external carotid artery branches	Pleomorphic adenoma Low and high grade malignant salivary neoplasms Acute or chronic parotitis
Visceral (VS)	Hyoid to mediastinum, anterior to PVS, medial to CS	Thyroid and parathyroid glands, larynx, hypopharynx, trachea, esophagus	Thyroid nodules, thyroid cancer, parathyroid adenoma, mucosal SCC, chondrosarcoma, diverticula
Carotid (CS)	Carotid sheath, enclosed by all three layers of DCF, skull base to aortic arch (SHN + IFN)	SHN: ICA, IJV, CN 9–12 IFN: CCA, IJV, CN 10 (vagus)	Vascular pathology related to carotid (aneurysm, dissection, arteritis) or jugular vein (thrombosis or thrombophlebitis) Nerve sheath tumors Paragangliomas
Retropharyngeal (RPS)	Skull base to T3, between visceral and alar fascia	Fat and lymph nodes	Metastatic lymph nodes (NPC, thyroid, hypopharynx, lymphoma) Suppurative lymph nodes (children) Effusion
Perivertebral (PVS)	Skull base to T4, posterior to RPS	Prevertebral muscles, vertebral bodies, scalene muscles, brachial plexus roots, phrenic nerve, vertebral artery and vein	Discitis/osteomyelitis, longus colli tendinitis, Primary bone tumors (chordoma, ABC, osteoma, giant cell) Vertebral metastases Sarcomas Nerve sheath tumors

SCC squamous cell carcinoma, *NPC* nasopharyngeal carcinoma, *ABC* aneurysmal bone cyst, *SHN* suprahyoid neck, *IFH* infrahyoid neck, *ICA* internal carotid artery, *CCA* common carotid artery, *IJV* internal jugular vein

> **Take-Home Messages**
> - The three layers of the deep cervical fascia define spaces, each with unique contents and pathology.
> - These spaces can be grouped as suprahyoid or infrahyoid, with some spaces, like the carotid and retropharyngeal spaces, spanning both levels.
> - Displacement of the parapharyngeal fat can help determine the site of origin of a suprahyoid mass.
> - The visceral space is the only space contained entirely in the infrahyoid neck, and it contains the thyroid and parathyroid glands as well as portions of the aerodigestive tract below the oropharynx.

References

1. Gamss C, Gupta A, Chazen JL, Phillips CD. Imaging evaluation of the suprahyoid neck. Radiol Clin N Am. 2015;53(1):133–44.
2. Warshafsky D, Goldenberg D, Kanekar SG. Imaging anatomy of deep neck spaces. Otolaryngol Clin N Am. 2012;45(6):1203–21.
3. Guidera AK, Dawes PJ, Fong A, Stringer MD. Head and neck fascia and compartments: no space for spaces. Head Neck. 2014;36(7):1058–68.
4. Parker GD, Harnsberger HR, Jacobs JM. The pharyngeal mucosal space. Semin Ultrasound CT MR. 1990;11(6):460–75.
5. Stambuk HE, Patel SG. Imaging of the parapharyngeal space. Otolaryngol Clin N Am. 2008;41(1):77–10.
6. Meltzer DE, Shatzkes DR. Masticator space: imaging anatomy for diagnosis. Otolaryngol Clin N Am. 2012;45(6):1233–51.
7. Kanekar SG, Mannion K, Zacharia T, Showalter M. Parotid space: anatomic imaging. Otolaryngol Clin N Am. 2012;45(6):1253–72.
8. La'porte SJ, Juttla JK, Lingam RK. Imaging the floor of the mouth and the sublingual space. Radiographics. 2011;31(5):1215–30.
9. Tessler FN, Middleton WD, Grant EG, et al. ACR thyroid imaging, reporting and data system (TI-RADS): white paper of the ACR TI-RADS Committee. J Am Coll Radiol. 2017;14(5):587–95.
10. Russ G, Bonnema SJ, Erdogan MF, Durante C, Ngu R, Leenhardt L. European thyroid association guidelines for ultrasound malignancy risk stratification of thyroid nodules in adults: the EU-TIRADS. Eur Thyroid J. 2017;6(5):225–37.
11. Hoang JK, Middleton WD, Tessler FN. Update on ACR TI-RADS: successes, challenges, and future directions, from the AJR special series on radiology reporting and data systems. AJR Am J Roentgenol. 2021;216(3):570–8. https://doi.org/10.2214/AJR.20.24608.
12. Kim DH, Kim SW, Basurrah MA, Lee J, Hwang SH. Diagnostic performance of six ultrasound risk stratification systems for thyroid nodules: a systematic review and network meta-analysis. AJR Am J Roentgenol. 2023;220(6):791–803. https://doi.org/10.2214/AJR.22.28556.
13. Loevner LA, Kaplan SL, Cunnane ME, Moonis G. Cross-sectional imaging of the thyroid gland. Neuroimaging Clin N Am. 2008;18(3):445–61. vii
14. Aiken AH. Imaging of thyroid cancer. Semin Ultrasound CT MR. 2012;33(2):138–49.
15. Phillips CD, Shatzkes DR. Imaging of the parathyroid glands. Semin Ultrasound CT MR. 2012;33(2):123–9.
16. Juneja R, Arora N, Meher R, et al. Laryngocele: a rare case report and review of literature. Indian J Otolaryngol Head Neck Surg. 2019;71(Suppl 1):147–51. https://doi.org/10.1007/s12070-017-1162-x.
17. Kuwada C, Mannion K, Aulino JM, Kanekar SG. Imaging of the carotid space. Otolaryngol Clin N Am. 2012;45(6):1273–92.
18. Bhatt AA. Non-traumatic causes of fluid in the retropharyngeal space. Emerg Radiol. 2018;25(5):547–51.
19. Mills MK, Shah LM. Imaging of the perivertebral space. Radiol Clin N Am. 2015;53(1):163–80.

Head and Neck Squamous Cell Cancer: Approach to Staging and Surveillance

Heejun (Tony) Kang, Tabassum A. Kennedy, and Eugene Yu

Abstract

This chapter addresses the rising global burden of Head and Neck Squamous Cell Cancer (HNSCC), a heterogeneous group of cancers in the upper aerodigestive tract. We focus on the pivotal role of imaging modalities like CT, MRI, PET/CT, and US in the early detection, accurate staging, and management of HNSCC. The discussion includes the nuances of TNM staging, key upstaging features, and the evolving role of advanced imaging techniques such as MR/PET. The chapter highlights significant updates in the AJCC/UICC eighth edition, particularly concerning HPV-related cancers and the depth of invasion in oral cavity SCC. Special attention is given to the challenges in diagnosing Neck Cancer of Unknown Primary (NCUP), underlining the importance of integrated imaging, clinical exam, and molecular markers. Overall, the chapter emphasizes the essential role of radiologists in the comprehensive management of HNSCC, combining imaging insights with clinical findings for optimal patient care.

Keywords

Head and Neck Cancer · Extranodal extension Perineural Spread (PNS) · NI-RADS (Neck Imaging Reporting and Data System) · HPV (Human Papillomavirus) · NCUP (Neck Cancer of Unknown Primary)

Learning Objectives

- Recognize the primary imaging modalities (CT, MRI, PET/CT) used in the diagnosis, staging, and surveillance of Head and Neck Squamous Cell Cancer (HNSCC), including their advantages and limitations.
- Understand the principles and components of TNM staging according to the AJCC/UICC eighth edition for HNSCC.
- Identify the anatomic boundaries and key upstaging features for different HNSCC sites: nasopharynx, oral cavity, oropharynx, and hypopharynx/larynx.
- Appreciate the implications of cervical lymphadenopathy in HNSCC, including the size criteria and features of abnormal lymph nodes, and the concept of perineural spread.
- Understand the importance of surveillance in managing HNSCC, including the guidelines from NCCN and NI-RADS, and the role of PET/CT in this context.

Head and Neck Squamous Cell Cancer (HNSCC) remains a significant global health burden with high morbidity and mortality rates. HNSCC encompasses a heterogeneous group of neoplasms arising from the squamous epithelium of the upper aerodigestive tract, which includes the oral cavity, oropharynx, nasopharynx, hypopharynx, and larynx. It is the sixth most common cancer worldwide with 890,000 new cases and 450,000 deaths in 2018 [1, 2]. The incidence of HNSCC continues to rise and is projected to increase 30% annually by 2030 [3].

Traditionally, the highest rates of HNSCC occurred in older males due to tobacco and alcohol use [4]. However, a rising number of cases have been associated with human papillomavirus (HPV) infection in both developing and developed countries. This trend particularly affects younger and healthier patients and is often associated with oropharyngeal sites [5].

H. (T). Kang (✉) · E. Yu
Department of Medical Imaging, University of Toronto, Toronto, ON, Canada
e-mail: heejun.kang@sunnybrook.ca; eugene.yu@uhn.ca

T. A. Kennedy
Department of Radiology, University of Wisconsin, Madison, WI, USA
e-mail: tkennedy@uwhealth.org

J. Hodler et al. (eds.), *Diseases of the Brain, Head and Neck, Spine 2024-2027*, IDKD Springer Series,
https://doi.org/10.1007/978-3-031-50675-8_17

Early detection and accurate staging of HNSCC are crucial for effective therapeutic strategy planning and prognostication. To this end, imaging plays a pivotal role. In the following sections, we will delve into the specifics of the imaging methods, the nuances of TNM (Tumor, Node, Metastasis) staging, anatomic boundaries of HNSCC, and key upstaging features. The aim of this chapter is to provide a comprehensive approach to the imaging and staging of HNSCC.

17.1 Imaging Methods

The choice of imaging modality in HNSCC is critical to accurately assess tumor extent, stage the disease, evaluate treatment response, and detect recurrence during surveillance. Computed tomography (CT), magnetic resonance imaging (MRI), and positron emission tomography/computed tomography (PET/CT) are all essential tools. Each provide a unique and complementary information that guide diagnosis, staging, treatment planning, and follow-up [3]. The selection depends on the location of the primary tumor, the suspected stage of disease, the patient's clinical condition, and the available resources.

17.1.1 Computed Tomography (CT)

CT is widely used due to its accessibility, relatively low cost, and speed of acquisition. It provides excellent spatial resolution and good contrast differentiation between soft tissue, bone, and air [6]. This makes it especially ideal for detecting bony invasion.

Current advancements in multidetector CT technology permit scans with a slice thickness of under 1 mm. Ideally, a slice thickness of 3 mm is preferred. The images should be both reconstructed and viewed in bone and soft tissue windows.

For oral cavity cancers, CT scans can assist in determining how deeply a tumor has infiltrated into the tongue's deep muscles and whether it has reached the mandible. The "puffed cheek" method can enhance the assessment of lesions within the oral cavity. This method entails patients self-inflating their oral cavity with air by blowing out their cheeks which can unmask a lesion along the buccal mucosa or gingiva. Dental fillings can lead to significant beam hardening artifacts that can obscure important details within the scan plane. This issue can be rectified by re-scanning with a tilted gantry angle or using metal suppression techniques, such as dual-energy CT [7].

For other types of head and neck cancers, CT scans are generally beneficial in identifying advanced stages of cancers that have infiltrated neighboring structures that are difficult to detect clinically. For laryngeal cancers, CT scans can shed light on the invasion of the pre-epiglottic space, paraglottic space, and subglottic extension. Recent advances in dual-energy CT technology has improved the accuracy for assessing cartilage invasion compared with conventional CT, a determinant for stage T4 disease [8].

However, CT may not clearly delineate early mucosal lesions or tumoral invasion into soft tissue structures, limiting its utility in certain scenarios and necessitating the use of MRI and/or PET/CT.

17.1.2 Magnetic Resonance Imaging (MRI)

MRI is superior in demonstrating the extent of soft tissue invasion and perineural spread (Table 17.1) [9]. Its high contrast resolution makes it particularly valuable for imaging complex anatomical areas such as the skull base, nasopharynx, and parapharyngeal spaces. MRI is particularly useful for evaluating perineural tumor extension and cartilage invasion, especially when the cartilage is not ossified. MRI is also excellent for detecting early tumoral changes following treatment, distinguishing between fibrosis and recurrence. Nonetheless, obtaining a high-quality, full-neck image is more challenging with MRI than with CT due to its high susceptibility to motion artifacts. This can become particularly troublesome in post-treatment patients who might find it difficult to remain still for an extended duration.

17.1.3 Positron Emission Tomography/ Computed Tomography (PET/CT)

PET/CT combines the anatomical detail of CT with the metabolic activity visualization of PET, providing both structural and functional information. It is particularly useful in initial staging, especially for nodal staging, detecting distant metastases, and identifying an unknown primary [10, 11]. Moreover, during post-treatment surveillance, PET/CT can differentiate post-treatment changes from residual or recurrent disease with a high degree of accuracy [12]. However, PET/CT is not without downsides. It is not ideal for detecting very small tumors or microinvasion due to low spatial resolution. Furthermore, considerations such as cost, availability, patient

Table 17.1 Standard MRI sequences

MRI sequence	Utility
Noncontrast T1-weighted imaging	It offers anatomical views and can help identify tumor margins and infiltration into bone, significantly contributing to staging the disease.
T2-weighted imaging with fat suppression (FS)	This is used for tumor identification and characterization and helps to identify neck lymph nodes. FS is generally used in this imaging to increase contrast although it can sometimes cause image artifacts.
Contrast-enhanced T1-weighted imaging with (FS)	This utilizes gadolinium-based contrast agents for characterizing lesions and assessing intracranial extension of disease.

preparation, extended examination time, and higher radiation dose present additional challenges that need to be weighed.

17.1.4 Ultrasound (US)

US is less frequently used for primary tumor evaluation due to its inability to penetrate bone and air-filled spaces. However, it can be valuable in specific circumstances. For instance, US is excellent for evaluating superficial structures such as thyroid and salivary glands and has high sensitivity for detecting cervical lymphadenopathy. Moreover, US is safe, cost-effective, and can be used for real-time image-guided biopsy of suspected lesions, providing a valuable adjunct.

17.1.5 Up and Coming: Magnetic Resonance/ Positron Emission Tomography (MR/ PET)

MR/PET is an emerging imaging modality that attempts to combine the strengths of MRI and PET. It offers the excellent soft tissue contrast resolution of MRI with the metabolic information of PET while reducing radiation exposure [3]. This hybrid imaging modality can potentially provide superior information for tumor characterization, staging, and treatment response evaluation. However, larger, multicenter trials are necessary to validate FDG PET/MRI's role in head and neck cancer. In addition, cost-related issues concerning purchase, maintenance, and reimbursement must also be addressed. Ultimately, practical standardized protocols are required for FDG PET/MRI to be adopted more broadly in the evaluation of head and neck cancers.

> **Key Point**
> - No single imaging modality can answer all clinical questions for HNSCC. Each method has its advantages and limitations.
> - The choice of modality should be tailored to the clinical question at hand, the anatomical location of the tumor, and the resources available.

17.2 TNM Staging

The eighth edition of the AJCC/UICC TNM classification system is an internationally recognized manual that provides a standardized language for discussing HNSCC [13]. The radiologist's primary role is to provide the necessary anatomic information related to tumor assessment based on imaging characteristics that will allow the clinician to assign a correct TNM stage.

The "T" refers to the primary tumor's size and extent. Its specific classification can range from T0, indicating no evidence of a primary tumor, to T4, which suggests a significantly advanced disease in terms of size and/or invasion into adjacent structures. The T classification varies depending on the site of the cancer; therefore, having ready access to the staging table is helpful for accurate classification.

The "N" represents the degree of regional lymph node involvement. It is well recognized that cervical lymph node metastasis significantly impacts the prognosis of HNSCC patients. Identification of extranodal extension (ENE) is particularly critical in upstaging tumors.

The "M" refers to the presence (M1) or absence (M0) of distant metastasis. HNSCC typically metastasizes to the lungs, followed by bone and liver [14].

17.2.1 Key Changes in the AJCC/UICC Eighth Edition

Oropharyngeal SCC (OPSCC): In the recent years, there has been a paradigm shift in the epidemiology with an increase in HPV-related (or p16-positivity as a surrogate) cases, particularly in younger individuals with little to no history of tobacco use [15]. These typically show excellent responses to treatment, even in patients with advanced stage disease. Given the distinct clinical and biological behavior of p16-positive OPC compared to p16-negative OPC, it has been recognized as a separate entity requiring a specific staging system. One key example is that for p16-positive OPC, the ipsilateral multiplicity of lymph node involvement is no longer considered, whereas it remains a significant factor in the staging of p16-negative OPC.

Oral Cavity SCC (OCSCC): The depth of invasion (DOI) is now included as a component in the T staging as it has critical prognostic factor. While it is a pathologic measurement, studies have shown that there is good radiologic-pathologic correlation and the radiographic measurement is predictive of outcome [16].

Extranodal Extension (ENE): ENE has been incorporated in the N category, except for tumors associated with HPV. Its presence now upstages nodal disease to N3b for p16 negative and non-EBV lymph node SCC.

> **Key Point**
> - For radiologists who interpret OPC staging scans and participate in tumor boards, it is crucial to have knowledge of the p16 and HPV status.
> - While the staging of ENE primarily relies on clinical assessment, radiology can supply supportive evidence especially when physical examination results are ambiguous.

17.3 Nasopharyngeal Carcinoma (NPC)

17.3.1 Anatomic Boundaries

The nasopharynx's anatomic boundaries consist of the anterior boundary (posterior nasal septum and choanae), the posterior boundary (vertebral bodies of C1-C2), and the lateral boundaries (tori tubarii, Eustachian tube orifices, and pharyngeal recess). The superior boundary is the base of the skull, specifically the undersurface of the sphenoid bone and basiocciput. The inferior boundary is the level of the soft palate, which separates the nasopharynx from the oropharynx.

This region is richly connected to adjacent critical structures like the skull base, paranasal sinuses, cavernous sinus, and the orbits. This has significant implications when it comes to the spread of malignancies and the subsequent impact on staging and treatment planning.

17.3.2 Key Upstaging Features

The involvement of the parapharyngeal space up categorizes the T classification from T1 to T2. There is considered parapharyngeal spread when the tumor invades laterally through the levator palatini muscle and pharyngobasilar fascia to involve the tensor palatini muscle and parapharyngeal fat space [17]. This can also act as a potential pathway for tumor extension from the nasopharynx to the deeper neck spaces, the skull base, and other vital structures. Tumors that invade the parapharyngeal space often present as a more advanced disease and require more aggressive management [17].

NPC often invades the skull base upon diagnosis, upgrading the disease from T2 to T3. The commonly invaded structures include the clivus, pterygoid bones, body of the sphenoid, and petrous apices. The tumor also frequently infiltrates the skull base foramina and fissures, such as the foramen rotundum, foramen ovale, foramen lacerum, vidian canal, pterygomaxillary and petroclival fissures, as well as the pterygopalatine fossa (PPF) (Fig. 17.1). This enables further spread to the orbit and intracranial structures by both direct and PNS, complicating treatment and worsening prognosis.

NPC also have a tendency for early nodal spread due to the rich lymphatic network. Cervical lymph node involvement is a common finding and can further upstage the disease. The nodal levels most frequently involved include retropharyngeal and levels II and III nodes.

17.4 Oral Cavity SCC (OCSCC)

The oral cavity includes various structures: lips, oral tongue, buccal mucosa, alveolar ridge, retromolar trigone, hard palate, and the floor of the mouth (FOM).

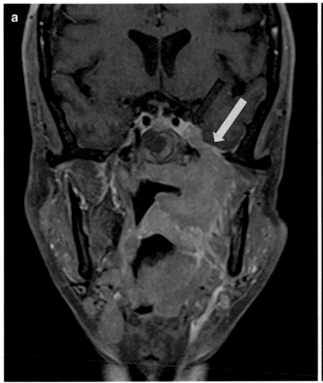
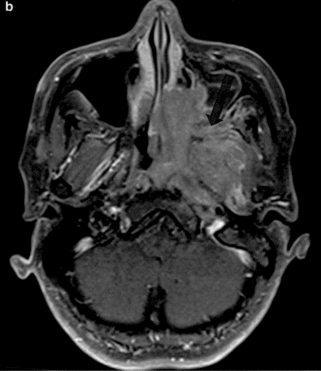

Fig. 17.1 Coronal (**a**) and axial (**b**) post-contrast T1-weighted fat-suppressed images show an enhancing left nasopharyngeal mass invading into the left pterygopalatine fossa (purple arrow), masticator space, and nasal cavity. There is perineural spread along the right V3 nerve into the left foramen ovale (yellow arrow) and cavernous sinus (red arrow)

17.4.1 Anatomic Boundaries

The oral cavity extends anteriorly from the lips to the junction of the hard and soft palate superiorly and to the line of the circumvallate papillae on the tongue inferiorly. The lateral borders are the buccal mucosa, extending posteriorly to the anterior tonsillar pillars.

The FOM, the area under the tongue, is a common site for oral cavity cancers. The hard palate, forming the roof of the mouth, divides the oral and nasal cavities. The tongue is divided into the anterior two-thirds (oral part) and the posterior one-third (base). The alveolar ridges contain the tooth sockets, and the retromolar trigone is the small area behind the wisdom teeth.

The oral cavity is richly supplied by branches of the external carotid artery, mainly the lingual artery.

17.4.2 Key Upstaging Features

Tumor thickness (TT) and the DOI are essential prognostic indicators in OCSCC [16]. Tumors that are thicker and invade deeper into the oral cavity tissues have a higher risk of metastasizing to the cervical lymph nodes and involving deep soft tissues. DOI refers to a specific pathological measurement taken during surgical resection, quantifying the extent the tumor has spread beneath the basement membrane [18]. This is distinct from TT, which measures the vertical dimension of the tumor from the surface to its deepest point. Exophytic tumors may have a large TT but can exhibit minimal DOI, as they may be broad but not deeply invasive. Conversely, endophytic tumors may demonstrate a large DOI even if the TT is smaller due to a reduced diameter. Tumors with a DOI of more than 5 mm are categorized as T2 or higher depending on other tumor characteristics. It is important to recognize that DOI is a pathologic measurement and because the primary treatment for oral cavity cancer is surgical resection, pathologic staging will typically be performed.

The inferior alveolar nerve is one of the branches of the mandibular nerve (V3), providing sensation to the lower teeth and the lower lip. It runs through the mandibular foramen and mandibular canal within the mandible and exits through the mental foramen. Its proximity makes it susceptible to invasion by OCSCC, especially those arising in the lower gingiva or the FOM (Fig. 17.2). Involvement of this nerve signifies a more advanced tumor and portends a worse prognosis. In many cases, it might escalate the category to T4, depending on other characteristics of the tumor. It also necessitates a more aggressive surgical approach, including a mandibulectomy. Damage to or resection of the inferior alveolar nerve may lead to chronic numbness or pain in the area, decreasing the patient's quality of life.

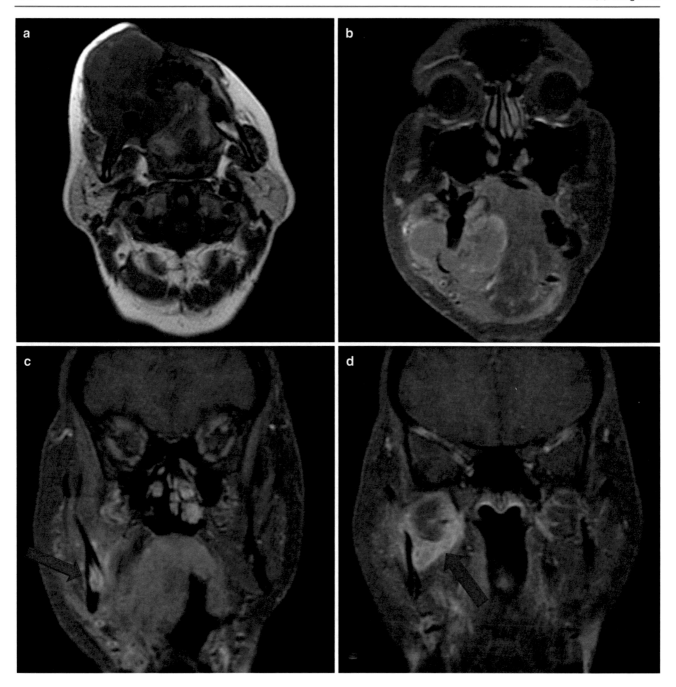

Fig. 17.2 Axial T1-weighted image (**a**) demonstrating a large T1 hypointense mass arising from the right mandibular gingiva invading into the mandible and surrounding soft tissues, including the mandibu-lar canal. Coronal post-contrast T2-weighted fat saturated images (**b–d**) showing perineural spread of tumor along the right inferior alveolar (red arrow) and V3 nerve (purple arrow)

17.5 Oropharyngeal SCC (OPSCC)

17.5.1 Anatomic Boundaries

The oropharynx is located at the central portion of the phar-ynx, extending from the soft palate superiorly to the level of the hyoid bone inferiorly. It plays a vital role in speech and swallowing and is delineated by several distinct structures. It includes the base of the tongue, the palatine tonsils, and the posterior pharyngeal wall, which forms the posterior bound-ary. The palatine tonsils are housed in the tonsillar fossa which is the space between the anterior tonsillar pillar, or the palatoglossal arch, and the posterior tonsillar pillar, or the palatopharyngeal arch.

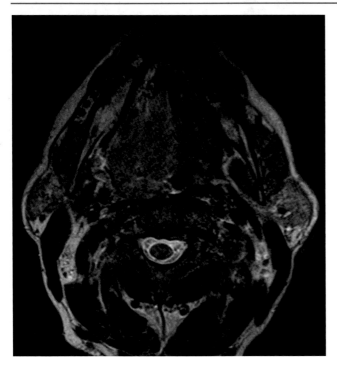

Fig. 17.3 Axial T1-weighted image shows a large right floor of mouth mass invading into the ipsilateral genioglossus and hyoglossus muscles with encasement of the right lingual artery. The tumor extends posteriorly into the right tonsil across the glossotonsillar sulcus

17.5.2 Key Upstaging Features

The extrinsic muscles of the tongue include the genioglossus, hyoglossus, styloglossus, and palatoglossus muscles. They are fundamental in orchestrating the movements of the tongue, assisting in functions like speech, mastication, and deglutition. In the context of OPSCC, the involvement of any one of the muscles serves as a sign of the tumor's spread and aggressiveness and up categorizes to T4 regardless of the p16 status. Imaging plays a particular role as it is difficult to determine their involvement clinically. CT and MRI may reveal irregularities, thickening, or a loss of symmetry that indicates malignant involvement (Fig. 17.3).

17.6 Hypopharynx/Larynx SCC

17.6.1 Anatomic Boundaries

The larynx serves as a complex organ for voice production, airway protection, and breathing. It spans from the epiglottis to the trachea and consists of three main parts: supraglottis, glottis, and subglottis. Supraglottis includes the epiglottis, aryepiglottic folds, arytenoids, and laryngeal ventricles. It is important to note that the anterior surface of the aryepiglottic folds resides in the larynx, while the posterior surface is part of the hypopharynx. Anteriorly, there is the triangular fat

containing space between the epiglottis and hyoid bone called the pre-epiglottic space. The glottis is home to the true vocal cords which comes together at the anterior commissure and posterior commissure. On either side of the larynx exists a fat-containing space called the paraglottic space. The subglottis extends from 1 cm below the lateral margin of the ventricle to the inferior margin of the cricoid cartilage.

The hypopharynx represents the lower part of the pharynx, bridging the oropharynx to the esophagus and larynx. It extends from the hyoid bone to the cricoid cartilage, containing subsites: pyriform sinuses, posterior pharyngeal wall, and post-cricoid region.

The pyriform sinuses are pear-shaped recesses on either side of the laryngeal opening. Lying between the thyroid cartilage and thyrohyoid membrane, they are considered a common location for hypopharyngeal carcinoma. The posterior pharyngeal wall is the back wall of the pharynx, descending from the level of the soft palate to the esophagus, behind the larynx. Its muscular layer helps in swallowing. The post-cricoid region lies behind the cricoid cartilage and continues as the esophagus. Although less common, tumors can arise in this location.

17.6.2 Key Upstaging Features

Invasion into the paraglottic space for all subtypes of laryngeal SCC is a poor prognostic factor and up categorizes the tumor to a T3 lesion. MRI is usually the preferred modality due to its excellent soft tissue contrast, allowing the precise delineation of the tumor from the surrounding fatty tissue. CT can also be valuable, especially in preoperative planning.

Involvement of cartilages and extralaryngeal extension are significant factors separating between T3 and T4a categories for both laryngeal and hypopharyngeal SCC (Figs. 17.4 and 17.5). This carries significant surgical implications, as these structures maintain the structural integrity of the larynx. Their invasion usually necessitates aggressive management, including total laryngectomy, which has serious consequence for patient's quality of life. Therefore, identifying cartilage involvement through imaging is crucial although it often challenging. Typically, MRI has higher sensitivity than CT, but motion artifact poses a serious problem. CT remains a preferred method for imaging the larynx and hypopharynx, but it may miss disease involvement of a non-ossified cartilage. Dual-energy CT seems to offer promising improvements in detecting cartilage invasion, especially in reducing overestimation of cartilage invasion, thereby preventing unnecessary total laryngectomy [19].

Prevertebral space involvement, or the fixation of a tumor to the prevertebral muscles, is clinically challenging to assess. The invasion of this space signals a very advanced

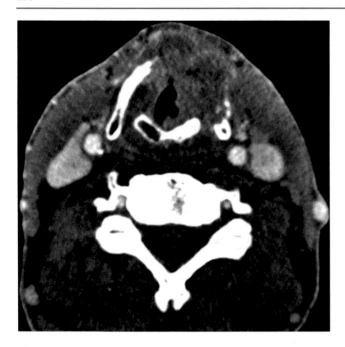

Fig. 17.4 Axial contrast-enhanced CT showing a heterogeneously enhancing left laryngeal mass invading into the overlying thyroid cartilage with infiltration of the strap musculature. The left aspect of the cricoid cartilage is sclerotic, also raising the possibility of involvement

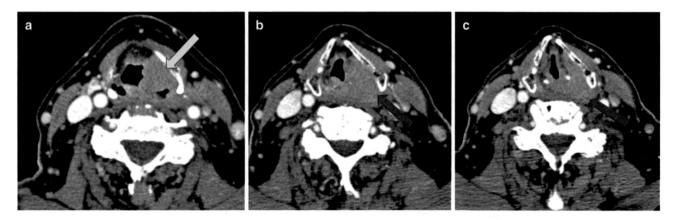

Fig. 17.5 Axial contrast-enhanced CT (**a–c**) demonstrating a left supraglottic/piriform sinus squamous cell carcinoma invading into the left paraglottic fat (yellow arrow). The tumor extends into the hypopharynx via the widened thyroarytenoid interval (red arrow)

disease, categorized as T4b, and generally indicates unresectability. The use of imaging to identify the preservation of the retropharyngeal fat plane offers a valuable diagnostic tool, as it can accurately predict the absence of direct tumor infiltration into the prevertebral space [20].

17.7 Cervical Lymphadenopathy

Identification of nodal metastases is critical in treatment and prognosis of HNSCC. A single lymph node metastasis decreases the 5-year survival rate to half. If there is an addi-

tional contralateral nodal metastasis, the survival rate is roughly halved again to 33% [21].

The mnemonic "CRISPS" can be used when assessing for cervical lymphadenopathy [14]:

Clustering: Clustering refers to a group of three or more abutting nodes without intervening fat planes measuring 8–15 mm long or 9–10 mm short axis in the jugulodigastric area and 8–9 mm elsewhere in the neck. It portends a poorer prognosis than isolated nodes.
Rounded shape: Typically, lymph nodes have an oblong or elongated shape when they are healthy. However, when

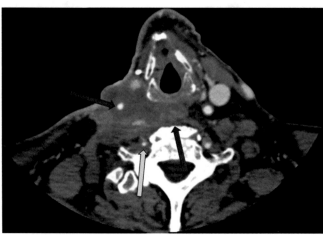
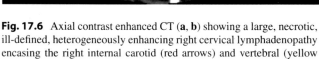
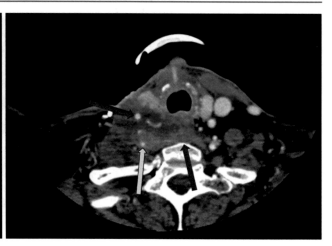

Fig. 17.6 Axial contrast enhanced CT (**a**, **b**) showing a large, necrotic, ill-defined, heterogeneously enhancing right cervical lymphadenopathy encasing the right internal carotid (red arrows) and vertebral (yellow arrows) arteries. The lesion is also inseparable from the prevertebral musculature raising the possibility of invasion (purple arrows)

they take on a more spherical or rounded shape, it often indicates a higher probability of metastasis.

Inhomogeneity: A metastatic lymph node is composed of a mix of tumor cells, native lymph node tissue, and areas of necrosis, leading to an internally heterogeneous appearance. If the heterogeneous area is larger than 3 mm, it is referred to as "central necrosis" and is one of the most reliable imaging indicators of metastatic disease.

Size: The size criteria and measurement techniques vary widely and may depend on the institution and clinicians' preference based on sensitivity and specificity. For example, at our institution, we use the largest long axis diameter on axial imaging greater than 15 mm in level I and II (jugulodigastric), and greater than 10 mm at other locations in the neck [22]. Other institutions may employ a 1-cm short axis cutoff [23]. It is important to understand that while size criteria can guide suspicion, it is not definitive. Approximately 20% of nodes larger than 1-cm short-axis diameter may show only hyperplasia, while 23% of nodes with ENE measure less than 1-cm [24]. The morphology and internal characteristics of a lymph node are arguably more reliable at identifying its pathological status.

Periphery: Any abnormalities along the borders of the lymph node can indicate underlying ENE, where the cancer cells breach the outer boundary of the lymph node. On imaging modalities, this often manifests as irregular nodal margins, capsular enhancement, and surrounding fat stranding (Fig. 17.6). Recognizing ENE is crucial at it indicates a more aggressive disease and increases the likelihood of recurrence by up to 10 times.

Sentinel node: The sentinel node is the first lymph node or group of nodes that cancer cells are most likely to spread to from the primary tumor. For majority of the oral cavity and oropharyngeal SCC, the jugulodigastric node serves as the sentinel node. Tongue-based SCC can occasionally bypass the level II nodes and spread to an ipsilateral level III or IV nodes. This information can increase the index of suspicion for nodal disease even when the appearance may be near normal.

> **Key Point**
> - Lymph node metastasis negatively impacts the prognosis in HNSCC.
> - "CRISPS" mnemonic guides cervical lymphadenopathy assessment, including clustering, rounded shape, inhomogeneity, size, periphery, and sentinel nodes.
> - Node morphology and internal characteristics are more telling than size alone, especially noting extracapsular spread.

17.8 Perineural Spread (PNS)

PNS involves the dissemination of the tumor along the nerve sheaths, but it is often loosely used to encompass neoplastic involvement along any or all compartments of a nerve. The significance of PNS on prognosis cannot be overstressed. It increases the probability of locoregional recurrence by 300% and decreases the 5-year survival rate by 30% [25]. Clinically, PNS can lead to functional deficits based on the nerve involved, sometimes leaving lastingdebilitation even after treatment. Therefore, the role of imaging becomes invaluable in detecting PNS.

Primary imaging features of PNS include nerve enhancement and thickening, as well as obliteration of perineural fat at foraminal openings. In advanced cases, bony erosion of the skull base foramina can be present. Secondary imaging features involve denervation atrophy of the muscles supplied by the nerves. Early on, T2-weighted MR images show muscle hyperintensity, resembling edema, and increased contrast enhancement due to increased perfusion. Over time, muscle atrophy with fatty replacement is evident.

The trigeminal nerves, particularly the maxillary and mandibular divisions, frequently become conduits for PNS due to their extensive network across the head and neck. Tumors from the facial region, as well as oropharyngeal and sinonasal cancers, can spread along the maxillary nerve. Furthermore, any skull base tumors that infiltrate the PPF can also extend to the brain through the foramen rotundum.

The mandibular nerve is often affected by masticator space and skull base tumors, such as NPC. Cancers of the submandibular gland, tongue, and mouth floor can invade the lingual or inferior alveolar nerve, and track back along the mandibular nerve and the foramen ovale, which is a portal for extending intracranially, particularly into the cavernous sinus.

Parotid gland tumors can affect the facial nerve, spreading cranially as far as the internal auditory canal. They can also infiltrate along the auriculotemporal nerve to involve the mandibular nerve. In addition, any tumors involving the PPF can also infiltrate the facial nerve along the vidian and greater superficial petrosal nerves.

> **Key Point**
> - PNS drastically affects outcomes, increasing locoregional recurrence and decreasing the 5-year survival rate.
> - Primary imaging features include nerve enhancement/thickening and secondary features, such as denervation atrophy.
> - The trigeminal nerves, especially the maxillary and mandibular divisions, frequently serve as pathways for PNS, affecting the course and treatment of various head and neck cancers.

17.9 Surveillance

HNSCC often recurs within the first 3 years after treatment, making this period crucial for clinical and imaging surveillance [26]. Despite development of evidence-based guidelines, none is universally accepted for surveillance timing and modality.

In general, there is a consensus that baseline post-treatment imaging should be performed within 6 months after therapy completion. This initial study could be challenging to interpret due to distorted anatomy after reconstruction flaps and radiation but will aid in reading subsequent follow-up studies. Thus, understanding the expected post-treatment findings is crucial to differentiate between treatment changes, residual tumor, and early recurrence. Ideally, the baseline scan should not show any signs of the remaining primary mass or abnormal lymph nodes.

The role of surveillance imaging for asymptomatic patients after initial post-treatment is less clear due to limited literature. However, given the high recurrence rates and difficulty identifying recurrences, many institutions routinely monitor advanced HNSCC for 2–3 years post-treatment [3].

In 2018, Neck Imaging Reporting and Data System (NI-RADS) was introduced to standardize surveillance imaging algorithm for HNSCC [27]. It offers standardized descriptions for the primary site and regional nodal basin. They include a recurrence suspicion level at each site, linked to management suggestions. NI-RADS enhances report consistency and communication, aiding clinical decisions. Studies confirm its reliability, with good interreader agreement and strong discriminatory ability in assessment categories.

Incorporating PET/CT in surveillance is increasingly popular due to its ability to detect metabolic changes before structural ones. It proves especially valuable in differentiating between post-treatment changes and tumor recurrence with studies showing specificity as high as 100% and NPV of 90–100% [3]. However, the interpretation requires caution. False positives can arise from inflammatory changes, especially when performed earlier than 12 weeks. Also, false negatives are possible with small lesions due to limited spatial resolution. Moreover, factors like cost, radiation exposure, and limited accessibility may limit its universal adoption. Regardless, in instances of clinical uncertainty, PET/CT remains a useful adjunct.

Ultimately, there is no rigid surveillance plan, and several factors must be considered. Firstly, the initial disease stage is pivotal; advanced stages necessitate more frequent monitoring. The type and intensity of treatment received play a role as well. Patients who undergo aggressive treatments, given their higher potential for complications, may be monitored more closely. The presence of residual symptoms, such as persistent pain or swelling, also directs the surveillance intensity.

Patient and clinician comfort is a nuanced yet essential aspect. Some patients may prefer more frequent check-ups for peace of mind, while others might find it anxiety-inducing. Tailoring surveillance to individual needs, balanced with evidence-based recommendations, is vital.

The overarching aim is to strike a balance between thoroughness and patient well-being. Over-surveillance may lead to unnecessary interventions, elevated healthcare costs, and undue anxiety. On the other hand, infrequent monitoring can miss early signs of recurrence. Thus, surveillance should be patient-centric, evidence-guided, and continuously evolving based on the latest research and individual patient progress.

> **Key Point**
> - HNSCC often re-emerges within 3 years, stressing early and robust post-treatment surveillance.
> - The 2018 NI-RADS system standardizes HNSCC surveillance, while PET/CT is emerging as a valuable tool for differentiating post-treatment changes from recurrences.
> - Surveillance must be tailored to individual patient needs and disease specifics, balancing evidence-based recommendations with patient well-being and comfort.

17.10 Neck Cancer of Unknown Primary (NCUP)

A challenging scenario in the realm of head and neck oncology is the diagnosis of cervical metastatic squamous cell carcinoma without an identifiable primary tumor, also known as NCUP. Approximately 3% of patients presenting with cervical lymphadenopathy, typically in the upper jugular chain, have no apparent primary tumor after a thorough clinical and radiographical evaluation [28].

The initial workup for NCUP involves a comprehensive clinical examination, office-based endoscopy, fine-needle aspiration (FNA) of the neck lymph node, and medical imaging. For a definitive diagnosis, operative panendoscopy with directed biopsies and palatine and/or lingual tonsillectomy are often required.

The HPV or EBV status obtained from the FNA sample is crucial, as over 90% of NCUP cases are related to HPV. Typically, HPV-related NCUP has its primary tumor in the base of the tongue and tonsillar fossa. Following this, EBV-related nasopharyngeal carcinoma is the next most common occult primary tumor. Advanced imaging, including CT, MRI, and PET/CT, often targets these areas for potential tumor detection in P16-positive cases (Fig. 17.7).

In contrast, a P16-negative status complicates the search. The primary tumor could be in numerous head and neck sites, or even more remotely in areas like the lungs. In these situations, a systematic and comprehensive evaluation is crucial.

PET/CT has a pivotal role in pinpointing unknown primaries. Particularly in the early stages, where anatomical changes may be subtle, the metabolic activity picked up by PET can guide the search.

When both advanced imaging and panendoscopy do not yield results, a "wait and watch" strategy might be adopted, especially if the lymph nodes have been surgically excised. Some primaries manifest later, while others never reveal themselves. The latter group, despite the mystery, often experiences favorable outcomes, paralleling those of known primary tumors.

> **Key Point**
> - NCUP denotes cervical metastatic squamous cell carcinoma where the primary tumor remains undetected.
> - Most NCUP cases are HPV-related, often originating from the base of the tongue or tonsillar fossa.
> - Advanced imaging (e.g., PET/CT) becomes instrumental in pinpointing these elusive primaries, especially given their metabolic activity.

Fig. 17.7 Patient initially presented with right cervical lymphadenopathy with the biopsy showing p16-positive squamous cell carcinoma. PET-CT (**a**) shows a small focal FDG avidity at the right tongue base in keeping with the primary site of tumor. On the corresponding CT (**b**) and MRI (**c** and **d**), only subtle soft tissue thickening and enhancement are appreciated (green arrows)

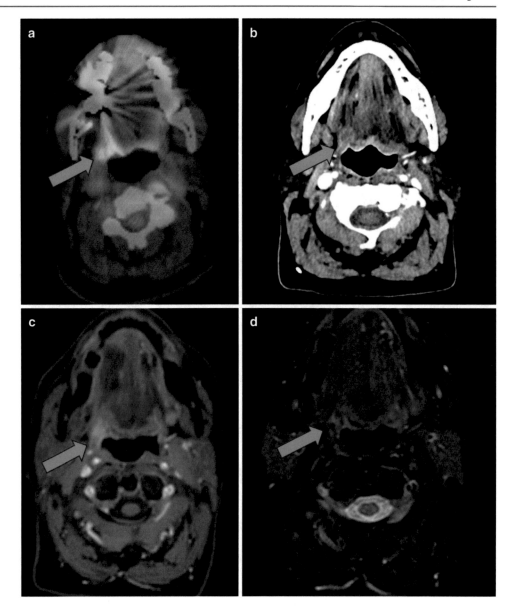

17.11 Concluding Remarks

Radiologists play a central role in the management of HNSCC. Advanced imaging techniques, from PET/CT to MRI, are crucial for accurate diagnosis and staging. It is vital to recognize key upstaging features such as PNS and ENE as they have a significant bearing on treatment and outcomes. Familiarity with the AJCC/UICC eighth edition and its updates aids in consistent and accurate reporting. The challenge of HNSCC with an unknown primary highlights the importance of integrating imaging with markers like P16. Ultimately, radiologists provide essential insights that influence patient management decisions in HNSCC.

Take-Home Messages

- Advanced imaging techniques are central to the precise staging and surveillance of HNSCC, with modalities like PET/CT offering a comprehensive insight into tumor behavior and spread.
- The refined criteria in AJCC/UICC eighth edition highlight the importance of specific anatomical and molecular markers, such as P16 status, in dictating prognosis and guiding therapeutic strategies.
- Invasion into critical structures, like the paraglottic space or cartilage, significantly impacts the upstaging and prognosis of HNSCC.
- Cervical lymphadenopathy and perineural spread are pivotal factors influencing disease spread and patient outcomes, requiring meticulous evaluation.
- In the challenging realm of HNSCC with unknown primary, an integrated approach using advanced imaging, molecular markers, and endoscopy is imperative for accurate diagnosis and treatment planning.

References

1. Sung H, Ferlay J, Siegel RL, Laversanne M, Soerjomataram I, Jemal A, et al. Global cancer statistics 2020: GLOBOCAN estimates of incidence and mortality worldwide for 36 cancers in 185 countries. CA Cancer J Clin. 2021;71(3):209–49.
2. Gormley M, Creaney G, Schache A, Ingarfield K, Conway DI. Reviewing the epidemiology of head and neck cancer: definitions, trends and risk factors. Br Dent J. 2022;233(9):780–6.
3. Mukherjee S, Fischbein NJ, Baugnon KL, Policeni BA, Raghavan P. Contemporary imaging and reporting strategies for head and neck cancer: MRI, FDG PET/MRI, NI-RADS, and carcinoma of unknown primary-AJR expert panel narrative review. Am J Roentgenol. 2023;220(2):160–72.
4. Wyss A, Hashibe M, Chuang SC, Lee YCA, Zhang ZF, Yu GP, et al. Cigarette, cigar, and pipe smoking and the risk of head and neck cancers: pooled analysis in the international head and neck cancer epidemiology consortium. Am J Epidemiol. 2013;178(5):679–90. https://pubmed-ncbi-nlm-nih-gov.myaccess.library.utoronto.ca/23817919/
5. Thomas SJ, Penfold CM, Waylen A, Ness AR. The changing aetiology of head and neck squamous cell cancer: a tale of three cancers? Clin Otolaryngol. 2018;43(4):999–1003. https://pubmed.ncbi.nlm.nih.gov/29770611/
6. Weissman JL, Akindele R. Current imaging techniques for head and neck tumors. Oncology. 1999;13(5):697–709.
7. Bannas P, Habermann CR, Jung C, Bley TA, Ittrich H, Adam G, et al. Diagnostic accuracy of state-of-the-art MDCT scanners without gantry tilt in patients with oral and oropharyngeal cancer. Eur J Radiol. 2012;81(12):3947–52. http://www.ejradiology.com/article/S0720048X11006486/fulltext
8. Kuno H, Onaya H, Iwata R, Kobayashi T, Fujii S, Hayashi R, et al. Evaluation of cartilage invasion by laryngeal and hypopharyngeal squamous cell carcinoma with dual-energy CT. Radiology. 2012;265(2):488–96.
9. Sakata K, Hareyama M, Tamakawa M, Oouchi A, Sido M, Nagakura H, et al. Prognostic factors of nasopharynx tumors investigated by MR imaging and the value of MR imaging in the newly published TNM staging. Int J Radiat Oncol Biol Phys. 1999;43(2):273–8.
10. Lonneux M, Hamoir M, Reychler H, Maingon P, Duvillard C, Calais G, et al. Positron emission tomography with [18F]fluorodeoxyglucose improves staging and patient management in patients with head and neck squamous cell carcinoma: a multicenter prospective study. J Clin Oncol. 2010;28(7):1190–5.
11. Zhu L, Wang N. 18F-fluorodeoxyglucose positron emission tomography-computed tomography as a diagnostic tool in patients with cervical nodal metastases of unknown primary site: a meta-analysis. Surg Oncol. 2013;22(3):190–4.
12. Wong ET, Dmytriw AA, Yu E, Waldron J, Lu L, Fazelzad R, et al. 18F-FDG PET/CT for locoregional surveillance following definitive treatment of head and neck cancer: a meta-analysis of reported studies. Head Neck. 2019;41(2):551–61. https://doi.org/10.1002/hed.25513.
13. Brierley JD, Gospodarowicz MK, Wittekind C. TNM classification of malignant tumours, 8th edition due December 2016. Union Int Cancer Control. 2017;1–272. https://www.wiley.com/en-gb/TNM+Classification+of+Malignant+Tumours%2C+8th+Edition-p-9781119263579
14. Dmytriw AA, El Beltagi A, Bartlett E, Sahgal A, Poon CS, Forghani R, et al. CRISPS: a pictorial essay of an acronym to interpreting metastatic head and neck lymphadenopathy. Can Assoc Radiol J. 2014;65(3):232–41. https://doi.org/10.1016/j.carj.2013.07.004.
15. Zanoni DK, Patel SG, Shah JP. Changes in the 8th edition of the American Joint Committee on Cancer (AJCC) Staging of Head and Neck Cancer: Rationale and Implications. Curr Oncol Rep. 2019;21(6):52. http://www.ncbi.nlm.nih.gov/pubmed/30997577
16. Weimar EAM, Huang SH, Lu L, O'Sullivan B, Perez-Ordonez B, Weinreb I, et al. Radiologic-pathologic correlation of tumor thickness and its prognostic importance in squamous cell carcinoma of the oral cavity: implications for the eighth edition tumor, node, metastasis classification. Am J Neuroradiol. 2018;39(10):1896–902.
17. Abdel Razek AAK, King A. MRI and CT of nasopharyngeal carcinoma. Am J Roentgenol. 2012;198(1):11–8.
18. Glastonbury CM. Critical changes in the staging of head and neck cancer. Radiol Imaging Cancer. 2020;2(1):1–8.
19. Kuno H, Sakamaki K, Fujii S, Sekiya K, Otani K, Hayashi R, et al. Comparison of MR imaging and dual-energy ct for the evaluation of cartilage invasion by laryngeal and hypopharyngeal squamous cell carcinoma. Am J Neuroradiol. 2018;39(3):524–31.
20. Imre A, Pinar E, Erdoan N, Ece AA, Olgun Y, Aladag I, et al. Prevertebral space invasion in head and neck cancer: negative predictive value of imaging techniques. Ann Otol Rhinol Laryngol. 2015;124(5):378–83.
21. Kao J, Lavaf A, Teng MS, Huang D, Genden EM. Adjuvant radiotherapy and survival for patients with node-positive head and neck cancer: an analysis by primary site and nodal stage. Int J Radiat Oncol Biol Phys. 2008;71(2):362–70.
22. Som PM, Curtin HD. Head and neck imaging. 2011;47.
23. Hoang JK, Vanka J, Ludwig BJ, Glastonbury CM. Evaluation of cervical lymph nodes in head and neck cancer with CT and MRI: tips, traps, and a systematic approach. Am J Roentgenol. 2013;200(1):W17–25.
24. Alsowey AM, Amin MI, Ebaid NY. Diagnostic accuracy, reliability, and reviewer agreement of a new proposed risk prediction model for metastatic cervical lymph node from head and neck squamous cell carcinoma using MDCT. Egypt J Radiol Nucl Med. 2022;53(1):1–10. https://doi.org/10.1186/s43055-022-00920-y.
25. Ong CK, Chong F-H. Imaging of perineural spread in head and neck tumours. Cancer Imaging. 2010;10:92–8.
26. Chang JH, Wu CC, Yuan KSP, Wu ATH, Wu SY. Locoregionally recurrent head and neck squamous cell carcinoma: incidence,

survival, prognostic factors, and treatment outcomes. Oncotarget. 2017;8(33):55600–12. https://pubmed.ncbi.nlm.nih.gov/28903447/

27. Aiken AH, Rath TJ, Anzai Y, Branstetter BF, Hoang JK, Wiggins RH, et al. ACR neck imaging reporting and data systems (NI-RADS): a white paper of the ACR NI-RADS committee. J Am Coll Radiol. 2018;15(8):1097–108. https://doi.org/10.1016/j.jacr.2018.05.006.

28. Strojan P, Ferlito A, Langendijk JA, Corry J, Woolgar JA, Rinaldo A, et al. Contemporary management of lymph node metastases from an unknown primary to the neck: II. A review of therapeutic options. Head Neck. 2013;35(2):286–93. https://doi.org/10.1002/hed.21899.

Part V

Spine, Spinal Cord, Plexus and Nerves

Evaluation of Myelopathy and Radiculopathy

18

Lubdha M. Shah and Jeffrey S. Ross

Abstract

Myelopathy and radiculopathy can be due to extrinsic causes, most often degenerative in origin. Imaging can elucidate an often-confusing clinical picture to guide management and provide prognostic information. For intrinsic causes of myelopathy, the differential diagnosis categories include demyelination, inflammation, infection, vascular, and neoplasm. The combination of clinical symptoms, timing of presentation, and imaging features can help narrow the differential diagnosis.

Keywords

Myelopathy · Radiculopathy · MRI · CT · Degenerative Inflammation · Demyelination · Infection · Neoplasm Vascular · Hematoma · Metabolic

Learning Objectives
- Explain the clinical differences between myelopathy and radiculopathy to help develop the appropriate differential diagnosis.
- Review the pathophysiology of degenerative changes that result in myelopathy and/or radiculopathy.
- Describe the etiologies that result in extrinsic myelopathy.
- Discuss differentiating imaging features of inflammatory, infectious, vascular, and metabolic spinal cord pathologies.

L. M. Shah (✉)
Department of Radiology, University of Utah,
Salt Lake City, UT, USA
e-mail: lubdha.shah@hsc.utah.edu

J. S. Ross
Department of Radiology, Mayo Clinic, Phoenix, AZ, USA
e-mail: Ross.Jeffrey1@mayo.edu

18.1 Clinical Presentation

Spinal cord lesions may result in the clinical findings of myelopathy, presenting as abnormalities in motor, sensory, and autonomic pathways which can be manifest as paresthesias, decreased dexterity, changes in mobility, or frequent falls. When a patient has a lesion either intrinsically or extrinsically affecting a spinal nerve or plexus, they may present with radiculopathy, which includes pain, weakness, reflex changes, and sensory loss in the specific nerve distribution. The lumbosacral cauda equina nerve roots are the peripheral transition distal to the conus medullaris of the central nervous system. As these two areas are in close-proximity, lesions in one area can affect the function of the other.

18.2 Myelopathy

Lesions that cause myelopathy may either be extrinsic compressive or intrinsic non-compressive to the spinal cord. Although many etiologies can have overlapping imaging appearances, clinical history and demographics are critical to narrow the possible etiologies. The pattern of spinal cord involvement is also important to consider and can help in developing a differential diagnosis.

Key Point
- When a patient presents with symptoms of myelopathy, it is important to consider both extrinsic compressive lesions, which may necessitate surgical intervention, and pathologies that involve the spinal cord parenchyma.

© The Author(s) 2024
J. Hodler et al. (eds.), *Diseases of the Brain, Head and Neck, Spine 2024-2027*, IDKD Springer Series,
https://doi.org/10.1007/978-3-031-50675-8_18

18.2.1 Extrinsic

Degenerative cervical myelopathy (DCM) is a very common cause of myelopathy due to extrinsic compression. DCM reflects age-related chronic spinal cord injury through degenerative changes of the spinal axis with both static and dynamic contributing factors. Disc degeneration includes loss of disc height, disc herniations, osteophyte formation, and thickening of the ligamentum flavum, which may result in loss of cervical lordosis. There may be instability or hypermobility due to the ligamentous laxity, which may put stress on the facet and uncovertebral joints with resultant hypertrophy. The osteophytes and buckled ligaments may cause static compression of the spinal cord, which is further exacerbated by the straightened or kyphotic alignment with stretching of the spinal cord while the hypermobility contributes to dynamic injury. Regional and local spinal cord perfusion are compromised in DCM. The blood–spinal cord barrier may be disrupted with chronic ischemia followed by an influx of inflammatory cells into the spinal cord parenchyma with subsequent inflammation [1].

DCM pathophysiology is reflected in the imaging appearance. Patients with DCM may have hyperintensity within the cord on T2WI (T2-weighted imaging) and, less commonly, hypointensity on T1WI (T1-weighted imaging) in the region of the compression. The prevalence of hyperintense signal on T2WI among patients with clinically confirmed DCM has been reported within the range of 58–85%. T2WI hyperintensity may be strongly hyperintense and well-circumscribed or less hyperintense and diffuse (without a clear margin). It is thought that these changes represent different states of pathology and have different recovery potentials [2]. DCM may also have a distinct pattern of contrast enhancement: a transverse axial or pancake-like enhancement at or just caudal to the site of maximal stenosis and at the rostrocaudal midpoint of a spindle-shaped T2 hyperintensity (Fig. 18.1). This enhancement can persist for months, even years, following surgical decompression [3]. Clinical correlation is essential for the diagnosis of DCM since cervical degenerative disc disease is ubiquitous. One study found that up to 60% of asymptomatic individuals older than 40 years of age can show degenerative changes on MRI [4], while another showed that up to 90% over the age of 60 years and associated with age and degeneration in other spinal segments [5].

Key Point
- DCM may have a distinct pancake-like enhancement at the site of maximal stenosis.

Epidural lesions such as spontaneous epidural hematoma (SEH) and epidural abscess may cause neurologic deficits due extrinsic compression. SEH is the atraumatic accumulation of blood in the epidural space due to multiple potential etiologies such as coagulopathy, anticoagulation, neoplasm, vascular malformation, hypertension, increased intra-abdominal or intra-thoracic pressure (such as straining, sneezing, lifting), and idiopathic (40–60% of cases). Patients with spontaneous spinal epidural hematoma typically present with acute onset of severe back pain and rapidly develop signs of compression of the spinal cord or cauda equina nerve roots. The pathophysiology is hypothesized to be due to venous bleeding [6] or, less likely, arterial bleeding. CT may reveal hyperdense blood products effacing the hypodense fat in the epidural space. Similarly on MRI, effacement of the T1 hyperintense epidural fat is a helpful clue to the epidural location. MR imaging appearance of SEH changes over time as the hemoglobin evolves (Table 18.1). SEH may demonstrate mild peripheral enhancement [7] (Fig. 18.2).

Epidural abscess may occur due to hematogenous dissemination, direct inoculation, or extension from contiguous infected tissues, such as discitis-osteomyelitis. Patients may present with neck or back pain and fever. The severity of neurological deficits depends on the extent of cord compression. An epidural abscess will show central nonenhancing fluid signal intensity, with irregular and thick peripheral enhancement. Diffusion-weighted imaging (DWI) can be extremely helpful in the diagnosis of spinal epidural abscess, as it is in the brain, showing markedly increased signal with infection (Fig. 18.3). Although blood products may also show increased signal on DWI [8], imaging clues such as paraspinal edema/enhancement/abscess or bone marrow edema/enhancement may point to infectious process. The appearance of epidural phlegmon is usually amorphous T1 isointense to hypointense, and T2 hyperintense fluid which effaces the epidural fat. Phlegmon shows diffuse enhancement while abscess will demonstrate peripheral enhancement.

Neoplastic lesions involving the extradural space, originating in the osseous structures or the epidural compartment, can compress the spinal cord and nerve roots. A pathologic fracture with retropulsion of bone can result in cauda equina syndrome (e.g., urinary retention urinary/fecal incontinence, saddle anesthesia, lower extremity weakness, back and/or leg pain). Imaging features on conventional MRI that favor a pathologic fracture include abnormal posterior element signal, epidural or paravertebral soft tissue mass, geographic replacement of normal marrow signal, irregular margins, and bowing of the posterior cortex [9] (Fig. 18.4). The acutely impacted spinal cord may exhibit intramedullary T2 hyperintensity due to edema.

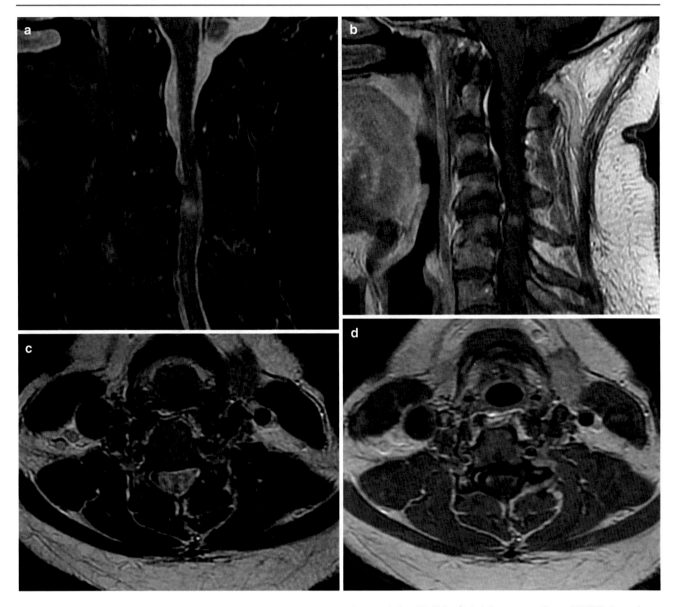

Fig. 18.1 (**a**) Sagittal and (**c**) axial T2WI shows focal intramedullary hyperintensity at the C5 level. (**b**) Sagittal contrast-enhanced T1WI demonstrates horizontal, "pancake-like" enhancement at this level, characteristic of DCM. (**d**) Axial contrast-enhanced T1WI shows irregular, peripheral enhancement

Table 18.1 MRI of spontaneous epidural hematoma

Age	MRI appearance
Acute	Nonspecific fluid intensity: T1 isointense, T2 heterogeneous hyperintense
Early subacute	T1 hyperintense, T2 hypointense
Late subacute	T1 hyperintense, T2 hyperintense
Chronic	T1 hypointense, T2 hypointense

Key Point
- MRI features of a pathologic fracture include abnormal posterior element signal, soft tissue mass, abnormal marrow signal, irregular margins, and bowing of the posterior cortex. On the other hand, an osteoporotic fracture shows normal posterior element signal intensity, retropulsion of the posterior cortex, linear horizontal hypointense T1/T2 band, fluid sign, and normal enhancement relative to adjacent vertebrae.

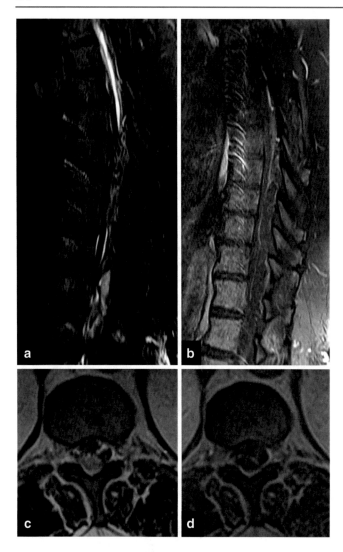

Fig. 18.2 (**a**) Sagittal STIR MRI shows heterogeneous hyper-/hypointense collection in the dorsal epidural space. (**c**) Axial T2WI demonstrates anterior displacement and mass effect on the thecal sac by the SEH. (**b**) Sagittal and (**d**) axial contrast-enhanced T1WI shows peripheral enhancement of the dorsal epidural collection

Intradural extramedullary lesions can also impinge upon the spinal cord, resulting in myelopathic symptoms. Meningiomas are common intradural extramedullary spinal lesions, which arise from the arachnoid meningothelial cells, are commonly in the thoracic segment (80%), and shows a female predilection [10]. Although the majority of meningiomas are World Health Organization grade I, they are symptomatic because of spinal cord or nerve root compression. Patients may experience gait ataxia, localized or radicular pain, and sensorimotor deficits. On MRI, meningiomas demonstrate T1 iso-/hypointensity, slight T2 hyperintensity, and avid enhancement (Fig. 18.5). Tapered enhancing margins, (dural tail) can be a helpful imaging clue. Susceptibility artifacts may be present if there is calcification. Densely calcified lesions may be confusing on post-contrast images as

they tend to show very little central enhancement. The compressed spinal cord will exhibit intramedullary T2 hyperintensity due to edema and gliosis in the setting of chronic impingement.

Ventral displacement of the spinal cord may reflect a variety of lesions which may be anterior or posterior to the cord. Primary posterior lesions include arachnoid web and arachnoid cyst. A ventral lesion is transdural cord herniation. Arachnoid webs are an intradural extramedullary transverse bands of arachnoid tissue that extends to the dorsal surface of the spinal cord, causing mass effect and dorsal cord indentation. Altered CSF flow dynamics from this web may result in cord edema which may eventually develop into syringomyelia. Patients may present with back pain and upper and lower extremity weakness and numbness. On MRI or CT myelogram, the arachnoid web causes a characteristic focal dorsal indentation of the dorsal spinal cord, "scalpel sign" [11] (Fig. 18.6a, b, c). Spinal cord herniation is considered when there is focal ventral protrusion of the spinal cord is a patient with back pain and motor and sensory deficits. The "C-shape" of the dorsal indentation favors spinal cord herniation [12] (Fig. 18.6d, e). Although most spinal cord herniation cases are idiopathic, other uncommon etiologies include prior trauma, dural rent due to disc protrusion, congenital dural defect, or inflammatory process leading to adhesion of the cord to the ventral dura.

18.2.2 Intrinsic

Non-compressive lesions affecting the spinal cord parenchyma can result in myelopathy. The MRI pattern, particularly on the T2WI sequences, can be helpful in developing differential diagnosis. However, the temporal presentation and clinical signs and symptoms are crucial to narrow the differential considerations. For example, infectious processes and vascular injuries tend to present acutely. On the other hand, if the patient's myelopathic symptoms are insidious in onset or progressive, differential considerations include metabolic or inflammatory processes and intramedullary neoplasm.

Demyelinating diseases may have characteristic imaging features on brain and spine MRI that may be helpful in distinguishing between the different demyelinating diseases (Fig. 18.7). Multiple sclerosis (MS) is the prototypical demyelinating disease, characterized by waxing and waning symptoms related to brain and spinal lesions. The spinal cord, particularly the cervical segment, is affected in more than 90% of patients with clinically definite MS. The classic spinal cord MS plaque is an ovoid T2 hyperintense lesion, spanning less than two vertebral bodies craniocaudally, affecting less than half the cross-section of the cord, and located in the posterior and posterolateral cord [13]. Active

Fig. 18.3 (a) Sagittal contrast-enhanced T1WI demonstrates a peripherally enhancing fluid collection in the patient with increasing upper back pain and mild leukocytosis. (b) Sagittal DWI shows hyperintensity in this collection due to the purulent material. (c) Axial contrast-enhanced T1WI and (d) T2WI show compression and anterior displacement by this epidural abscess

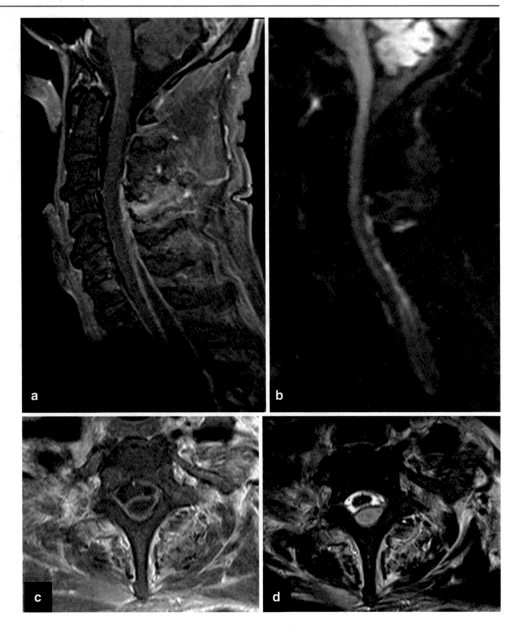

lesions may show mild swelling, and transient breakdown of the blood–cord barrier can result in lesion enhancement of the lesion. Chronic disease may result in spinal cord atrophy with focal areas of gliosis due to axonal loss.

Other demyelinating lesions involve longer segments of the spinal cord. Acute disseminated encephalomyelitis (ADEM) is a monophasic illness that may occur after viral illness or vaccination due to autoimmune reaction to myelin basic protein. ADEM lesions are poorly marginated, longer in the craniocaudal extent, involve a greater cross-section of the spinal cord, variably enhance, and tend to involve the thoracic spinal cord.

Neuromyelitis optica spectrum disorder (NMOSD) is a demyelinating process that involves the optic nerves and spinal cord, with brain involvement concentrated in the distribution of the aquaporin four channels (e.g., hypothalamus,

periaqueductal gray matter, area postrema). The spinal cord lesions are classically greater than three vertebral bodies in craniocaudal extent (longitudinally extensive), involve the central gray matter and greater than 2/3 of the cord cross-section, and frequently extend cephalad to the medulla [14]. Some lesions have heterogeneous internal foci of T2 hyperintensity, described as "bright spotty lesions" [15]. There may be variable enhancement and tumefactive cord expansion.

Myelin Oligodendrocyte Glycoprotein IgG Associated Disease (MOGAD) is a distinct severe demyelinating pathology related to a glycoprotein on the myelin surface, which may be confused with NMOSD. Children older than 9 years of age and adults present with optic neuritis, usually bilateral, longitudinally extensive transverse myelitis, and brainstem lesions [16]. Conus medullaris predilection [17], central

Fig. 18.4 (**a**) Sagittal T2WI and (**b**) contrast-enhanced T1WI show multiple osseous metastases involving the lower thoracic and lumbar spine with a pathological fracture of T12. (**c**) Axial T2WI and (**d**) axial contrast-enhanced T1WI demonstrate bowing of the posterior cortex and the epidural extension causing severe narrowing of the spinal subarachnoid space and compression of the distal spinal cord

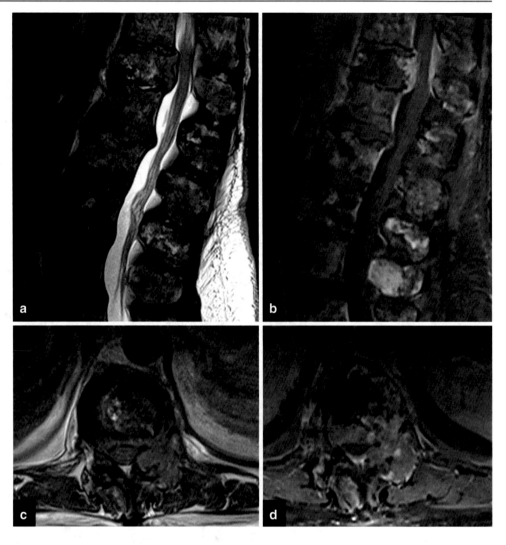

grey matter involvement, and lack of enhancement are more characteristic features of MOGAD.

Sarcoidosis is chronic idiopathic, multisystem inflammatory disorder which can involve the central nervous system in up 25% of patients [18], with intramedullary involvement in less than 1% of cases [19]. T2WI demonstrates mildly enlargement of the spinal cord with extensive hyperintensity. On contrast-enhanced T1WI, there may be linear leptomeningeal enhancement along pial surface in early phases. Intramedullary involvement occurs due to centripetal spread through perivascular spaces. Central canal enhancement with a "trident sign" can be seem with subacute myelitis and manifest as dorsal cord involvement with central and lateral extensions [20] (Fig. 18.8).

Key Point
- Neurosarcoidosis can have a characteristic pattern of central and lateral enhancement, "trident sign" due to centripetal spread through perivascular spaces.

Infectious myelopathies may result from direct invasion by the pathogen or as a parainfectious immune-mediated process. Contrast-enhanced MRI will reveal patterns of spinal cord abnormality including central (segmental or longitudinally extensive), eccentric tract-specific (lateral columns, posterior columns), ventral horn, and irregular/mass-like, which may help to narrow the differential diagnosis. Overlapping imaging patterns may be seen, and, in some cases, the spinal cord may appear normal on MRI.

Numerous viruses can cause infectious myelitis, some of which are particularly neurotropic such as herpesviruses, flaviviruses, and enteroviruses. Several enteroviruses are implicated in myelitis (e.g., enterovirus 71, coxsackieviruses, echovirus, and poliovirus) and have a predilection for ventral horn cell involvement. On MRI, there will be abnormal signal within the ventral nerve roots (unilateral or bilateral). With enterovirus 71, MRI typically shows segmental or longitudinally extensive T2 hyperintensity centered in the ventral horns with variable enhancement (Fig. 18.9). A central longitudinally extensive transverse myelitis pattern may also be seen less frequently and portends a worse prognosis [21].

Fig. 18.5 (a) Sagittal T2WI shows a mildly hypointense, well-circumscribed intradural extramedullary lesion anteriorly displacing the mid-thoracic spinal cord. (c) Axial T2WI demonstrates marked compression of the spinal cord by this lesion. (b) Sagittal and (d) axial contrast-enhanced T1WI display the avid enhancement of the meningioma

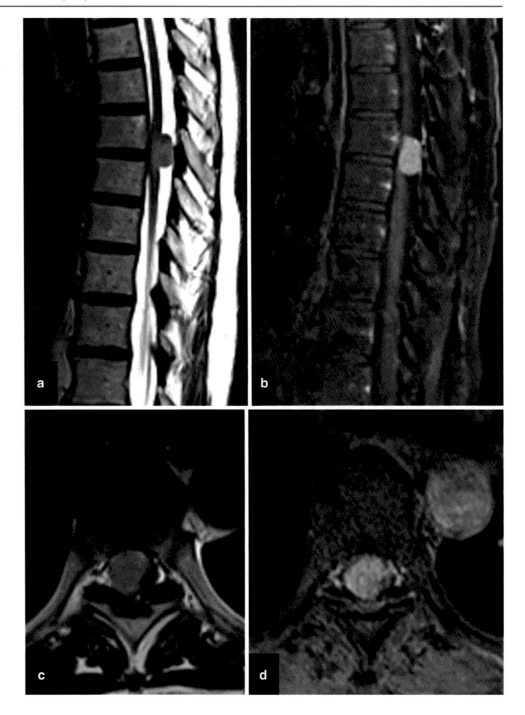

Similarly, enterovirus D68 infections result in confluent longitudinally extensive T2 hyperintensity of the cervical spinal cord gray matter, with involvement of dorsal pontine tegmentum and ventral pons. Central intramedullary and nerve root enhancement has also been described [21]. Approximately 5–10% of neuroinvasive cases of West Nile virus (WNV) are associated with myelitis, presenting with acute flaccid paralysis. The MRI appearance in WNV is quite variable and may be unremarkable. WNV also has a predilection for ventral horn cell involvement, which may present as abnormal signal within the ventral cord, sometimes with associated ventral nerve root enhancement.

Other neurotropic viruses can have distinct patterns of spinal cord involvement. MRI in patients with Human Immunodeficiency Virus (HIV) demonstrates symmetric nonenhancing T2 hyperintensity within the posterior columns, most commonly involving the thoracic spinal cord (Fig. 18.10). The pathologic process is vacuolar myelopathy and parallels the AIDS dementia complex spectrum, i.e., seen in later stages of the disease. The posterior column

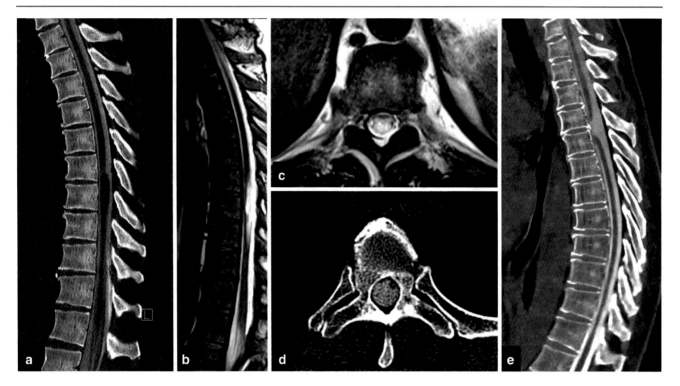

Fig. 18.6 (a) Sagittal CT myelogram and (b) sagittal T2WI demonstrates the dorsal indentation in the mid-thoracic spine (scalpel sign) due to an arachnoid web. (c) Axial T2WI shows intramedullary edema. (d) Axial CT myelogram demonstrates ventral herniation of the spinal cord through a dural defect. (e) Sagittal CT myelogram shows the "C-shaped" morphology suggestive of cord herniation

involvement explains the symptoms of a slowly progressive spastic paraparesis, impaired vibratory and position sense, and urinary urgency. In patients with varicella zoster virus myelitis, MRI reveals T2 hyperintensity in the dorsal horn and posterior column. The virus enters the spinal cord dorsal root and posterior column sand can extend vertically. Patients present with a skin rash then after a few days to weeks, the myelopathic symptoms begin. The skin rash is typically at the level of the spinal cord lesions.

Arterial vascular pathologies of the spinal cord can cause neurologic deficits. Clinical presentation of spinal cord ischemia is usually abrupt and depends mainly on the location and extent of the infarction. The maximal symptomatology is reached within 12 h for 50% of patients and within 72 h for most patients [22]. Spinal cord infarctions, predominantly in the anterior spinal artery distribution, are commonly due to atherosclerosis, hypertension, diabetes, fibrocartilaginous emboli, and other various vaso-occlusive etiologies. Acutely, DWI will show hyperintensity with corresponding hyperintensity on the apparent diffusion coefficient (ADC) images in the affected region. There will be hyperintense signal on T2WI and STIR and isointensity on T1WI. When the anterior spinal artery territory is affected, abnormal signal is seen in the ventral horns and the adjacent white matter (Fig. 18.11). Associated edema results in slight cord enlargement. Patchy enhancement may be seen in the subacute phase due to breakdown of the blood–cord barrier.

Spinal vascular malformations can present with acute or progressive symptoms, depending on the type of vascular shunt. Multiple different naming conventions have been applied to the wide variety of spinal vascular malformations, but in general the most common types can be defined as (1) Spinal dural arteriovenous fistula (SDAVF); (2) Glomus arteriovenous malformations (AVM); and (3) Perimedullary AVFs. SDAVFs are slow-flow lesions and account for 70% of all spinal vascular shunts. Classically, the presentation is that of an older male (55–60 years) with a history of nonspecific progressive myelopathic symptoms. Most (~80%) of SDAVFs are observed along the posterior lower thoracic cord surface between levels T6 and L2. The anomalous intradural communication between a dural artery and radicular vein within the intervertebral foramen results in engorged venous collaterals, producing the angiographic "single coiled vessel" appearance (Fig. 18.12). On T2WI, there are prominent serpentine flow voids overlying the posterior spinal cord. Venous congestion results in intramedullary edema/ T2 hyperintensity and mild cord expansion. Deoxyhemoglobin in dilated capillaries may produce a T2 hypointense rim [23]. There may be patchy intramedullary enhancement due to breakdown of the blood–cord barrier. Patients with a spinal glomus AVM may present with acute or subacute symptoms related to subarachnoid or cord hemorrhage. Similarly, patients with an intradural perimedullary AVF can present with acute neurologic deficits due to subarachnoid hemor-

Fig. 18.7 (**a**) Sagittal STIR MRI and (**d**) contrast-enhanced T1WI of the cervical spinal cord show the ovoid lesion of MS, spanning <2 vertebral bodies in length. The lesion demonstrates well-defined enhancement. (**b**) Sagittal T2WI and (**e**) contrast-enhanced T1WI of the cervical spinal cord in a patient with ADEM shows a long segment of intramedullary T2 hyperintensity and patchy, ill-defined enhancement, respectively, and mild cord expansion. This patient had viral prodrome and rapidly processive extremity weakness. (**c**) Sagittal T2WI and (**f**) contrast-enhanced T1WI of the thoracic spinal cord demonstrates a heterogeneously T2 hyperintense lesion involving the mid-thoracic cord with avid "mass-like" enhancement in this patient with NMOSD

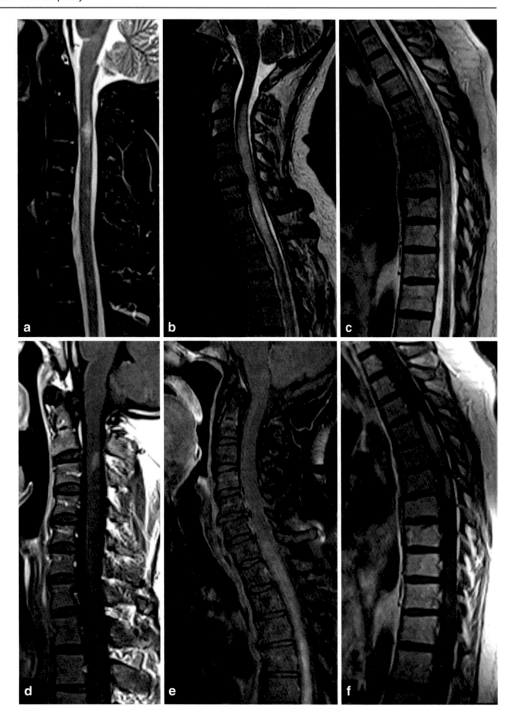

rhage or myelopathy related to venous congestion. The spinal glomus AVM nidus shows variable enhancement and may be partially or completely intramedullary with surrounding T2 hyperintensity. There may be radicular venous intra- and perimedullary flow voids and subarachnoid or parenchymal hemorrhage. With intradural perimedullary AVFs, MRI demonstrates prominent perimedullary flow voids typically along the ventral cord surface. Arterial and venous ectasia may cause cord compression. There is variable intramedullary T2 hyperintensity and pial enhancement.

Cavernous malformations are intramedullary lobulated dilated sinusoidal channels of dense capillary-like vessels without intervening neural tissue. While half of the patients with cavernous malformations present with progressive deterioration due to microhemorrhage, gliosis, microcirculatory changes, and partial thrombosis, the other half may have an acute or recurrent presentation due to larger hemorrhage

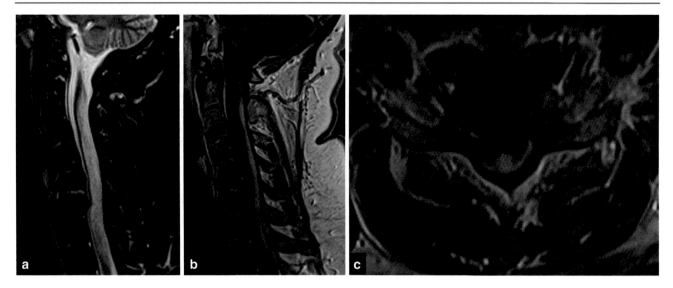

Fig. 18.8 (a) Sagittal STIR MRI shows long segmental of cervical cord intramedullary hyperintensity with mild expansion. (b) Sagittal contrast-enhanced T1WI demonstrates intramedullary enhancement along the dorsal aspect of the cord. (c) Axial contrast-enhanced T1WI illustrates dorsal cord enhancement with central and lateral extensions (trident sign), a finding highly suggestive of neurosarcoidosis

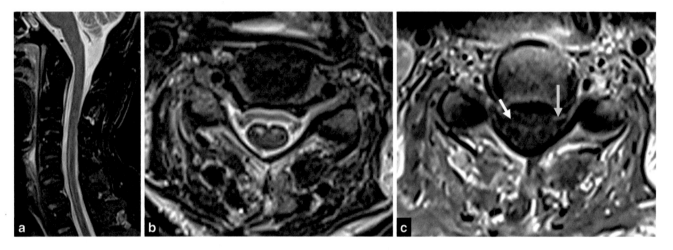

Fig. 18.9 (a) Sagittal STIR MRI shows a long segment of hyperintensity in the ventral cord. (b) Axial T2WI demonstrates hyperintensity in the ventral horns in this patient with enterovirus 71 myelitis. (c) Axial contrast-enhanced T1WI illustrates enhancement in the ventral horns (white arrow) and linear enhancement along the left ventral nerve root (yellow arrow)

within or beyond the capsule of the lesion. The average estimated annual hemorrhage risk of 2.1% [24]. On MRI, spinal cavernous malformations have the typical appearance of circumscribed, multilobulated lesions with heterogeneous T1 and T2 signal intensity and T2 hypointense rim. The heterogenous signal intensities are due to the various ages of blood by-products as well as calcifications and fibrosis (Fig. 18.13).

A variety of metabolic lesions can present with myelopathic symptoms. Subacute combined degeneration (SCD) is the term given for vitamin B12 deficiency that can produce paresthesias initially followed by sensory disturbances, weakness, and spasticity and primarily involves the dorsal and lateral spinal columns. As this is a treatable condition and the symptoms are potentially reversible, awareness of the imaging features is critical. B12 is important for all methylation reactions, including those needed for myelin phospholipids; therefore, its deficiency results in unstable myelin. On MRI, there may be modest expansion of the cervical and thoracic spinal cord and increased signal intensity on T2-weighted images, primarily in the dorsal columns in an inverted "V" configuration (Fig. 18.14). Rarely, there may be mild enhancement due to breakdown of the blood–cord barrier [25]. Other deficiency-related metabolic diseases that can cause T2 hyperintensity in the dorsal and possible lateral columns include acquired copper, folate, vitamin E deficiency, nitrous oxide toxicity (such in substance abuse with inhalation of whipped cream chargers), and intrathecal methotrexate [26].

Fig. 18.10 (**a**) Sagittal STIR MRI show intramedullary hyperintensity in the posterior cord. (**b**) Axial T2WI demonstrates abnormal signal in the posterior and lateral columns related to HIV vacuolar myelopathy

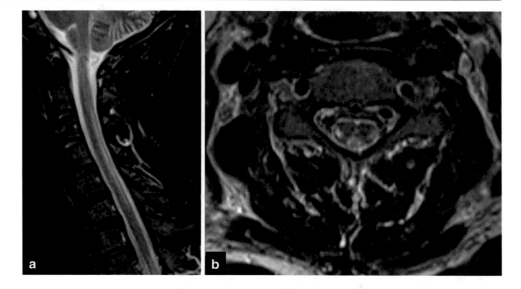

Fig. 18.11 (**a**) Sagittal STIR MRI and (**b**) DWI show anterior cervical cord hyperintensity in this patient with acute onset of extremity weakness related to spinal cord infarction. (**c**) Axial GRE and (**d**) DWI demonstrate hyperintensity in the ventral horns, reflecting anterior spinal artery territory of the ischemic injury

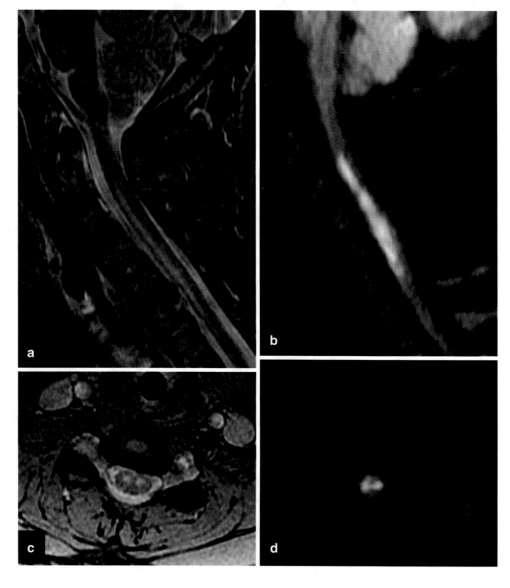

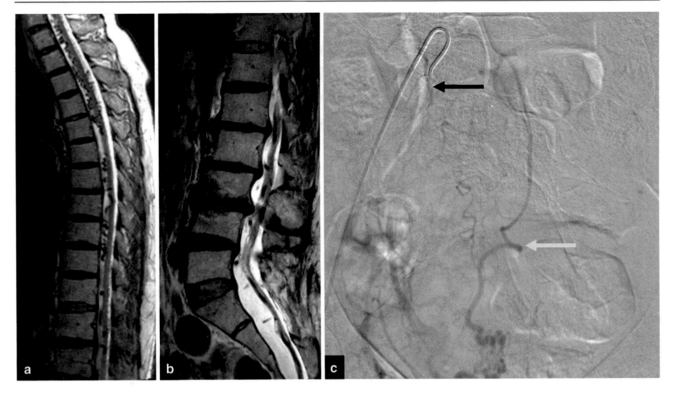

Fig. 18.12 Sagittal T2WI of the (**a**) thoracic and (**b**) lumbar spine demonstrates prominent, serpentine vessels overlying the spinal cord and the cauda equina nerves. (**c**) Frontal digital subtraction angio-graphic image shows SDAVF arising from lateral sacral arteries (black arrow). Venous drainage is to a dilated perimedullary vein coursing superiorly (yellow arrow)

Fig. 18.13 (**a**) Sagittal and (**b**) axial T2WI show a heterogenous intramedullary lesion with a T2 hypointense rim in the distal spinal cord related to a cavernous malformation. Recent intralesional hemorrhage results in mild cord expansion and edema

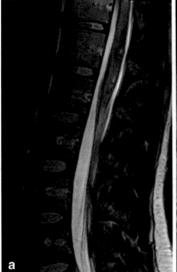 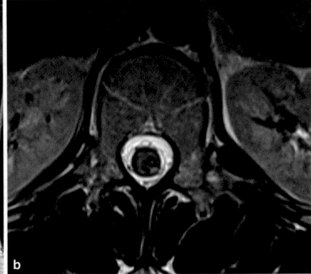

Key Point
- SCD has the classic appearance of an inverted "V" on T2-weighted MRI.

Imaging features that suggest intramedullary neoplasm as the cause of a patient's subacute/ chronic or progressive neu-rologic symptoms include abnormal cord signal intensity with focal cord expansion, focal/nodular cord enhancement, hemorrhage, and cord cyst formation. The common primary

Fig. 18.14 (a) Sagittal and (b) axial T2WI show hyperintensity in the posterior cervical cord, specifically involving the posterior columns, in this patient with leg and arm numbness due to SCD

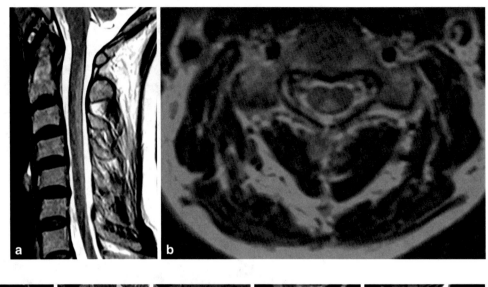

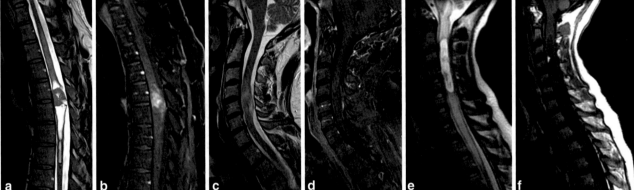

Fig. 18.15 (a) Sagittal T2WI and (b) contrast-enhanced T1WI shows an intramedullary expansile mass with central, irregular enhancing nodularity and polar cysts. The inferior hemosiderin cap favors ependymoma. (c) Sagittal T2WI and (d) contrast-enhanced T1WI demonstrates an intramedullary infiltrative mass with ill-defined patchy enhancement, features which suggest astrocytoma. (e) Sagittal T2WI and (f) contrast-enhanced T1WI shows a hemangioblastoma with the characteristic punctate enhancing nodule along the anterior cord associated with a large cyst and extensive edema

intramedullary neoplasms to consider are ependymoma, astrocytoma, and hemangioblastoma. In patients with history of malignancy, metastases should be in the differential diagnosis.

Ependymoma is the most frequently encountered glial tumor in adults, while astrocytoma is the most common glial tumor in the pediatric population. Ependymomas are sharply defined, variable enhancing, encapsulated tumors, which are usually central in location. These tumors commonly demonstrate peritumoral cystic change and hemorrhage. The hemosiderin "cap" sign is seen in 20–30% of cases and is a helpful clue to the diagnosis [27]. In contradistinction, astrocytomas have a poorly defined, infiltrative appearance often involving multiple vertebral body levels and sometimes the entire spi-

nal cord [27]. There is often patchy enhancement and peritumoral edema. Hemangioblastomas are nonglial tumors with the typical appearance of an avidly enhancing nodule with or without an associated tumor cyst or syrinx formation. Large hemangioblastomas may show adjacent serpentine flow voids from prominent feeding vessels (Fig. 18.15). Intramedullary spinal cord metastasis may show features on postgadolinium images to help distinguish them from primary cord masses: the "rim" sign (more intense thin rim of peripheral enhancement around an enhancing lesion) and the "flame" sign (ill-defined flame-shaped region of enhancement at the superior/inferior lesion margins) (Fig. 18.16). Either or both signs have high specificity (97% and 100%, respectively) [28].

Fig. 18.16 (a) Sagittal contrast-enhanced T1WI and (b) T2WI demonstrate an intramedullary spinal cord metastasis. The lesion shows more intense thin rim of peripheral enhancement and ill-defined flame-shaped region of enhancement at the inferior margin. Extensive intramedullary T2 hyperintensity extends superiorly due to cord edema

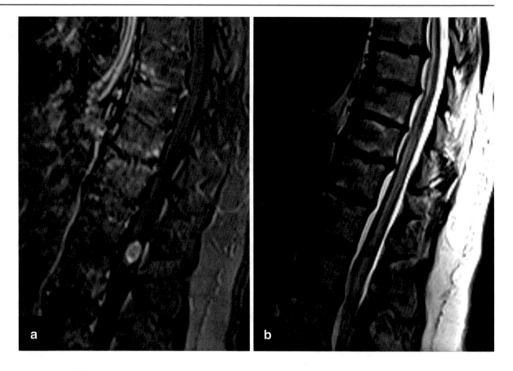

18.3   Radiculopathy

When evaluating the imaging for a patient with radiculopathy, degenerative changes affecting spinal nerves are the leading consideration followed by infectious and inflammatory processes. Pathologies involving the brachial and lumbosacral plexus can also present as radiculopathy.

Degenerative lesions, such as disc herniations (protrusion, extrusion) and endplate osteophytes can impinge on the exiting nerve roots in the neural foramina and on the transiting nerve roots in the subarticular zones. Patients will present with radicular symptoms in a distinct nerve distribution. Other degenerative processes that cause nerve impingement include synovial cysts (Fig. 18.17), facet or uncovertebral osteophytes, and segmental motion with instability. The latter may not be appreciated on supine imaging and upright radiographs with axial loading provides complementary functional information. Findings of degenerative isthmic spondylothesis and facet hypertrophy with facet effusions suggests segmental motion [29].

Inflammatory lesions that involve the cauda equina nerves can present with neurological symptoms that can be difficult to differentiate clinically from myelopathy. One such entity that is a common cause of acute flaccid paralysis is acute inflammatory demyelinating polyneuropathy (AIDP)/ Guillain-Barré syndrome. AIDP is an immune-mediated polyradiculoneuropathy that presents with acute ascending limb weakness associated with reduced reflexes. There is often history of a preceding infective illness [30]. Extremity weakness progresses, which can last up to 4 weeks before

reaching plateau. The disease may progress in some patients, causing autonomic dysfunction, bulbar weakness, and respiratory insufficiency. Acutely, the cauda equina nerves may show thickening and enhancement on MRI, which has a sensitivity of 83% [31]. Classically, there may be anterior root involvement although both anterior and posterior roots may be involved. Chronic inflammatory demyelinating polyneuropathy (CIDP) is an indolent demyelinating pathology with symptoms beyond 8 weeks. Patients may present with posterior column sensory signs (e.g., ataxia, vibratory, or proprioceptive loss). On MRI, the brachial plexus, lumbosacral plexus, and cauda equina nerves may be diffusely enlarged and show mild enhancement (Fig. 18.18). Additionally, the muscles, supplied by the nerves, will demonstrate denervation changes: mild enhancement and T2 hyperintensity acutely/ subacutely and fatty atrophy chronically.

Neoplastic processes from primary or secondary tumors can metastasize to the leptomeninges, resulting in leptomeningeal carcinomatosis. The subarachnoid spread of malignant cells may be "drop metastases" from primary CNS tumors or via hematogenous spread. The imaging appearance of leptomeningeal metastatic disease is variable, from thin and linear to thick and nodular enhancement (sugar coating).

Spinal nerve sheath tumors as schwannoma and neurofibroma can be intradural extramedullary in location or may involve the brachial and lumbosacral plexi. Schwannomas are often solitary and sporadic, presenting initially with radicular pain followed by motor weakness, voiding difficulty, and myelopathy. These globular, well-defined, encap-

Fig. 18.17 (a) Sagittal and (b) axial T2WI show a synovial cyst with the classic T2 hypointense rim, protruding anteromedially from the left L3/L4 facet joint. The impinges on the transiting L4 nerve as well as compresses the thecal sac

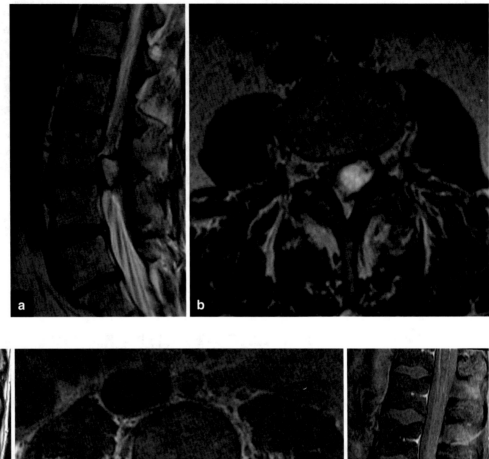

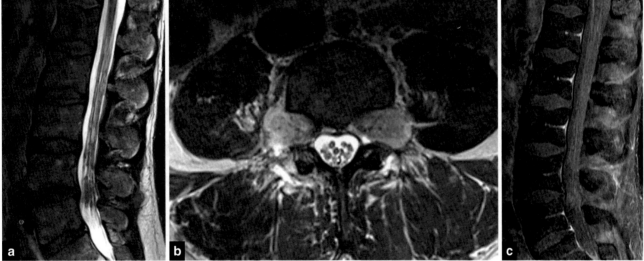

Fig. 18.18 (a) Sagittal and (b) axial T2WI shows thickened cauda equina nerves. The exiting nerves are mildly T2 hyperintense and markedly enlarged. (c) Sagittal contrast-enhanced T1WI demonstrates mild enhancement of the thickened cauda equina nerves

sulated tumors arise from Schwann cells of a sensory nerve root. Most spinal schwannomas are intradural extramedullary in location with adjacent osseous remodeling. Schwannomas and neurofibromas can appear very similar on MRI: T1 isointense, T2 hyperintense, enhancement. Some distinguishing features of schwannomas are hemorrhage, intrinsic vascular changes (thrombosis, sinusoidal dilatation), cyst formation, and fatty degeneration. Neurofibromas are often asymptomatic but may present with pain and/or radicular sensory changes. These lesions are hypodense on CT and cause smooth scalloping of the adjacent bone. On T2WI, neurofibromas may show a target sign: central low signal of collagenous stroma with hyperintense rim (Fig. 18.19).

Malignant peripheral nerve sheath tumors are rare and often associated with neurofibromatosis 1 (25–50% of cases) [32]. Clinical presentation includes new pain, weakness, and rapidly growing mass. On imaging, it can be difficult to differentiate malignant peripheral nerve sheath tumors from neurofibromas, particularly in patients with neurofibromatosis 1. MRI features that suggest malignant peripheral nerve sheath tumor are increased largest dimension of the mass,

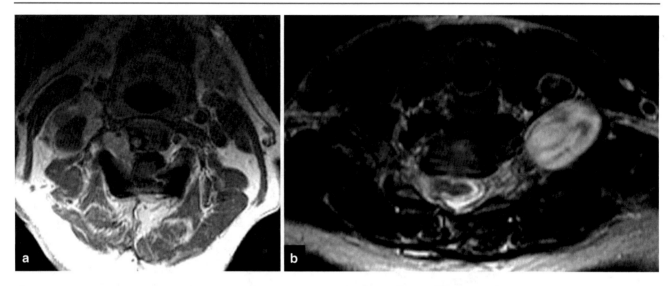

Fig. 18.19 (**a**) Axial contrast-enhanced T1WI of a dumbbell-shaped schwannoma shows heterogeneous enhancement with central cystic change and peripheral thick enhancement. (**b**) Axial T2WI of an extra-dural neurofibroma demonstrates hyperintensity with internal curvilinear hypointensity related to collagenous stroma

Fig. 18.20 (**a**) Coronal contrast-enhanced T1WI and (**b**) STIR MRI show an intensely enhancing malignant nerve sheath tumor arising from the lower left brachial plexus infiltrating along the trunks, divisions, and cords

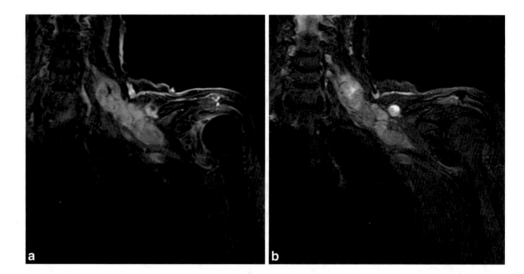

presence of peripheral enhanced pattern, presence of perilesional edema-like zone, presence of intratumoral cystic lesion, and heterogeneity on the T1-weighted images (particularly in patients with neurofibromatosis 1) (Fig. 18.20). One study found the presence of two or more of the four features suggests malignancy with a sensitivity of 61% and a specificity of 90% [32]. FDG-PET uptake can be an essential component of diagnosis of malignant transformation of peripheral nerve sheath tumors.

Key Point
- Intradural extramedullary nerve sheath tumors can press upon spinal nerves and/or the spinal cord and result in radicular and myelopathic symptoms, respectively.

18.4 Concluding Remarks

A spectrum of spine pathologies can result in myelopathy and/or radiculopathy. Integrating the clinical features, temporal course, and anatomic distribution with the imaging characteristics, particularly on MRI, is important in narrowing the differential diagnosis or establishing a definitive diagnosis.

Take-Home Messages

- Extrinsic lesions such as DCM, meningiomas, and epidural hematoma can cause neurologic symptoms due to compression of the spinal cord.
- Imaging findings can be valuable in differentiating between lesions that cause ventral cord displacement: cord herniation, arachnoid web, and arachnoid cyst.
- The MRI pattern combined with the temporal presentation and clinical signs and symptoms can help narrow the differential considerations of intrinsic spinal cord lesions.
- Breakdown of the blood–cord barrier resulting in spinal cord enhancement can be seen a variety of pathologies including infections, inflammation, demyelination, and neoplastic.
- Clues to the diagnosis of spinal cord pathology may lie in the surrounding soft tissues or bones.

References

1. Wilson JRF, Badhiwala JH, Moghaddamjou A, Martin AR, Fehlings MG. Degenerative cervical myelopathy; a review of the latest advances and future directions in management. Neurospine. 2019;16(3):494–505.
2. Vedantam A, Rajshekhar V. Does the type of T2-weighted hyperintensity influence surgical outcome in patients with cervical spondylotic myelopathy? A review. Eur Spine J. 2013;22(1):96–106.
3. Flanagan EP, Krecke KN, Marsh RW, Giannini C, Keegan BM, Weinshenker BG. Specific pattern of gadolinium enhancement in spondylotic myelopathy. Ann Neurol. 2014;76(1):54–65.
4. Boden SD, McCowin PR, Davis DO, Dina TS, Mark AS, Wiesel S. Abnormal magnetic-resonance scans of the cervical spine in asymptomatic subjects. A prospective investigation. J Bone Joint Surg Am. 1990;72(8):1178–84.
5. Matsumoto M, Okada E, Ichihara D, et al. Age-related changes of thoracic and cervical intervertebral discs in asymptomatic subjects. Spine. 2010;35(14):1359–64.
6. Holtas S, Heiling M, Lonntoft M. Spontaneous spinal epidural hematoma: findings at MR imaging and clinical correlation. Radiology. 1996;199(2):409–13.
7. Fukui MB, Swarnkar AS, Williams RL. Acute spontaneous spinal epidural hematomas. AJNR Am J Neuroradiol. 1999;20(7):1365–72.
8. Atlas SW, DuBois P, Singer MB, Lu D. Diffusion measurements in intracranial hematomas: implications for MR imaging of acute stroke. AJNR Am J Neuroradiol. 2000;21(7):1190–4.
9. Mauch JT, Carr CM, Cloft H, Diehn FE. Review of the imaging features of benign osteoporotic and malignant vertebral compression fractures. AJNR Am J Neuroradiol. 2018;39(9):1584–92.
10. Koeller KK, Shih RY. Intradural extramedullary spinal neoplasms: radiologic-pathologic correlation. Radiographics. 2019;39(2):468–90.
11. Reardon MA, Raghavan P, Carpenter-Bailey K, et al. Dorsal thoracic arachnoid web and the "scalpel sign": a distinct clinical-radiologic entity. AJNR Am J Neuroradiol. 2013;34(5):1104–10.
12. Schultz R Jr, Steven A, Wessell A, et al. Differentiation of idiopathic spinal cord herniation from dorsal arachnoid webs on MRI and CT myelography. J Neurosurg Spine. 2017;26(6):754–9.
13. Kearney H, Miller DH, Ciccarelli O. Spinal cord MRI in multiple sclerosis--diagnostic, prognostic and clinical value. Nat Rev Neurol. 2015;11(6):327–38.
14. Pekcevik Y, Mitchell CH, Mealy MA, et al. Differentiating neuromyelitis optica from other causes of longitudinally extensive transverse myelitis on spinal magnetic resonance imaging. Mult Scler. 2016;22(3):302–11.
15. Yonezu T, Ito S, Mori M, et al. "Bright spotty lesions" on spinal magnetic resonance imaging differentiate neuromyelitis optica from multiple sclerosis. Mult Scler. 2014;20(3):331–7.
16. Dos Passos GR, Oliveira LM, da Costa BK, et al. MOG-IgG-associated optic neuritis, encephalitis, and myelitis: lessons learned from neuromyelitis optica spectrum disorder. Front Neurol. 2018;9:217.
17. Ciccarelli O, Cohen JA, Reingold SC, et al. Spinal cord involvement in multiple sclerosis and neuromyelitis optica spectrum disorders. Lancet Neurol. 2019;18(2):185–97.
18. Bathla G, Singh AK, Policeni B, Agarwal A, Case B. Imaging of neurosarcoidosis: common, uncommon, and rare. Clin Radiol. 2016;71(1):96–106.
19. Hashmi M, Kyritsis AP. Diagnosis and treatment of intramedullary spinal cord sarcoidosis. J Neurol. 1998;245(3):178–80.
20. Zalewski NL, Krecke KN, Weinshenker BG, et al. Central canal enhancement and the trident sign in spinal cord sarcoidosis. Neurology. 2016;87(7):743–4.
21. Talbott JF, Narvid J, Chazen JL, Chin CT, Shah V. An imaging-based approach to spinal cord infection. Semin Ultrasound CT MR. 2016;37(5):411–30.
22. Novy J, Carruzzo A, Maeder P, Bogousslavsky J. Spinal cord ischemia: clinical and imaging patterns, pathogenesis, and outcomes in 27 patients. Arch Neurol. 2006;63(8):1113–20.
23. Hurst RW, Grossman RI. Peripheral spinal cord hypointensity on T2-weighted MR images: a reliable imaging sign of venous hypertensive myelopathy. AJNR Am J Neuroradiol. 2000;21(4):781–6.
24. Badhiwala JH, Farrokhyar F, Alhazzani W, et al. Surgical outcomes and natural history of intramedullary spinal cord cavernous malformations: a single-center series and meta-analysis of individual patient data: clinic article. J Neurosurg Spine. 2014;21(4):662–76.
25. Larner AJ, Zeman AZ, Allen CM, Antoun NM. MRI appearances in subacute combined degeneration of the spinal cord due to vitamin B12 deficiency. J Neurol Neurosurg Psychiatry. 1997;62(1):99–100.
26. Marelli C, Salsano E, Politi LS, Labauge P. Spinal cord involvement in adult-onset metabolic and genetic diseases. J Neurol Neurosurg Psychiatry. 2019;90(2):211–8.
27. Koeller KK, Rosenblum RS, Morrison AL. Neoplasms of the spinal cord and filum terminale: radiologic-pathologic correlation. Radiographics. 2000;20(6):1721–49.
28. Rykken JB, Diehn FE, Hunt CH, et al. Rim and flame signs: postgadolinium MRI findings specific for non-CNS intramedullary spinal cord metastases. AJNR Am J Neuroradiol. 2013;34(4):908–15.

29. Aggarwal A, Garg K. Lumbar facet fluid-does it correlate with dynamic instability in degenerative spondylolisthesis? A systematic review and meta-analysis. World Neurosurg. 2021;149:53–63.

30. Jacobs BC, Rothbarth PH, van der Meche FG, et al. The spectrum of antecedent infections in Guillain-Barre syndrome: a case-control study. Neurology. 1998;51(4):1110–5.

31. Gorson KC, Ropper AH, Muriello MA, Blair R. Prospective evaluation of MRI lumbosacral nerve root enhancement in acute Guillain-Barre syndrome. Neurology. 1996;47(3):813–7.

32. Wasa J, Nishida Y, Tsukushi S, et al. MRI features in the differentiation of malignant peripheral nerve sheath tumors and neurofibromas. AJR Am J Roentgenol. 2010;194(6):1568–74.

Spinal Trauma and Spinal Cord Injury (SCI)

19

Luc van den Hauwe and Adam E. Flanders

Abstract

The imaging methods for evaluating patients with acute spinal trauma has dramatically changed in the last decade especially with the development of thin section multidetector computed tomography (MDCT) and isotropic datasets that provide high-resolution sagittal and coronal reformats. MDCT allows for a comprehensive assessment of spinal column injury that has largely supplanted radiography except in the pediatric population. MRI has become the procedure of choice for evaluation of the spinal cord and surrounding soft tissues when there is a suspected SCI.

Keyword

Trauma · Spinal injury · Spinal cord injury · MRI · CT · Vertebral body fractures · Ligamentous injury Traumatic disc herniation · SWICORA · Neurological deficits · BASIC · Diffusion tensor imaging

Learning Objectives
- To understand the prevalence and clinical consequences of spinal trauma.
- To appreciate the utility of radiography, computed tomography (CT), and magnetic resonance imaging (MRI) in the evaluation of spinal trauma and spinal cord injury (SCI).
- To comprehend the grading systems used in spinal trauma.

- To appreciate the soft tissue components of spinal trauma and how they differ in the pediatric population.
- To understand the imaging features of SCI and traumatic vascular injury.

19.1 Imaging Modalities for Spinal Trauma

The majority of the spinal injuries (60%) affect young healthy males between 15 and 35 years of age with cervical spine injuries to be most common. The main cause for spinal injuries is blunt trauma most often due to motor vehicle accidents (48%) followed by falls (21%), and sports-related injuries (14.6%). Assault and penetrating trauma account for approximately 10–20% of the cases. Injuries to the spinal column and the spinal cord are a major cause of disability with important socioeconomic consequences and the costs incurred over a lifetime can easily exceed one million US dollars per patient excluding financial losses related to lost wages and productivity. Over the past several decades, the mean age of the spinal cord injured patient has increased which is attributed to a greater proportion of injuries related to falls in the elderly. Cervical spine injuries remain most frequent, and nearly one third of cervical injuries occur in the cranio-cervical junction (CCJ) [1]. Almost half of the spinal injuries result in neurological deficits, often severe and sometimes fatal [2]. Survival is inversely related to the patient's age, and neurologic level of injury, with lower overall survival for high quadriplegic patients compared to low quadriplegia and paraplegic injuries. Mortality rate of SCI during the initial hospitalization approximates 10% [3]. Injury to the spinal cord occurs in 10–14% of spinal fractures and dislocations with injuries of the cervical spine being by far the most common cause of neurological deficits (40% of cervical injuries) [4, 5]. The majority of injuries to the spinal

L. van den Hauwe
Department of Radiology, Antwerp University Hospital—University of Antwerp, Antwerp, Belgium

A. E. Flanders (✉)
Department of Radiology, Division of Neuroradiology, Thomas Jefferson University, Philadelphia, PA, USA
e-mail: adam.flanders@jefferson.edu

© The Author(s) 2024
J. Hodler et al. (eds.), *Diseases of the Brain, Head and Neck, Spine 2024-2027*, IDKD Springer Series,
https://doi.org/10.1007/978-3-031-50675-8_19

cord (85%) occur at the time of trauma, whereas in a minority of cases (5–10%) the SCI occurs in the immediate post-injury period due to delayed instability [6].

In the emergency setting, the appropriate selection of imaging for spinal trauma depends upon several factors such as modality availability, the patient's clinical and neurological status, type of trauma (blunt, single or multi-trauma), and associated comorbidities. Clinical factors should help determine the necessity and type of imaging. Factors to consider include the quality and severity of pain, limitations in motion or the presence of permanent or transient neurological deficits. MRI is reserved for those patients with post-traumatic myelopathy (spinal cord dysfunction) or in the instance whereupon a patient's symptoms cannot be explained by findings on radiographs or CT, or in some instances when a reliable neurologic exam cannot be obtained.

19.1.1 Plain Film Radiography

With the exception of pediatric trauma, in most settings, radiography has been supplanted by MDCT. In the rare circumstance where MDCT is not available, the initial imaging modality is radiography. A minimum of a lateral and antero-posterior view must be obtained for the spinal axis with the addition of an open-mouth odontoid view for the cervical spine. Often additional views such as oblique views and/or the swimmer's view are performed in an attempt to clear the cervicothoracic junction.

19.1.2 Computed Tomography (CT)

MDCT of the spinal axis has been shown to be more efficient and safer by virtually eliminating the need for repeat radiographs and unnecessary patient transfers in the setting of an unstable spine. Moreover, the diagnostic quality of radiography varies considerably, is more time consuming to acquire, and may be difficult to perform in a medically unstable patient. Submillimeter axial partitions from multi-detector computed tomography (MDCT) is the preferred method for evaluating the spine for bony injury. Multi-planar reformatted (MPR) sagittal and coronal datasets are derived from the isotropic axial dataset. The entire spinal axis can be reliably and expeditiously evaluated in this manner [7–13]. Moreover in the instance of polytrauma, spine images can be reconstructed directly from chest, abdomen, and pelvis datasets with sensitivity that is equivalent to a dedicated spine CT study without having to rescan the patient thereby minimizing radiation dose to the patient and table time. A high-resolution CT imaging protocol begins with submillimeter overlapping partitions to create an isotropic dataset that yields identical spatial resolution in any reconstructed plane. Axial data can be reformatted into thicker sections for diag-nostic display. Multi-planar reformatted (MPR) sagittal and coronal images of the entire spine are typically produced automatically from the scanning console or from a nearby workstation. Reconstructions are performed with both bone and soft tissue algorithms.

Most trauma centers employ dedicated acute (multi-) trauma protocol(s) which include MDCT of the brain, cervical spine, thorax, abdomen, and pelvis, with reformatted images of the thoracic and lumbar spine. Some protocols include a concurrent CT angiogram of the supra-aortic vessels. This both expedites the data acquisition for medically unstable patients and serves to minimize radiation dose since the body imaging data can be reconstructed off-line into targeted spine reconstructions. CT has a higher sensitivity to fractures (especially involving the posterior elements) than radiography. While MDCT excels at delineating bony injury, it also can detect many soft tissue abnormalities such as disc herniation, paravertebral soft tissue and epidural hematoma. A diagnostic quality MDCT excludes any significant soft tissue injury in the vast majority of cases and no further imaging is required if the CT is normal unless there is an unexplained neurologic deficit.

19.1.3 Magnetic Resonance Imaging (MRI)

The greatest impact that MRI has made in the evaluation of spinal trauma has been in assessment of the soft tissue component of injury. MRI is today considered the method of choice for assessing the spectrum of soft tissue injuries associated with spinal trauma. This includes damage to the intervertebral discs, ligaments, vascular structures, and spinal cord [14–16]. No other imaging modality has been able to faithfully reproduce the internal architecture of the spinal cord, and it is this particular feature that is unique to MRI. Any patient who has a persistent neurologic deficit after spinal trauma should undergo an MRI in the acute period to exclude direct damage/compression to the spinal cord. MRI provides unequivocal evidence of not only SCI but will also reliably demonstrate disc injuries/herniations, paraspinal soft tissue edema (ligament strain/failure), epidural hematomas, and vascular injury. In addition, MRI provides the most reliable assessment of chronic SCI and the imaging analogs of post-traumatic progressive myelopathy (PTPM) which is often manifested with imaging as syrinx formation, myelomalacia, and cord atrophy. The extent with which MRI is able to determine spinal instability is overstated as MRI is unable to provide a reliable assessment of ligamentous integrity in most cases. In fact, MRI falsely overestimates the soft tissue component of injury [17]. MRI can sometimes prove useful in categorizing acute from chronic vertebral compressive injuries where the former will demonstrate marrow edema on T2W images.

At minimum, an acute spinal trauma MR imaging protocol of the cervical spine should include 3 mm thick sagittal T1-weighted (T1W), T2-weighted (T2W), and short tau inversion recovery (STIR) sequences or DIXON technique and axial T2*-weighted gradient echo (GRE) images that are no more than 3 mm thick and less than 3 mm when employing a 3D acquisition. Heavily T2W sagittal 3D acquisitions such as single-shot fast spin echo (FSE) with yield isotropic datasets that can be reformatted into axial images. These are useful for identifying nerve root avulsion and root diverticula; however, the contrast resolution for this method is insufficient to detect SCI or paraspinal ligamentous/muscle injury. In the thoracic and lumbar spine, 4 mm thick sagittal T1W, T2W, and STIR sequences and axial 4 mm thick T1W, T2W. Fat-saturated T2W images are valuable to evaluate for ligamentous and soft tissue injuries, and T2* GRE can be used in the thoracic spine to evaluate for small spinal cord hemorrhages associated with SCI.

> **Key Point**
> - Radiography has largely been supplanted by MDCT except in the pediatric population for evaluation of bony injury.
> - A negative MDCT virtually excludes any significant soft tissue injury and obviates the need for MRI unless there is objective evidence of neurologic injury.
> - MRI is the exam of choice to exclude SCI/compressive entities leading to neurologic dysfunction, and MRI is the most sensitive imaging modality to assess for any soft tissue component of injury.

19.2 Different Grading Systems to Evaluate Spinal Injuries

There are different classic grading scales for determining spinal instability of thoracolumbar injuries based upon the McAfee (two-column) and Denis three column concept [18, 19]. The Magerl classification relies exclusively on CT findings [20]. In recent years, a new grading scale that is based on CT and magnetic resonance (MR) imaging findings, like the thoracolumbar injury classification and severity score (TLICS) has been developed by the Spine Trauma Group [21] to overcome some of the perceived difficulties regarding the use of other thoracolumbar spinal fracture classification systems for determining treatment. Also for the grading of the cervical spine a new grading scale and score system—the cervical spine Subaxial Injury Classification and Scoring (SLIC) system [21] has been developed and is gaining acceptance among spine surgeons. The AO spine classification system provides a comprehensive classification schema for upper cervical, subaxial cervical, thoracolumbar and sacral injuries [22].

19.2.1 Injuries to the Vertebral Column

Classically, injuries to the spinal column are categorized by mechanism of injury and/or by instability. *Instability* is defined by White and Punjabi as abnormal translation between adjacent vertebral segments with normal physiologic motion. Unrecognized instability after trauma is a potential cause of delayed SCI . This is why early stabilization of the initial injury is an imperative to appropriate clinical management. The simplest method to test for instability in a controlled environment is by performing flexion and extension lateral radiography to produce a visible subluxation at a suspected level, but this is rarely performed in practice and has been replaced largely by the excellent sensitivity of even subtle injuries on using multi-detector CT (MDCT) and magnetic resonance imaging (MRI).

Classically, from a biomechanical point of view, the thoracolumbar spine can be divided into three osteo-ligamentous columns: anterior-, middle-, and posterior column [18]. Although this biomechanical model is often inferred for cervical injuries, there is no similar established model in the cervical spine. The anterior column includes the anterior longitudinal ligament and anterior two-thirds of the vertebral body and disc including the annulus fibrosus. The middle column is composed of the posterior third of the vertebral body and disc including annulus fibrosus, and posterior longitudinal ligament. Finally, the posterior column is composed of the pedicles, articular processes, facet capsules, laminae, ligamentum flavum, spinous processes, and the interspinous ligaments. The mechanism of injury will result in several different types of traumatic injuries to the cervical, thoracic, and lumbar vertebral column and spinal cord, which may result in stable or unstable spine injuries.

Because of the distinct anatomic differences and the resultant injury patterns, injuries to the cervical spine are divided into injuries to the upper cervical spine (C0–C2) and subaxial cervical injuries (C3–C7). There are separate classification schemes for fractures to the occipital condyles/skull base (Anderson and Montesano) and for the axis (C2). Injuries may also be categorized by stability or mechanism. The mechanism of injury to the cervical column can be divided into four major groups: hyperflexion, hyperextension, rotation, and vertical compression with frequent variations that include components of the major groups (e.g., flexion and rotation). Hyperflexion injuries can produce an array of findings including anterior subluxation, bilateral interfacetal dislocation, simple wedge fracture, fracture of the spinous process, teardrop fracture, and odontoid (dens) fracture. Of these the simple wedge fractures and isolated spinous process fractures are considered initially stable, while the other fractures are considered unstable such as the bilateral interfacetal dislocation and the teardrop fracture. Occipital condyle, atlas (C1), and odontoid fracture may be considered stable or unstable depending on the type of fracture type. Hyperextension mechanism is less frequent than the hyperflexion and result in the following types of injuries: dislocation, avulsion fracture or fracture of the posterior arch of C1, teardrop fracture of C2, laminar fracture, and traumatic spondylolisthesis of C2 (Hangman's fracture). Most of these injuries with the exception of Hangman's fracture are defined as stable fractures; however, this does not imply that these injuries should go untreated. Hyperextension injuries in the lower cervical spine are often associated with central cord syndrome, especially in patients with pre-existing cervical spondylosis and usually produce diffuse pre-vertebral soft tissue swelling. Vertical compression of the atlas (C1) may result in a Jefferson fracture in which there is failure of the anterior and posterior arch and is always unstable. An uncommon site for injuries is the cranio-cervical junction (CCJ) involving the atlantoaxial joint, which is the most mobile portion of the cervical spine; the majority of head rotation takes place at C1–C2 and the majority of head flexion is supported by the occipital condyles. This junction relies on a complex ligamentous framework for stability. CCJ injuries range from the severe atlanto-axial disassociation to more subtle traumatic rotatory subluxation which is a pure soft tissue injury more commonly reported in children with torticollis.

Fractures in the lower thoracic and lumbar spine differ from those in the cervical spine. The thoracic and lumbar fractures are often complex and due to a combination of mechanisms. An important factor that affects the distribution of injuries is the location of the center of gravity which is located anterior to the thoracic spine (from the normal kyphosis) and directly over the lumbar spine (secondary to the normal lordosis). In addition, the thoracic cage confers substantial biomechanical protection to the thoracic spine. Therefore, statistically, most injuries occur at the most mobile portion or the thoracolumbar junction where the thoracic cage ends. When injuries occur in the upper or middle thoracic spine, it is usually a result of major trauma, for example, high velocity trauma such as motor vehicle accidents. The most common fracture, at the thoracolumbar junction, is the simple compression- or wedge fracture (50% of all fractures) which is considered stable. The remaining types of fractures among those the so-called seat belt injury, which can be divided into three subtypes: type I (Chance fracture) involves the posterior bony elements, type II (Smith fracture) involves the posterior ligaments, and, in type III the annulus fibrosus is ruptured allowing for subluxation are considered unstable fractures [23]. With the advent of the three-point restraint system in motor vehicles, these severe hyperflexion-distraction injuries have become uncommon.

The most common of all thoracolumbar fracture—the burst fracture account for 64%–81% of all thoracolumbar fractures. The burst fracture, which can be divided into five subtypes, is associated with high incidence of injuries to the spinal cord, conus medullaris, cauda equina, and nerve roots [24]. Burst fracture involving anterior and middle column can be incorrectly categorized as a compression fracture on radiographs alone and is better evaluated by MDCT.

> **Key Point**
> - Nomenclature of spinal fractures differs by location (e.g., skull base/cranio-cervical junction, upper cervical/lower cervical, thoracolumbar, sacrum).
> - Classification systems for spinal fractures are generally based upon injury mechanism, stability, anatomic and biomechanical differences in unique areas of the spine.
> - The burst subtype is the most common thoracolumbar fracture.

19.3 Soft Tissue Injuries

19.3.1 Traumatic Disc Herniation and Ligamentous Injury

Traumatic disc injuries are caused by distraction and shearing with failure of the intervertebral disc. A direct injury to the disc is more common than post-traumatic disc extrusion. Traumatic disc herniation should be considered when the disc exhibits high signal on T2W images especially when traumatic vertebral body fractures and/or ligamentous injury is present at the same level [13]. Extruded disc material may extend into the epidural or pre-vertebral space.

Up to 25% of all cervical injuries will demonstrate signal changes in the posterior ligamentous complex. This finding does not equate with instability. When there is a gap between parts of the vertebrae or by discontinuity in the ligament or adjacent structures on fat suppressed T2W or STIR images, a ligamentous injury is suspected. Ligamentous injury without underlying fracture in the cervical spine is rare by can occur with severe hyperflexion sprain [25]. Disruption of the anterior longitudinal ligament (ALL) is generally associated with hyperextension mechanisms with co-existent edema of the pre-vertebral muscles and anterior aspect of the intervertebral discs. Rupture of the ALL may be visualized as focal interruption of the normal linear band of hypointense signal of the ligament on T1W images. Alternatively, hyperflexion and distraction forces may cause disruption of the posterior ligamentous complex which is manifested by increased distance between spinous processes and increased signal in the interspinous region on MR sagittal STIR sequences. Abnormal angulation, distraction, and subluxation is often recognized on initial CT study.

19.3.2 Whiplash-Associated Disorders

Whiplash injuries represent a separate, relatively common entity (1–4/1000), resulting from an acceleration-deceleration mechanism of injury to the neck, typically from rear-end vehicle collisions. Whiplash injury is among the leading automotive related injuries with respect to burden on patients, the healthcare system and insurance organizations [26]. The pathogenesis of whiplash complaints is still poorly understood. Injury to longitudinal ligaments, facet joints, intervertebral discs, spinal cord, and muscles have been described as possible sources of (chronic) pain. More recently, with the development of more detailed MRI techniques, morphologic changes of the ligaments and membranes of the craniovertebral junction, especially the alar and transverse ligaments have been described [27].

Whiplash-associated disorders (WAD) is a clinical diagnosis and describes a variety of clinical manifestations, such as neck pain immediately or 24 h after trauma, neck stiffness, headache, dizziness, vertigo, auditory and visual disturbances, concentration, and psychological problems. Imaging findings include osseous injuries such as bone contusions and occult fractures, ligamentous injuries (most common finding), and tears. Disc lesions and post-traumatic herniation also can occur [28]. MRI signal changes of the alar and transverse ligaments may be observed. Whether these signal abnormalities are responsible for complaints of patients having WAD remains controversial, as these signal abnormalities have also been observed in asymptomatic individuals and were not significantly associated with clinical testing and prognosis of acute whiplash injury. A recent meta-analysis could not show any association between MRI signal changes in alar and transverse ligaments and WAD [27].

Key Point
- Mechanism of injury can often be inferred on MRI as the majority of soft tissue damage will occur ventral the spine (hyperextension) or in the posterior ligamentous complex (hyperflexion).
- Edema in the soft tissues does not equate with ligamentous instability or rupture. Focal discontinuity of a ligament is more pathognomonic.

19.4 Injuries to the Spinal Cord

A majority (80%) of patients with (SCI) harbor multisystem injuries [29]; typically associated injuries include other bone fractures (29.3%) and brain injury (11.5%) [30]. Nearly all SCI damage both upper and lower motor neurons because they involve both the gray matter and descending white matter tracts at the level of injury. The American Spinal Injury Association (ASIA) has suggested a comprehensive set of standardized clinical measurements which are based upon a detailed sensory and motor examination of all dermatomes and myotomes [31]. The neurologic deficit that results from injury to the spinal cord depends primarily upon the extent of damage at the injury site and the cranial-caudal location of the damage (i.e., the neurologic level of injury or NLI); anatomically higher injuries produce a greater neurologic deficit (e.g., cervical injury = quadriparesis, thoracic injury = paraparesis). These comprehensive set of standardized clinical measurements have been adopted worldwide. Functional transection of the spinal cord is a more frequent manifestation of SCI compared to true mechanical transection which is relatively rare and confined mostly to penetrating type injuries or extensive fracture-dislocations/translocations. SCI is further categorized clinically into anterior cord syndrome, Brown-Sequard syndrome, central cord syndrome, conus medullaris syndrome, and cauda equina syndrome depending upon the site of injury and the neurologic pattern of injury. Spontaneous neurologic recovery after overall is relatively poor and largely depends upon the severity of neurologic deficit identified at the time of injury. Of the different spinal cord syndromes, the anterior cord syndrome has the worst prognosis of all cord syndromes, especially if no recovery is noticed during the first 72 h after injury.

19.4.1 Spinal Cord Hemorrhage

Post-traumatic spinal cord hemorrhage or hemorrhagic contusion is defined as the presence of a discrete area of hemorrhage within the spinal cord after an injury. The most common location for hemorrhage to accumulate is within the central gray matter of the spinal cord and centered at the point of mechanical impact [32–34]. Experimental and autopsy pathologic studies have shown correlation with hemorrhagic necrosis of the spinal cord while true hematomyelia will rarely be found [35]. There are significant clinical implications if there is identification of frank hemorrhage in the cervical spinal cord following trauma on an MRI examination. Originally, it was thought that detection of intramedullary hemorrhage was predictive of a complete

Fig. 19.1 Acute hemorrhagic spinal cord injury. (**a**) Sagittal STIR sequence shows that there is a flexion type injury of C5 with acute ventral angulation. The spinal cord is markedly swollen with edema spanning the entire length of the spinal cord. There is a central hemorrhagic focus which is of low signal intensity that spans from C4 to C6. Note the disruption of the posterior spinal soft tissues. (**b**) Axial GRE image at the C4 level shows that the hypointense hemorrhage is confined to the central gray matter

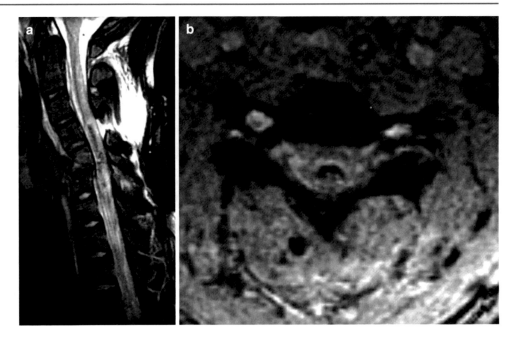

injury. However, the increased sensitivity and spatial resolution of current MRI techniques has shown that even small amounts of hemorrhage are identifiable in incomplete lesions. Therefore, the basic construct has been altered such that the detection of a sizable focus of blood (>4 mm in length on sagittal images) in the cervical spinal cord is often indicative of a complete neurological injury [36]. The anatomic location of the hemorrhage closely corresponds to the neurological level of injury and the presence of frank hemorrhage implies a poor potential for neurological recovery (Fig. 19.1). The cross-sectional involvement of injury on axial T2WI as described in the BASIC score has been shown to correlate both with severity of initial injury and neurologic recovery [32–34, 37–41].

19.4.2 Spinal Cord Edema

Spinal cord edema is defined as a focus of abnormal high signal intensity seen on MRI T2W images [34]. Presumably, this signal abnormality reflects a focal accumulation of intracellular and interstitial fluid in response to injury [33, 34, 42–44]. Edema is usually well defined on the mid-sagittal T2W image while the axial T2W images offer additional information in regard to involvement of structures in cross-section. Spinal cord edema involves a variable length of spinal cord above and below the level of injury, with discrete boundaries adjacent to uninvolved parenchyma and is invariably associated with some degree of spinal cord swelling. The length of spinal cord affected by edema is directly proportional to the degree of initial neurologic deficit [32, 41]. Notable is that spinal cord edema can occur without MRI evidence of intramedullary

hemorrhage. Cord edema alone connotes a more favorable prognosis than cord hemorrhage [37].

> **Key Point**
> - Length and location of spinal cord hemorrhage and edema provide a surrogate for neurologic deficit (ASIA impairment scale (AIS) and NLI).
> - The combination of intramedullary hemorrhage and/or edema correlates with neurologic function and capacity to recover after SCI.

19.5 Blunt Cerebrovascular Injury

Blunt cerebrovascular injury (BCVI) to the carotid arteries (CAs) and/or vertebral arteries (VAs) is a relatively rare but potentially devastating finding in patients with a high-impact trauma to the cervical spine and/or head. Most complications of BCVI occur hours to days after the initial trauma so early identification and prompt anticoagulation is important to reduce the incidence of postinjury ischemic stroke (Fig. 19.2).

Cervical spine fractures have the strongest association with BCVI, and specific cervical spine fractures are highly predictive of BCVI. These include fractures located at the upper cervical spine (C1-C3), subluxation, or involvement of the transverse foramina [45]. Nearly all VAIs are associated with cervical spine subluxations and fractures involving the transverse foramen [47]. Other mechanisms of BCVI include hyperflexion, a direct blow and strangulation. In the context

Fig. 19.2 Traumatic thrombosis/dissection of the bilateral vertebral arteries. (**a**) Sagittal T2WI in a 32y/o male after a skate-boarding accident. Traumatic subluxation of C2–C3 with circumferential disruption of the disco-ligamentous complex and spinal cord compression/edema. (**b**) Axial T2WI at the C2–C3 level show high signal in both foramen transversarium from clot/slow flow in both vertebral arteries

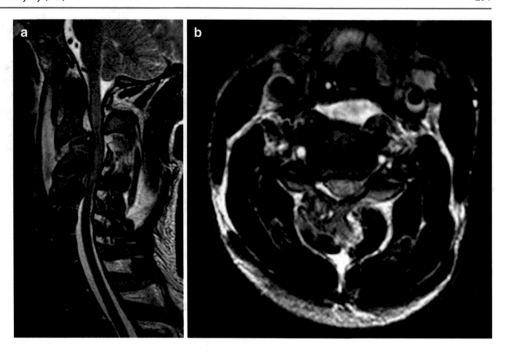

of a carotid artery injury, it is thought that cervical hyperextension and contralateral rotation lead to stretching of the internal carotid artery (ICA) over the C1-C3 transverse processes, precipitating a vessel wall injury [46].

According to the Denver criteria and Western Trauma Association (WTA) guidelines, radiologic risk factors associated with BCVI include high-energy injury mechanisms with Le Fort II or III fracture patterns; basilar skull fracture with carotid canal involvement; cervical vertebral body or transverse foramen fracture, subluxation, or ligamentous injury; any fracture at C1 through C3; closed head injuries with diffuse axonal injury and a Glasgow Coma Score of less than 6; clothesline-type injuries with associated swelling and/or pain; or near-hanging with anoxia. Urgent screening for BCVI should be performed in these patients that may be still neurologically asymptomatic at this time [46].

With the widespread use of MDCT scanners, CT angiography (CTA) has emerged as the first-line screening modality for BCVI. CTA is a cost-effective screening tool in high-risk populations, ultimately preventing the most strokes at a reasonable cost [46].

Several grading systems for BCVI exist, based on imaging findings. The Denver grading scale (aka the Biffl scale) is a widely accepted and commonly used system. In grade I injury, subtle vessel wall irregularities, a dissection/intramural hematoma with less than 25% luminal stenosis is observed. In grade II injury, an intraluminal thrombus or raised intimal flap is visualized, or a dissection/intramural hematoma with greater than 25% luminal narrowing. Grade III injury corresponds to traumatic pseudoaneurysms, observed as a variable-sized outpouching of the vessel wall. Grade IV injury represents a complete vessel occlusion, usu-

ally tapering in the CA and quite abrupt in the VA. Vessel transection represents a grade V injury, observed as free contrast extravasation into the surrounding tissues, or into the adjacent vein in the form of an arteriovenous fistula (AVF) [46, 47].

> **Key Point**
> - Occult vertebral artery injury (dissection or occlusion) can occur in association with spinal trauma even without the presence of SCI, neurologic deficit, or fracture.

19.6 Injuries to the Pediatric Spine and Spinal Cord

Spinal injuries are generally less common in the pediatric population compared to adults with cervical spine injuries being most frequent spine injury of all spine injuries occurring in up to 40–60% of all injuries in children. The etiology varies depending on the age of the child. The most common cause of pediatric cervical spine injury is a motor vehicle accident, but also obstetric complication, fall, and child abuse are known causes. In the adolescent, sports and diving accidents are other well-known causes. The specific biomechanics of the pediatric cervical spine leads to a different distribution of injuries and distinct radiological features and represent a distinct clinical entity compared to those seen in adults. Young children have a propensity for injuries to the CCJ (i.e., C0–C2) whereas older children are prone to lower cervical injuries similar to those seen in adults. The spinal cervical injuries in children less than 8 years of age demonstrate a high incidence of subluxation without fractures. The biomechanical differences are explained by the relative ratio of the size of the cranium to the body in the young child, lack of ligamentous stability, poor muscle strength and increased forces relative to the older child and adult. Children can manifest an SCI with otherwise normal radiographs the so-called SCIWORA (without radiographic abnormality) compared to adults. This is especially evident in children younger than 9 years of age where there is a high incidence of reported complete cord injuries associated with SCIWORA. Suggested mechanisms of the SCIWORA include hyperextension or flexion injuries to the immature and the inherently elastic spine, which is vulnerable to external forces and allows for significant intersegmental movement and transient soft disc protrusion, resulting in distraction injuries, and/or ischemic injury of the spinal cord [48]. The elasticity of the spine allows it to stretch up to 5 cm before rupture, whereas the spinal cord, which is anchored to the brachial plexus superiorly and the cauda equina inferiorly, ruptures after 4–6 mm of traction [49]. As MRI is readily capable of detecting the soft tissue injury component, the concept of SCIWORA is less relevant.

The imaging algorithm for pediatric spinal trauma is somewhat different than that for adults. MDCT is used more judiciously due to radiation exposure considerations and places lower dose radiography is preferred. MRI is always used if there is a consideration of a pure soft tissue injury or neurologic deficit.

> **Key Point**
> - Patterns of spinal injury in the pediatric population is different than adults primarily due to biomechanical differences.

19.7 Neurologic Recovery After Spinal Cord Injury

Although there are no pharmacologic "cures" for SCI, spontaneous neurologic recovery after injury can occur, and it largely depends upon the severity of the initial neurologic deficit, the neurologic level of injury, patient age, and comorbidities. Very few patients with a neurologically complete (i.e., no motor or sensory function below the injury level) actually regain any useful function below the injury level although most patients will spontaneously improve by one neurologic level (e.g., a C5 level spontaneously descends to a C6 level). Even these small improvements can have a sub-

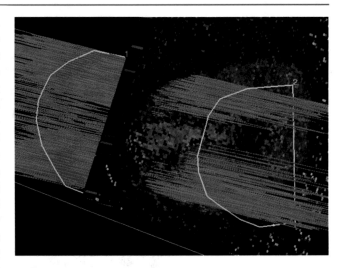

Fig. 19.3 Disruption of the lateral cortical spinal tracts on tractography. Diffusion tractography performed on a lesioned rat spinal cord at 9.4 T shows disruption of the fiber tracts in the lateral column following a lesion in the lateral funiculus. (Image courtesy of Eric D. Schwartz MD)

stantial impact on a patient's capacity to function independently.

The role of MRI to predict capacity for spontaneous neurologic recovery after cervical SCI has been evaluated. Although there is considerable overlap in results some general characterizations about the MRI appearance of SCI and neurologic recovery are evident. Intramedullary hemorrhage 4 mm or greater is equated with a severe neurologic deficit and a poor prognosis. Cord edema alone is indicative of a mild to moderate initial neurological deficit and a better capacity for spontaneous neurological improvement. The length of the cord lesion may also correlate with the initial deficit and in the neurological outcome. Newer MRI techniques such as diffusion tensor imaging (DTI) (Fig. 19.3) have shown great promise not only in stratification of neurologic injury but has also been shown to have benefits in predicting recovery [50–52]. As novel pharmacologic therapies for SCI are developed and tested, MRI will likely play a more essential role in characterizing the injury and helping to select patients for clinical trials.

> **Key Point**
> - MRI findings of SCI have shown promise as a surrogate for the neurologic examination; better prognostic information is attained when MR imaging patterns are used in combination with the clinical examination.
> - Newer physiologic techniques like DTI hold promise to better stratify patients for selection of novel therapies.

19.8 Concluding Remarks

The demographic of adult spinal trauma SCI and has changed over the last several decades noting a considerable increased prevalence in the elderly. Safety measures in sports and motor vehicles have drastically reduced the incidence of SCI in the young adult and middle age population. Imaging algorithms for spinal trauma have also changed in the past few decades with greater reliance on MDCT over radiography in adults and greater emphasis towards minimizing radiation dose in the injured pediatric population. While there have been tremendous improvements in orthopedic stabilization methods through novel instrumentation/fusion techniques, there are still no known cures for paralysis. While SCI was previously considered to be a fatal disease with patient succumbing to injury at the scene or from long term complications, most SCI patients now survive and many return to meaningful lives while living with their disability. This is principally attributed to revolutionary improvements in rehabilitation and chronic care for the SCI patient.

Take-Home Messages
- Spinal trauma and SCI are prevalent worldwide.
- Spinal trauma is now more common in the elderly due to falls.
- MDCT has supplemented radiography.
- MRI reveals the soft tissue components of injury including damage to the spinal cord.
- MRI offers the capacity to predict the severity of neurologic injury and prognostic information to help guide treatment and select patients for novel therapies.

References

1. Riascos R, Bonfante E, Cotes C, Guirguis M, Hakimelahi R, West C. Imaging of atlanto-occipital and atlantoaxial traumatic injuries: what the radiologist needs to know. Radiographics. 2015;35(7):2121–34. https://doi.org/10.1148/rg.2015150035.
2. Hill MW, Dean SA. Head injury and facial injury: is there an increased risk of cervical spine injury? J Trauma. 1993;34:549–54.
3. Pope AM, Tarlov AR. Disability in America: toward a national agenda for prevention. Washington, DC: National Academy Press; 1991.
4. Riggins RS, Kraus JF. The risk of neurological damage with fractures of the vertebrae. J Trauma. 1997;17:126–30.
5. Castellano V, Bocconi FL. Injuries of the cervical spine with spinal cord involvement (myelic fractures): statistical considerations. Bull Hosp J Dis Orthop Inst. 1970;31:188–98.
6. Rogers WA. Fractures and dislocations of the cervical spine; an end-result study. J Bone Joint Surg. 1957;39:341–51.
7. Diaz JJ Jr, Gillman C, Morris JA Jr, et al. Are five-view plain films of the cervical spine unreliable? A prospective evaluation in blunt trauma in patients with altered mental status. J Trauma. 2003;55:658–63.
8. Griffen MM, Frykberg ER, Kerwin AJ, et al. Radiographic clearance of blunt cervical spine injury: plain radiograph or computed tomography scan? J Trauma. 2003;55:222–6.
9. Holmes JF, Mirvis SE, Panacek EA, for the NEXUS Group, et al. Variability in computed tomography and magnetic resonance imaging in patients with cervical spine injuries. J Trauma. 2002;53:524–9.
10. Kligman M, Vasili C, Roffman M. The role of computed tomography in cervical spine injury due to diving. Arch Orthop Trauma Surg. 2001;121:139–41.
11. Schenarts PJ, Diaz J, Kaiser C, et al. Prospective comparison of admission computed tomographic scan and plain films of the upper cervical spine in trauma patients with altered mental status. J Trauma. 2001;51:663–8.
12. Berne JD, Velmahos GC, El Tawil Q, et al. Value of complete cervical helical computed tomographic scanning in identifying cervical spine injury in the unevaluable blunt trauma patient with multiple injuries: a prospective study. J Trauma. 1999;47:896–902.
13. Van Goethem JW, Maes M, Özsarlak Ö, et al. Imaging in spinal trauma. Eur Radiol. 2005;15(3):582–90.
14. Flanders AE, Schaefer DM, Doan HT, et al. Acute cervical spine trauma; correlation of MR imaging findings with degree of neurological deficit. Radiology. 1990;177:25–33.
15. Sliker CW, Mirvis SE, Shanmuganathan K. Assessing cervical spine stability in obtunded blunt trauma patients; review of medical literature. Radiology. 2005;234:733–9.
16. Wilmink JT. MR imaging of the spine: trauma and degenerative disease. Eur Radiol. 1999;9:1259–66.
17. Hogan GJ, Mirvis SE, Shanmuganathan K, Scalea TM. Exclusion of unstable cervical spine injury in obtunded patients with blunt trauma: is MR imaging needed when multi-detector row CT findings are normal? Radiology. 2005;237:106–13.
18. Denis F. The three column spine and its significance in the classification of acute thoracolumbar spinal injuries. Spine. 1983;8(8):817–31.
19. Mcafee PC, Yuan HA, Fredrickson BE, et al. The value of computed tomography in thoracolumbar fractures. An analysis of one hundred consecutive cases and a new classification. J Bone Joint Surg Am. 1983;65(4):461–73.
20. Magerl F, Aebi M, Gertzbein SD, et al. A comprehensive classification of thoracic and lumbar injuries. Eur Spine J. 1994;3(4):184–201.
21. Lee JY, Vaccaro AR, Lim MR, et al. Thoracolumbar injury classification and severity score: a new paradigm for the treatment of thoracolumbar spine trauma. J Orthop Sci. 2005;10(6):671–5.
22. Kepler CK, Vaccaro AR, Koerner JD, Dvorak MF, Kandziora F, Rajasekaran S, Aarabi B, Vialle LR, Fehlings MG, Schroeder GD, Reinhold M, Schnake KJ, Bellabarba C, Cumhur Öner F. Reliability analysis of the AOSpine thoracolumbar spine injury classification system by a worldwide group of naïve spinal surgeons. Eur Spine J. 2016;25(4):1082–6.
23. Rogers LF. The roentgenographic appearances of transverse or chance fractures of the spine: the seat belt fracture. Am J Roentgenol. 1971;111:844–9.
24. Gertzbein SD. Scoliosis Research Society: multicenter spine fracture study. Spine. 1992;17:528–40.
25. Diaz JJ, Aulino JM, Collier B, et al. The early work-up for isolated ligamentous injury of the cervical spine; does computed tomography scan have a role. J Trauma. 2005;59:897–904.
26. Sarrami P, Armstrong E, Naylor JM, Harris IA. Factors predicting outcome in whiplash injury: a systematic meta-review of prognostic factors. J Orthopaed Traumatol. 2017;18:9–16.

27. Li Q, Shen H, Li M. Magnetic resonance imaging signal changes of alar and transverse ligaments not correlated with whiplash-associated disorders. A meta-analysis of case-control studies. Eur Spine J. 2013;22:14–20.
28. Boban J, Thurnher MM, Van Goethem JW. Spine and spinal cord trauma. In: Barkhof F, et al., editors. Clinical neuroradiology. Springer Nature Switzerland AG; 2018.
29. Burney RE, Maio RF, Maynard F, et al. Incidence, characteristics, and outcome of spinal cord injury at trauma centers in North America. Arch Surg. 1993;128:596–9.
30. Dawodu ST. Spinal cord injury - definition, epidemiology, pathophysiology. In: Emedicine, ed. 2009.
31. American Spinal Injury Association. International standards for neurological classifications of spinal cord injury. Revised edition. Chicago, IL: American Spinal Injury Association; 2000. p. 1–23.
32. Bondurant FJ, Cotler HB, Kulkarni MV, et al. Acute spinal cord injury. A study using physical examination and magnetic resonance imaging. Spine. 1990;15(3):161–8.
33. Flanders AE, Spettell CM, Friedman DP, Marino RJ, Herbison GJ. The relationship between the functional abilities of patients with cervical spinal cord injury and the severity of damage revealed by MR imaging. AJNR Am J Neuroradiol. 1999;20(5):926–34.
34. Kulkarni MV, McArdle CB, Kpanicky D, et al. Acute spinal cord injury: MR imaging at 1.5 T. Radiology. 1987;164(3):837–43.
35. Schouman-Claeys E, Frija G, Cuenod CA, et al. MR imaging of acute spinal cord injury: results of an experimental study in dogs. AJNR Am J Neuroradiol. 1990;11(5):959–65.
36. Boldin C, Raith J, Fankhauser F, Haunschmid C, Schwantzer G, Schweighofer F. Predicting neurologic recovery in cervical spinal cord injury with postoperative MR imaging. Spine (Phila Pa 1976). 2006;31(5):554–9.
37. Flanders AE, Spettell CM, Tartaglino LM, Friedman DP, Herbison GJ. Forecasting motor recovery after cervical spinal cord injury: value of MR imaging. Radiology. 1996;201(3):649–55.
38. Cotler HB, Kulkarni MV, Bondurant FJ. Magnetic resonance imaging of acute spinal cord trauma: preliminary report. J Orthop Trauma. 1988;2(1):1–4.
39. Sato T, Kokubun S, Rijal KP, et al. Prognosis of cervical spinal cord injury in correlation with magnetic resonance imaging. Paraplegia. 1994;32(2):81–5.
40. Marciello MA, Flanders AE, Herbison GJ, et al. Magnetic resonance imaging related to neurologic outcome in cervical spinal cord injury. Arch Phys Med Rehabil. 1993;74(9):940–6.
41. Talbott JF, Whetstone WD, Readdy WJ, Ferguson AR, Bresnahan JC, Saigal R, Hawryluk GW, Beattie MS, Mabray MC, Pan JZ, Manley GT, Dhall SS. The brain and spinal injury center score: a novel, simple, and reproducible method for assessing the severity of acute cervical spinal cord injury with axial T2-weighted MRI findings. J Neurosurg Spine. 2015;23(4):495–504.
42. Goldberg AL, Rothfus WE, Deeb ZL, et al. The impact of magnetic resonance on the diagnostic evaluation of acute cervicothoracic spinal trauma. Skelet Radiol. 1988;17(2):89–95.
43. Wittenberg RH, Boetel U, Beyer HK. Magnetic resonance imaging and computer tomography of acute spinal cord trauma. Clin Orthop Relat Res. 1990;260:176–85.
44. Schaefer DM, Flanders A, Northrup BE, et al. Magnetic resonance imaging of acute cervical spine trauma. Correlation with severity of neurologic injury. Spine. 1989;14(10):1090–5.
45. Kopelman TR, Leeds S, Berardoni NE, et al. Incidence of blunt cerebrovascular injury in low-risk cervical spine fractures. Am J Surg. 2011;202:684–8; discussion 688–689
46. Rutman AM, Vranic JE, Mossa-Basha M. Imaging and management of blunt cerebrovascular injury. Radiographics. 2018;38:542–63.
47. Cothren CC, Moore EE, Biffle WL, et al. Cervical spine fracture patterns predictive of blunt vertebral artery injury. J Trauma. 2003;55:811–3.
48. Kriss VM, Kriss TC. SCIWORA (spinal cord injury without radiographic abnormality) in infants and children. Clin Pediatr (Phila). 1996;35:119–24.
49. Manary MJ, Jaffe DM. Cervical spine injuries in children. Pediatr Ann. 1996;25:423–8.
50. Poplawski MM, Alizadeh M, Oleson CV, Fisher J, Marino RJ, Gorniak RJ, Leiby BE, Flanders AE. Application of diffusion tensor imaging in forecasting neurological injury and recovery after human cervical spinal cord injury. J Neurotrauma. 2019;36:3051–61. https://doi.org/10.1089/neu.2018.6092.
51. Shanmuganathan K, Zhuo J, Chen HH, Aarabi B, Adams J, Miller C, Menakar J, Gullapalli RP, Mirvis SE. Diffusion tensor imaging parameter obtained during acute blunt cervical spinal cord injury in predicting long-term outcome. J Neurotrauma. 2017;34:2964–71.
52. Dvorak MF, Fischer CG, Fehlings MG, Rampersaud YR, Öner FC, Aarabi B, Vaccaro AR. The surgical approach to subaxial cervical spine injuries: an evidence-based algorithm based on the classification system. Spine. 2007;32(23):2620–9.

Masses in and Around the Spine

20

Jan E. Vandevenne and Adrian Kastler

Abstract

The anatomical spaces in and around the spine encompass the paraspinal compartment, the vertebral compartment and the epidural compartment. Tumors in these compartments may easily spread via adipose corridors, direct contact or hematogenous pathways. Classifications such as the Weinstein-Boriani-Biagini, SINS, and ESCC or Bilsky score are used to grade these tumors. Imaging features of main tumoral and pseudotumoral masses are described and shown in this review. Detection of masses beyond the spine and even beyond the paraspinal space can be of utmost importance and examples are shown why radiologists should avoid tunnel view into the spinal canal.

Keywords

Detection · Paraspinal space · Epidural space · Vertebral tumor

Learning Objectives
- To understand that important diagnostic errors occur if the radiologist does not actively search for lesions beyond the spinal canal and vertebrae.
- To understand the anatomy of the paraspinal space, the intercostal space, the epidural space, and the vertebrae together with the interconnecting pathways.
- To understand imaging features of common masses in and around the spine.

J. E. Vandevenne (✉)
Department of Radiology, Ziekenhuis Oost-Limburg, Faculty of Medical and Life Sciences, University of Hasselt, Genk, Belgium
e-mail: jan.vandevenne@zol.be

A. Kastler
Department of Neuroradiology, University Hospital of Grenoble, Grenoble, France

It is the role of the radiologist to detect each mass imaged in and around the spine. Subsequently, the radiologist defines the compartments involved by the mass and furthermore describes the features of the mass in an attempt to understand its aggressiveness and to provide a differential diagnosis. These are the main tasks for the radiologist to provide added value to clinical and surgical management of the patient. Some masses may be well-suited for biopsy or treatment by interventional radiologists.

This text will focus on masses located in the paraspinal soft tissues and within the bony spine. Regarding the spinal canal, masses in the extradural space will be discussed but the intradural masses are beyond the scope of this chapter.

Rather than giving a complete overview of all possible masses, this text will focus on hints to ease detection of masses, on understanding the compartments involved by the tumor, on describing specific features to recognize masses and on pointing out the role of interventional radiology for some masses.

20.1 Detection of Masses in and Around the Spine

Masses within the vertebra and spinal canal are clearly depicted and easily detected on MRI by radiologists and clinicians. Rather than only focusing the eyes on the intraspinal structures or bony spine (tunnel view), radiologists should scrutinize all image series for lesions in the paravertebral soft tissues and even beyond, such as in the retroperitoneum, the lungs and the soft tissues of the neck. Although many of these lesions are benign or anatomical variations, some are of utmost importance and change the clinical management of patients.

When reading CT or MRI scans, the radiologist should take time to look at the paraspinal soft tissues and beyond the spine [1–4]. A CT or MRI of the lumbar spine typically will demonstrate an aneurysm of the abdominal aorta or a renal tumor, often not seen by the clinician but it should be reported and clearly communicated by the radiologist. An MRI of the cervical spine may reveal the pancoast tumor, but only if the radiologist specifically looks at the outer most lateral sagittal T1-weighted images of the C-spine where the lung apices are visualized. Even the localizer images of CT or MRI may demonstrate the presence of a malignant tumor outside the spine (Figs. 20.1 and 20.2).

When reading plain radiography of the thorax, one should specifically look at the spinal elements including the paraspinal lines and soft tissue, both on the lateral and the frontal view. It may reveal a paraspinal mass only visible by displaced paraspinal lines (Fig. 20.3).

Key Point Objectives
- Extraspinal masses may change the clinical pathway for your patient, but only if the radiologist picks up the extraspinal lesion (cave satisfaction of search).

Fig. 20.1 (**a**, **b**) Detection of a clinically significant mass. Tunnel vision into the spinal canal by physicians may obviate the timely diagnosis of a renal cell carcinoma (**a**). Not looking at the scout images of an MRI of the spine may obviate the timely diagnosis of a lung adenocarcinoma (**b**)

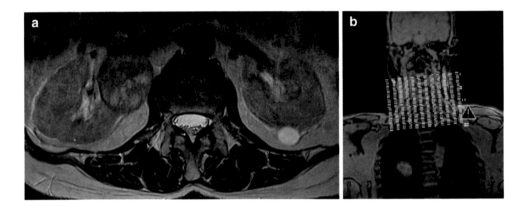

Fig. 20.2 (**a**, **b**) Detection of a clinically significant mass. Failure to evaluate upper and lower corners of the images may result in missed diagnosis of a vertebral artery aneurysm (**a**). Failure to evaluate the outer most lateral sagittal T1-weighted image of the C-spine may result in missed diagnosis of a pancoast tumor (**b**)

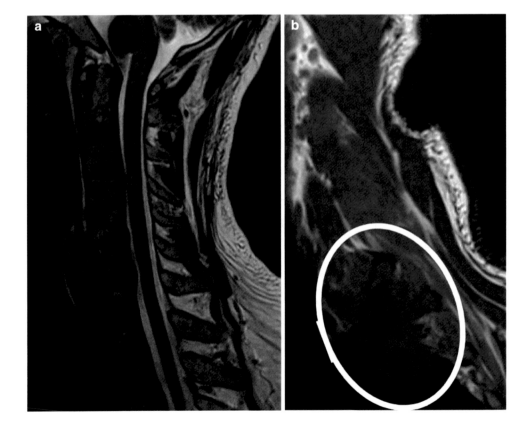

Fig. 20.3 (**a**, **b**) Detection of a paraspinal mass on radiography. Actively looking for abnormal paraspinal lines when reading non-spinal radiographies may improve detection of paraspinal masses, such as a tuberculosis abscess

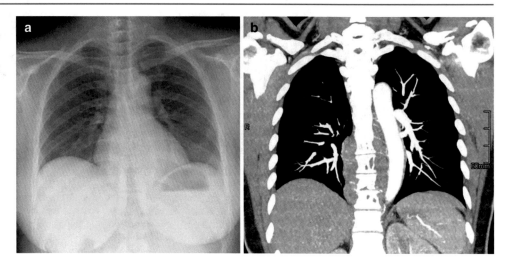

20.2 Anatomical Compartments in and Around the Spine: Paraspinal, Vertebral, and Epidural

The paraspinal compartment extends from the parietal fascia ventrally to the paraspinal muscle aponeurosis dorsally and from the skull base to the coccyx. It consists of soft tissues and surrounds the vertebrae and proximal part of the ribs [5].

The main soft tissue structure of the paraspinal compartment is muscle. Superficial muscles such as trapezius, latissimus dorsi, and levator scapulae do not belong to the paraspinal compartment because these are located superficial to the paraspinal aponeurosis. Deep to the paraspinal aponeurosis and thoracolumbar fascia (posterior layer) are the muscles of the epiaxial paraspinal compartment such as erector spinae and multifidi. Anterior to the transverse processes, muscles such as psoas and quadratus lumborum in the lumbar spine and longus colli in the cervical spine are present in the hypaxial paraspinal compartment. At the thoracic spine, no muscle is present anterior to the transverse processes and disease may more easily spread anteriorly to the parietal fascia (pleura). Open connection exists between the paraspinal soft tissues anterior (hypaxial) and posterior (epiaxial) to the transverse processes at all spinal levels. At the lumbar level, the middle layer of the thoracolumbar fascia forms an intermuscular septum at the level of each transverse process but in between the processes a narrow communication persists. This explains the often dumbbell shape of soft tissue tumors extending in the muscles anterior and posterior to the transverse process.

The paraspinal compartment is not well enclosed as it communicates with the epidural space of the spinal canal and the intercostal spaces; anteriorly, it is intimately related to the posterior mediastinum, pleura, and retroperitoneum. Moreover, the extensive vascular network and neural structures together with fat planes make passageways for infec-

tious and tumoral lesions to extend into or outside the paraspinal compartment. As such, spread of disease may easily occur by locoregional contiguity and by hematogeneous or perineural dissemination. Thorough radiological description of the tumoral spread and relation to neural and vascular structures is key information for surgeons.

The vertebral compartment contains the vertebrae and discs. Primary or secondary vertebral tumors may readily extend through the relative thin cortical bone and the periost into the epidural space or the paraspinal soft tissue. The Batson plexus consisting of the internal venous vertebral plexus, the basivertebral veins, and the external venous vertebral plexus connects intravertebral lesions to the paraspinal soft tissues (or vice versa), and to segmental veins towards the azygos and caval veins permitting hematogeneous spread.

The spinal epidural space lies outside the dura mater and within the spinal canal, and it extends from the foramen magnum to the sacrum. It contains epidural fat, spinal nerves, epidural veins and arteries, and meningovertebral ligaments. This space is connected to the vertebral body via the basivertebral veins and extends to the paraspinal compartment via the intervertebral foramina.

From the above paragraphs, it may be evident that extracompartmental extension frequently occurs in particular for tumors with aggressive behavior or malignant nature. The radiologist who is knowledgeable of the routes of spread will be able to guide the clinician and surgeon in their management decisions. The paraspinal compartment contains the adipose tissue corridor between the paraspinal muscles and along paraspinal vessels and nerves. It connects to the epidural space and the intercostal spaces. Contralateral spread may take place via the epidural space, throughout the bone or via the soft tissues anteriorly to the vertebrae (Fig. 20.4). Craniocaudal extension may easily occur within the epidural space and via the longitudinally oriented muscles and fat planes of the paraspinal compartment.

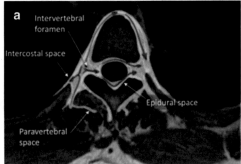
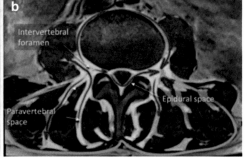

Fig. 20.4 Anatomy of the paraspinal space on axial T1WI (**a**, **b**). The green line surrounds the epiaxial paraspinal space and the green dashed line the hypaxial paraspinal space. Red arrows show the possible path-ways involved in paraspinal tumor spread along fat planes (shown in yellow). Note: epiaxial lesions are located posterior to and hypaxial lesions anterior to the transverse process. (From [5], licensed under CC-BY 4.0)

Key Point Objectives
- Anatomical compartments in and around the spine are not well compartmentalized and lesions can easily spread between vertebral body, epidural space, and paraspinal space.

20.3 Grading of Masses in and Around the Spine

Once a mass is detected by imaging, grading of the mass is necessary. Grading includes looking for features that show the aggressiveness of the tumor and defining the compartments involved. Grading can be helpful for characterization of a mass, and grading is of high importance to direct clinical and surgical management.

Radiography may provide insight into the overall morphology of the spine, is the best modality to evaluate spinal alignment in standing position (as required for the SINS classification, see below), and shows if the lesion will be visible on intra-operative radiography.

CT demonstrates the matrix of the tumoral mass (osteoid, chondroid, dystrophic) and the bony changes such as lytic, mixed and osteoblastic, expansile or exostosis, scalloping or foraminal enlargement, and periosteal reaction. Slow-growing lytic lesions are often surrounded with a thin sclerotic margin while fast-growing aggressive lesions have a wide transitional zone with ill-defined bone destruction, and moth-eaten cortical permeation.

MRI is the modality of choice to define size and extent of the tumoral mass. Bone involvement, spinal canal, and soft tissue involvement are well visualized due to excellent contrast resolution. It allows for tumor staging and detection of neurovascular involvement. T1-weighted sequences and T2-weighted sequences with fat saturation both in sagittal and axial planes are preferred.

20.3.1 Weinstein-Boriani-Biagini Classification

After describing the compartments involved and the craniocaudal segments involved, the radiologist can use the Weinstein-Boriani-Biagini classification regarding tumor extension in the axial plane to help the surgeon in treatment planning (Fig. 20.5). This classification divides spinal and paraspinal regions into five concentric layers regarding depth of tumor involvement (from paraspinal soft tissue, superficial bone, deep bone, epidural, to intradural involvement) while location is determined using a clockwise 12-sector grid. Surgical resection strategies may involve complete vertebral corporectomy, sagittal hemicorporectomy, or posterior arch resection.

20.3.2 Spinal Instability Neoplastic Score (SINS)

Vertebral lesions may lead to instability of the spine. Radiography, CT and MRI can be used to evaluate stability and fracture risk. The Spine Instability Neoplastic Score (SINS) assesses six variables: location of lesion, type of pain, type of bony lesion, radiographic spinal alignment, degree of vertebral body collapse, and involvement of posterolateral spinal elements (Table 20.1). The scores for each variable are added resulting in a final score between 0 and 18. A score of 0–6 denotes stability, a score of 7–12 denotes indeterminate (possibly impending) instability, and a score of 13 to 18 denotes instability [7].

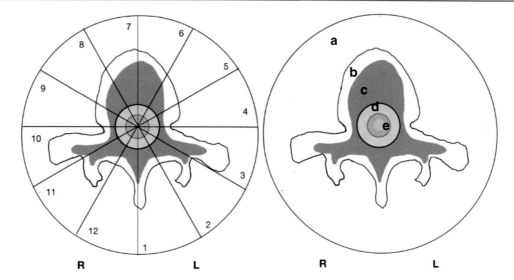

Fig. 20.5 Weinstein-Boriani-Biagni (WBB) classification: a surgical staging system that divides the vertebra into 12 equal radiating zones in an axial plane (1–12) and into five concentric layers regarding depth of tumor involvement (**a–f**); it is used to establish feasibility criteria and strategy for tumor resection [6]. (**a**) Extraosseous soft tissue; (**b**) Intraosseous (superficial); (**c**) Intraosseous (deep); (**d**) Extraosseous (epidural); (**e**) Extraosseous (intradural); (**f**) Vertebral artery involvement (not shown). (Medical art licensed under CC-BY 4.0 by Annick Gryspeirt)

Table 20.1 Spinal Instability Neoplastic Score (0–6: stable; 13–18: unstable)

Spinal instability neoplastic score (SINS) component	Score (0–18)
Location	
Junctional (occiput-C2, C7–Th2, Th11–L1, L5–S1)	3
Mobile spine (C3–C6, L2–L4)	2
Semi rigid (Th3–Th10)	1
Rigid (S2–S5)	0
Pain	
Mechanical pain[a]	3
Occasional pain but not mechanical	1
Pain-free lesion	0
Bone lesion	
Lytic	2
Mixed (lytic/blastic)	1
Blastic	0
Radiographic spinal alignment	
Subluxation/translation present	4
De novo deformity (kyphosis/scoliosis)	2
Normal alignment	0
Vertebral body collapse	
>50% collapse	3
<50% collapse	2
No collapse with >50% of body involved	1
None of the above	0
Posterolateral involvement of spinal elements[b]	
Bilateral	3
Unilateral	1
None of the above	0

[a] Pain improvement with recumbency and/or pain with movement/loading of spine
[b] Facet, pedicle, or costovertebral joint fracture or replacement with tumor

20.3.3 Epidural Spinal Cord Compression (ESCC) Scale, Bilsky Score

Vertebral body metastatic disease may extend in the epidural space and may compress the spinal cord in particular after vertebral body collapse. The Epidural Spinal Cord Compression (ESCC) score, also known as the Bilsky score and based on MRI only, helps to determine the management strategy regarding radiotherapy and surgery [8]. Grade 0 (bone only disease), grade 1a and 1b (epidural extension without or with deformation of the thecal sac) can be treated with radiotherapy. Treatment strategy for grade 1c (deformation of the tecal sac with spinal cord abutment) remains controversial. Grade 2 and 3 (spinal cord compression with and without visible cerebrospinal fluid around the cord) require surgical decompression except for highly radiosensitive tumors (Fig. 20.6). For other neoplasms involving the epidural space, grade 1–3 can be used to express the degree of spinal cord compression.

> **Key Point Objectives**
> - Radiologists add value to patient management decisions by grading the tumors according to established scales and scores.

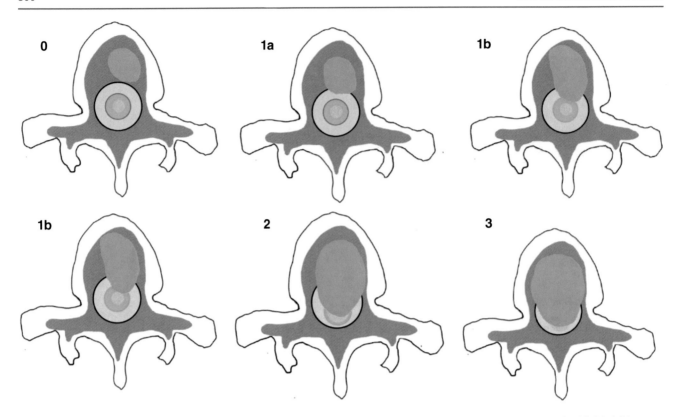

Fig. 20.6 Epidural spinal cord compression (ESCC) scale (Bilsky score) used to describe metastatic tumor extension from the vertebral body into the spinal canal and to assess the degree of spinal cord compromise. Low grade includes bone only disease (grade 0), epidural impingement without deformation of thecal sac (grade 1a), deformation of the thecal sac without spinal cord abutment (grade 1b), and deformation of the thecal sac with spinal cord abutment (grade 1c); high grade includes spinal cord compression with cerebrospinal fluid visible somewhere around the cord (grade 2) and spinal cord compression without cerebrospinal fluid visible (grade 3). Orange color represents tumor extending from vertebral body, yellow color represents the epidural space, and blue color represents the cerebrospinal fluid in the thecal sac (medical art licensed under CC-BY 4.0 by Annick Gryspeirt)

20.4 Characterization of Masses in and Around the Spine

20.4.1 Mass in the Paraspinal Space

To characterize the detected mass, clinical information should be considered together with the imaging findings [5, 9–11]. Clinical info should mention age and medical data including oncologic history, neurofibromatosis, chronic anemia such as in sickle cell disease or thalassemia, immunosuppression (lymphoma), trauma, infectious lab findings or endemic areas for infections such as tuberculosis, brucellosis, echinococcosis, and cysticercosis.

Image analysis starts with locating the epicenter of a mass: within the bone, in the epidural space, in the paraspinal compartment anterior or posterior to the transverse process (hypaxial or epiaxial, respectively). Extramedullary hematopoiesis and nerve sheath tumors will almost invariably present anterior to the transverse processes. Lipomas and liposarcomas may arise anterior or posterior to the transverse process. Posterior to the transverse process, benign tumors such as fibromatosis, hemangioma, epidermoid cyst,

and hibernoma are found together with malignant sarcomas such as synovial sarcoma, malignant peripheral nerve sheath tumor (MPNST), synovial sarcoma, leiomyosarcoma, and undifferentiated sarcoma.

Tumors located at the aponeurosis of the paraspinal muscles include desmoid and nodular fasciitis. At the boundaries of the paraspinal region, invading tumors from the skin appendages or tumors arising from anteriorly through the parietal fascia in the thorax and abdomen should be considered. Lipomas and pseudotumors such as hematoma and abscesses may occur at any site. Tables, flowcharts, and case examples are shown in the following sections (Figs. 20.7, 20.8, 20.9, and 20.10).

20.4.2 Mass Within the Vertebra

Diagnosis of vertebral masses may be quite challenging and several classifications can be used to distinguish vertebral tumors such as neoplastic vs. non-neoplastic, malignant vs. benign tumor, primitive vs. secondary, and the origin of a tumor, hematopoietic vs. osteogenic vs. chondrogenic vs.

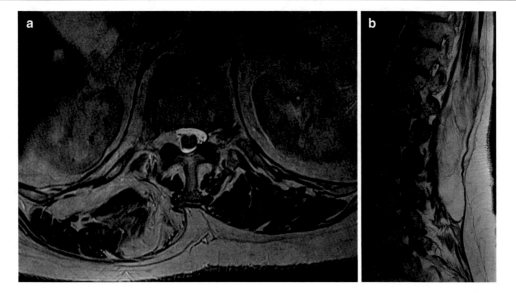

Fig. 20.7 As well known from soft tissue tumor MR imaging, masses containing fat, methemoglobin, protein-rich fluid or melanin will show high T1 signal intensity; hypercellular or myxoid lesions demonstrate fluid intensities; fibrous tumors with predominant collagen present with low signal intensity both on T1- and T2-weighted images; fluid-fluid levels can be a sign of blood-filled cavities. Post-contrast T1-weighted images help to separate solid fromSpinal massesparaspinal space cystic lesions, to estimate vascularity of the mass and identify tumor necrosis. (**a, b**) Lipoma or low-grade liposarcoma in the epiaxial paraspinal space, involving and enlarging the intermuscular fat planes and extending into the intervertebral foramen with some compression of the thecal sac, i.e., Bilsky grade 1b (**a**). The lesion is almost homogeneously hyperintense on T1WI inferring the diagnosis of lipoma, but because of its size (see longitudinal extension) low-grade liposarcoma should be suspected (**b**)

Fig. 20.8 (**a–d**) GLI1 fusion soft tissue sarcoma in a middle-aged woman, located in the hypaxial paraspinal space in the upper thoracic spine and extending through the intervertebral foramen (Bilsky grade 1C). Because of the widened intervertebral foramen, the initially small mass was in follow-up as a benign peripheral nerve sheath tumor (**a**). Progressive growth, bone involvement (vertebral body and facet), necrotic and solid components lead to suspicion of malignancy and subsequent surgery (**b–d**)

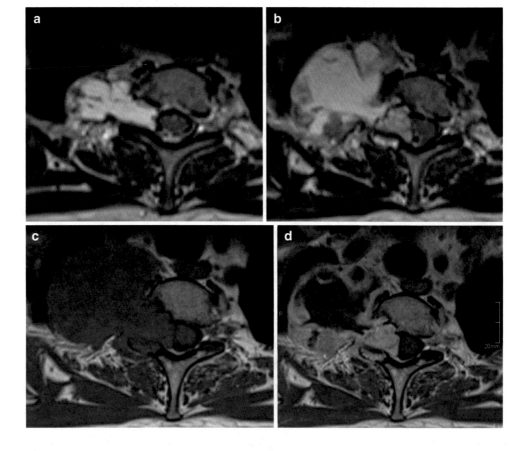

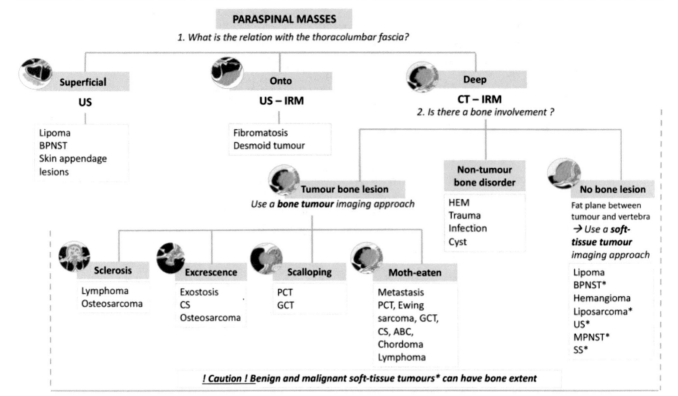

Fig. 20.9 Flowchart for paraspinal masses. Stars represent soft tissue tumors with bone involvement. BPMNST, benign peripheral nerve sheath tumor; MPNST, malignant peripheral nerve sheath tumor; ABC, aneurysmal bone cyst; CS, chondrosarcoma; GCT, giant cell tumor; PCT, plasma cell tumor; US, undifferentiated sarcoma; and SS, synovial sarcoma. (From [5], licensed under CC-BY 4.0)

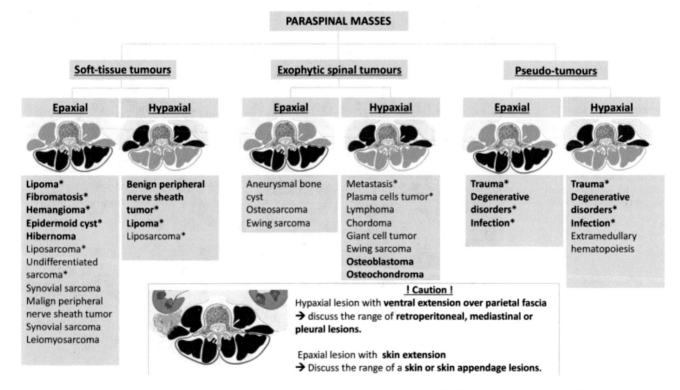

Fig. 20.10 Overview of paraspinal masses. Stars represent the more common lesions. Words in bold represent benign lesions. BPMNST, benign peripheral nerve sheath tumor; MPNST, malignant peripheral nerve sheath tumor; ABC, aneurysmal bone cyst; CS, chondrosarcoma; GCT, giant cell tumor; PCT, plasma cell tumor. (From [5], licensed under CC-BY 4.0)

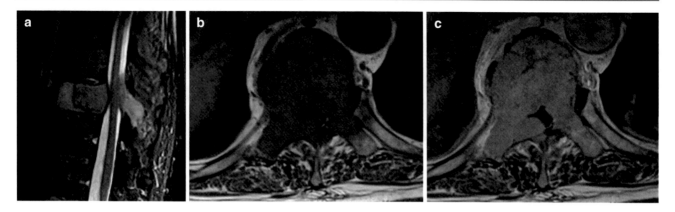

Fig. 20.11 (a–c) Metastasis. Aggressive bone lesion with involvement of vertebral body and lamina, cortical permeation, and extension in the spinal canal. Intermediate to high signal on T2WI and homogeneous low signal on T1WI with avid enhancement are seen (a–c). At the pos-terior border of the vertebral body, the posterior longitudinal ligament is lifted by the metastasis, known as "draped curtain" sign. (b, c) The epidural space involvement has resulted in spinal cord compression (Bilsky grade3)

vascular origin, etc. Therefore, final diagnosis must be made after assessment of both available imaging data (MRI and CT) and setting (age, sex, location, and clinical presentation) in order to accurately diagnose a vertebral mass. Typical presentation of specific lesions may result in "do-not-touch" lesions, meaning that a biopsy is not necessary; in unresolved cases, a biopsy may be deemed necessary for diagnosis.

20.4.2.1 Vertebral Metastasis

Arguments in favor of metastatic spine disease usually include multi-level lesions and presence of primary tumor known to be associated with bone metastasis (lung, breast, prostate, kidney, thyroid are the most common). Diagnosis of metastatic disease may be challenging in the case of a solitary mass with no known cancer setting, often requiring biopsy. Imaging features of metastatic disease include highly lytic lesions, highly sclerotic lesions, or mixed presentations. Osteolytic lesions are hyperintense on T2WI, iso- to hypointense on T1 with strong enhancement after IV contrast (Fig. 20.11), which correlates on CT with hypodense lesions that have indistinct borders often with permeation of cortical bone as in the Lodwick classification [12]. Local extension to surrounding soft tissues should be looked for, and the classic "draped curtain" presentation in the epidural space may be present. Metastatic disease may also present as a highly sclerotic bone lesion (hyperdense on CT, low signal on T1WI and T2WI) in primary tumors such as prostate, breast, transitional cell, and medullary thyroid carcinomas, lung adenocarcinoma, carcinoid, lymphoma (ivory vertebra), and small cell lung cancer. Bone metastases may have a mixed presentation of both lytic and sclerotic areas (e.g., 25% of breast carcinoma, 15% of prostate carcinoma, 15% of lung carcinoma, testicular tumors, cervix carcinoma, gastrointestinal cancer). Metastases may affect all bony segments of the vertebra.

20.4.2.2 Primary Malignant Tumors of the Vertebrae

These tumors are rare and present mainly in patients over 30 years of age and mainly involve the vertebral body. However, osteosarcoma, chondrosarcoma, and Ewing sarcoma are often seen in younger ages and have a propensity to occur in the posterior elements of vertebra before extending towards the vertebral body. Longitudinal extension to adjacent vertebral levels is most often seen in lymphoma followed by chordoma and chondrosarcoma [13–15].

Epidemiology, preferred location, and involvement of adjacent vertebra together with some imaging examples are shown (Table 20.2, Figs. 20.11, 20.12, 20.13, 20.14, and 20.15).

20.4.2.3 Primary Benign Tumors of the Vertebrae

These tumors may be classified according to tissue of origin such as osteogenic, chondrogenic, vascular, osteoclastic giant-cell rich, notochordal, mesenchymal, or hematopoetic [16, 17]. Characteristic imaging features often allow a specific diagnosis based on imaging and will avoid the need for biopsy (Table 20.3). Some imaging examples are shown (Figs. 20.16, 20.17, and 20.18).

20.4.3 Mass in the Epidural Space

Epidural masses are relatively limited in origin as they can either be derived from vascular or fat tissue. However, many tumoral or pseudotumoral lesions may invade or compromise the epidural space (Table 20.4). Some imaging examples are shown (Figs. 20.19, 20.20, and 20.21).

Table 20.2 Epidemiology, preferred location, and extension of primary malignant tumors of the vertebrae

Tumor type	Mean age (y)	Spine location	Axial location and longitudinal extension
Ewing sarcoma	19.3	S > L > T > C	Posterior elements
Osteosarcoma	38	T + L > S, C	Posterior elements (extension in body)
Chondrosarcoma	45	T > C > L	All + adjacent levels
Lymphoma	40–60	All	Body + adjacent levels
Chordoma	50–60	Skull base, S (C, T, L)	Body + adjacent levels
Plasmacytoma	>60	T	Body (extension in pedicle and in disk)
Multiple myeloma	Rare under 30	All	Body (extension in pedicle and in disk)

C cervical, *T* thoracic, *L* lumbar, *S* sacral

Fig. 20.12 (**a–d**) Chordoma of the sacrum. On MRI, the lesion is iso- to hyperintense on T2WI (**a**), iso- to hypointense on T1WI (**b**, **c**). It demonstrates avid inhomogeneous enhancement referred to as "honeycomb-like" in T1WI with fat saturation (**d**). It demonstrates features of an aggressive tumor, with cortical disruption, soft tissue invasion, and longitudinal extension. Diagnosis usually requires biopsy

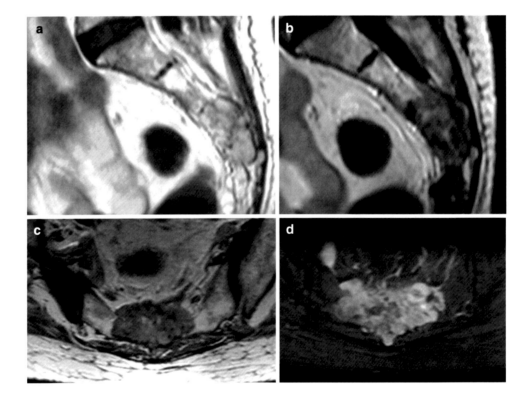

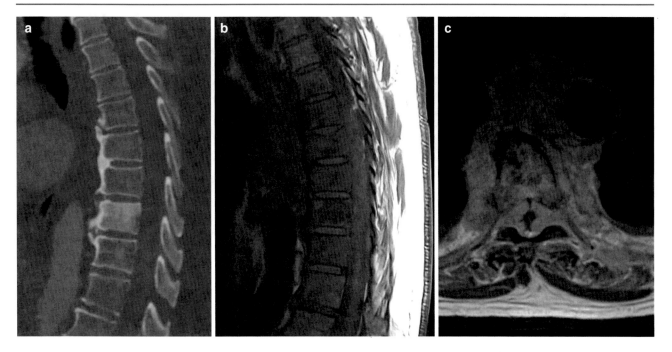

Fig. 20.13 (a–c) Diffuse large B-cell lymphoma of the thoracic spine in an elderly patient presenting with chronic dorsal pain and claudication. CT demonstrates an ivory vertebra together with paraspinal soft tissue mass (a). MRI shows the soft tissue extension in the hypaxial paraspinal space towards the posterior mediastinum, in the intercostal spaces, and in the epidural space with compression of the spinal cord, i.e., Bilsky grade 3 (b, c). Longitudinal extension in both the paravertebral space and the intradural space is seen together with vertebral involvement over at least 6 levels

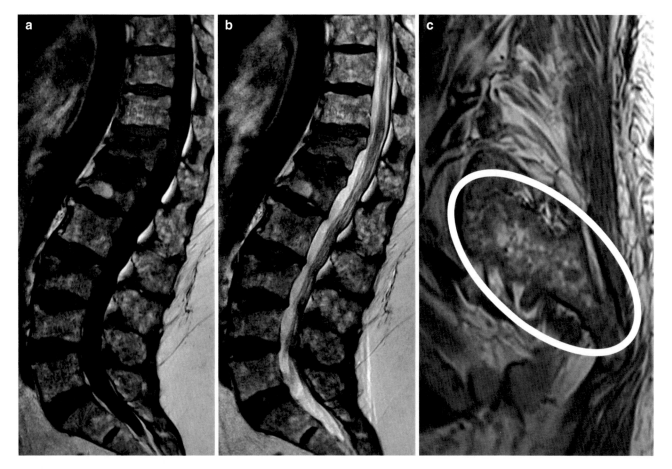

Fig. 20.14 (a–c) Multiple myeloma. When reading spine MRI exams, the astute radiologist will report the possibility of multiple myeloma in case of an elderly patient with multiple consecutive vertebral compression fractures, diffusely heterogeneous bone marrow, and in particular "red bone marrow" nodules in the normally fatty sacral wings of the elderly (c). Note: always look at the sacral wings in the outer most sagittal T1 images

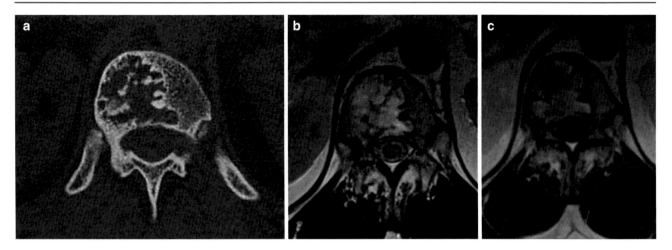

Fig. 20.15 (**a–c**) Plasmacytoma with mini-brain appearance. Example of a solitary plasmacytoma in a 31-year-old man presenting with low back pain. The CT image demonstrates an irregular shaped lytic lesion of the vertebral body, with cortical thickening correlating to linear hypointense struts in T1 and T2 imaging resembling the cortical gyration of a mini-brain

Table 20.3 Primary benign tumors: CT and MR characteristics and treatment modalities

Tumor type	CT features	MRI features (high and low refer to signal intensity)	Treatment
Osteoma	Dense sclerotic, round shape, sometimes with spicula	Low on all sequences	Not needed
Osteoid osteoma (OO)	Posterior elements, central nidus lucent or sclerotic with lucent rim, broad and dense sclerotic reactive zone	Nidus is low on T1 and high on T2, avidly enhancing; broad, enhancing reactive zone (not malignant!) nidus easily missed on MRI, CT is preferred	Surgical curettage or percutaneous ablation
Osteoblastoma	Like osteoid osteoma, osteoid forming tumor of larger size of nidus: >1.5 cm with variable mineralization	Low on T1, high on T2, variable enhancement peritumoral oedema and periosteal reaction fluid-fluid levels if associated ABC	Surgery
Hemangioma	Hypodense with coarse vertical trabeculae (white polka dots/corduroy sign)	Typical (fatty stroma): High on T1, high on T2 atypical (vascular): Iso or low on T1, high on T2	Not needed
Aggressive Hemangioma	Like hemangioma but with bone destruction	idem to atypical hemangioma, avid enhancement, use fat saturation to see extraosseous extension/cord compression	Optional: Embolization, vertebroplasty, surgery
Fibrous dysplasia	Expansile, ground-glass matrix; cystic areas may appear lytic (rare in spine, polyostotic)	Low on T1, low to intermediate on T2, cystic areas are high on T2, enhancement variable	Not needed
Osteochondroma	Continuity of bony cortex and medullary space from lesion into normal bone	Bone marrow signal, cortical bone signal cartilage cap (high on T2)	Optional (resection)
Chondroblastoma	Osteolytic, thin sclerotic rim, may involve cortical bone, variable intralesional calcification (chondroid matrix)	Iso on T1, heterogeneous on T2 and after contrast lobular matrix, low T1 and T2 rim, bone marrow and soft tissue edema with enhancement	Surgery (curettage)
Simple bone cyst	Radiolucent, thin sclerotic rim	Fluid signal intensity	Not needed
Aneurysmal bone cyst (ABC)	Balloon-like expansile, lytic with bony septa, thin cortical shell may focally disrupt	Fluid-fluid levels (lower layer is low on T2) solid ABC exist	Optional: Biopsy, surgery, or calcitonin/corticoid injection
Benign notochordal tumor	Sclerotic, may involve entire vertebra preserved trabecula, no cortical destruction	Hypo or iso, some high foci on T1 (entrapped fat) high on T2, may sometimes enhance	Not needed, MRI follow-up to exclude chordoma
Giant cell tumor	Lytic, expansile, cortical disruption, thin/disrupted sclerotic margins and trabecula, locally aggressive lesion	Soft tissue component, sharp margin, thin curvilinear bands (residual trabecula) fluid-fluid levels if associated ABC	Surgery (resection)
Eosinophilic granuloma (Langerhans histiocytosis)	Lucent lytic lesion, bone destruction locally aggressive lesion, vertebra plana	Low or iso on T1, high on T2, diffusely enhancing	Conservative, surgery

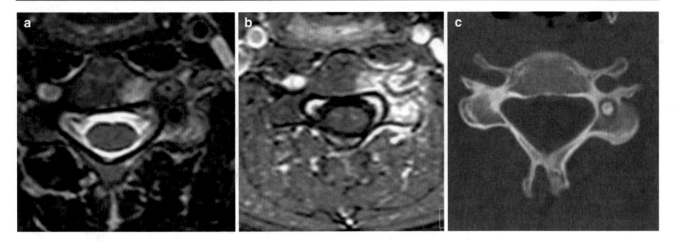

Fig. 20.16 (**a–c**) Osteoid osteoma in a child with inflammatory pain responding to salicylic acid and non-steroidal anti-inflammatory drugs. Use of these drugs are a diagnostic test for osteoid osteoma. On MRI, a hypointense sclerotic center with extensive surrounding inflammation (reactive zone) on T2WI (**a**) and strong enhancement after IV contrast on T1WI with fat suppression (**b**) is seen. CT to better advantage shows the typical sclerotic rounded center with a hypodense rim representing the osteoid nidus (**c**)

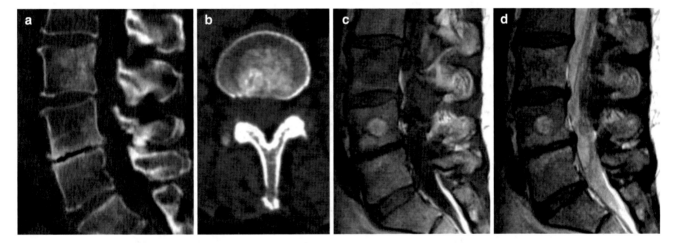

Fig. 20.17 (**a–d**) Benign Notochordal Cell Tumor (BNCT) in an asymptomatic young adult. Sclerotic lesion on CT involving a large central area of the L3 body showing visible, undestructed bone trabeculae (**a**, **b**). On MRI, the lesion is hypointense on T1WI (**c**) and hyperin- tense on T2WI (**d**). No contrast enhancement (not shown). Incidentally, a vertebral hemangioma is present in the L4 body, hyperintense on T1 and T2 due to fatty content. Modic type 2 changes are present at level L4-L5

Fig. 20.18 (**a–d**) Giant cell tumor in the cervical spine of a young adult. Benign locally aggressive tumor presenting as a lytic expansile lesion with cortical disruption and soft tissue invasion. CT demonstrates the osteolysis but also a thin sclerotic rim in the vertebral body (narrow transition zone) and a thin cortical shell that is rather eroded and displaced than destructed: signs of an expansile erosive lesion but not permeative (**a, b**). The characteristic finding on MRI is the heterogeneous to low signal on T2WI representing hemorrhagic components (**c**). The lesion is hypointense on T1 and avidly enhances after IV contrast administration (**d**)

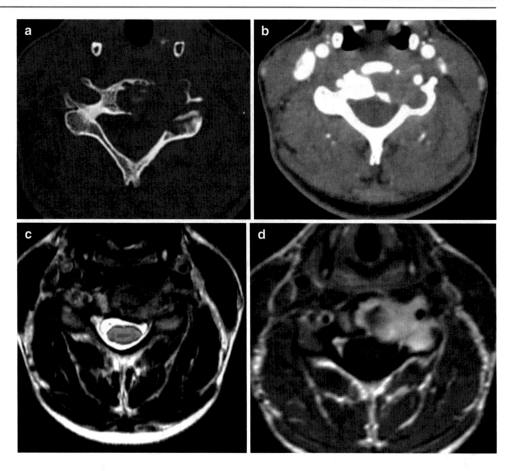

Table 20.4 Masses in the epidural space

Degenerative	Disc herniation, ligamentum flavum degeneration (mucoid and cystic change, calcification, hypertrophy), facet arthropathy, intraspinal synovial facet cyst, frictional bursitis de novo in Baastrup, ossification of posterior longitudinal ligament (OPLL), retrodental pseudotumor of transverse ligament
Infectious	Pyogenic abscess, tuberculous abscess, fungal infection
Neoplastic benign	Lipoma/lipomatosis, angiolipoma, cavernous hemangioma, schwannoma, neurofibroma, meningioma, paraspinal arteriovenous malformation/fistula, arachnoid cyst, dermoid, epidermoid cyst, extramedullary hematopoiesis
Neoplastic malignant	Lymphoma, metastasis, neuroendocrine spinal tumor (paraganglioma)
Congenital	Neurenteric cyst (more frequently intradural), meningeal cyst
Other	Epidural hematoma (spontaneous, post-traumatic, post-surgery), pseudomeningocele, postoperative fibrosis, early postoperative pseudomass (débris), dilated venous plexus as collateral pathway in inferior vena cava obstruction, Hirayama's disease

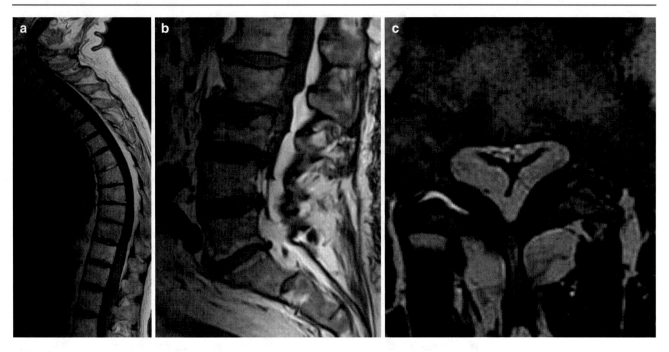

Fig. 20.19 (**a–c**) Epidural lipomatosis on T1WI, often seen in overweight patients or secondary to steroids intake. In the thoracic spine, excessive fat is usually present in the posterior epidural space (**a**), while in the lumbar spine excessive fat surrounds the thecal sac resulting in a Y shaped compression (**b, c**)

Fig. 20.20 (**a–d**) Epidural hematoma can occur after trauma, secondary to a vascular abnormality or anti-coagulant therapy, or spontaneously as in this case. Blood signal on MRI will vary according to age of the hematoma. An epidural hematoma posteriorly in the spinal canal is shown with intermediary signal on non-contrast T1WI (**a**, **c**) and typical hypointense signal on T2WI (**b**, **d**). No contrast enhancement was present (not shown)

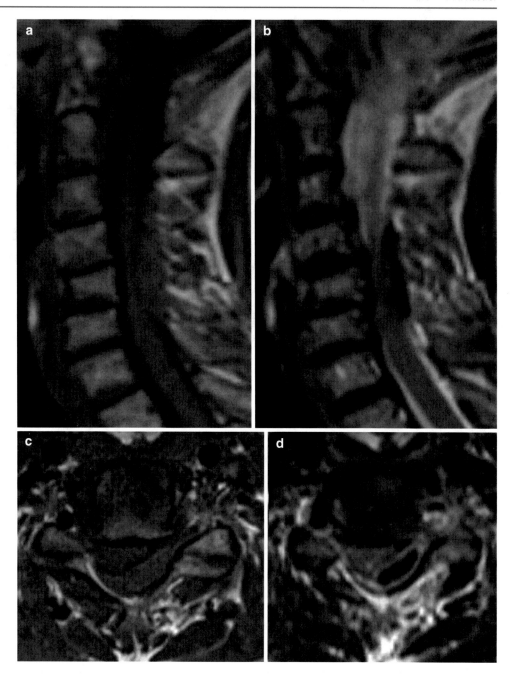

Fig. 20.21 (**a**, **b**). Cavernous hemangioma is rare in the epidural space and presents with typical low signal on T2, hypo-intense to iso-intense signal on T1 and with avid enhancement (**a**, **b**). A specific characteristic of cavernous hemangioma is the possible multilevel extension and the association with an osseous malformation such as a vertebral hemangioma (**b**)

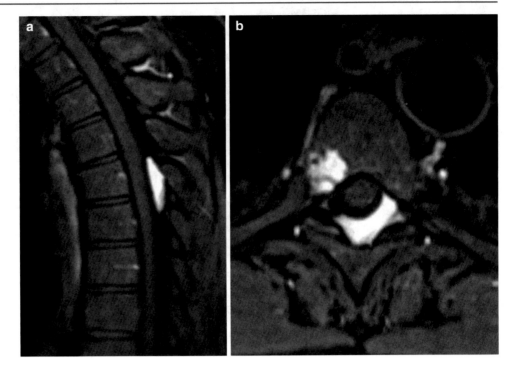

20.5   Concluding Remarks

Important tumoral or infectious lesions may be missed if the extraspinal soft tissues are not scrutinized by the radiologist. Once a lesion is detected, the compartment of origin and the extension to neigboring compartments needs to be determined using established classifications. Many lesions can be correctly diagnosed based on imaging features alone, however when in doubt follow-up imaging or a biopsy can be deemed necessary.

> **Take-Home Messages**
> - Beware of satisfaction of search and use your radiological skills to detect extraspinal lesions on every CT and MRI of the spine you read.
> - Add value by correctly grading and characterizing masses in and around the spine.

References

1. Reid A, Weig E, Dickinson K, Zafar F, Abid R, VanBeek M, Ferguson N. Hiding in plain sight: a retrospective review of unrecognized tumors during dermatologic surgery. Cureus. 2022;14(3):e23487. https://doi.org/10.7759/cureus.23487.
2. Busby LP, Courtier JL, Glastonbury CM. Bias in radiology: the how and why of misses and misinterpretations. Radiographics. 2018;38(1):236–47. https://doi.org/10.1148/rg.2018170107.
3. Ivan CV, Mullineux JH, Shah V, Verma R, Rajesh A, Stephenson JA. Peripheral vision: abdominal pathology missed outside the Centre of gaze. Br J Radiol. 2018;91(1091):20180142. https://doi.org/10.1259/bjr.20180142.
4. Kulkarni TG, Das K. Poster: "ECR 2017/C-2433/The CT and MRI scout views: don't forget to look!"
5. Creze M, Ghaouche J, Missenard G, Lazure T, Cluzel G, Devilder M, Briand S, Soubeyrand M, Meyrignac O, Carlier RY, Court C, Bouthors C. Understanding a mass in the paraspinal region: an anatomical approach. Insights Imaging. 2023;14(1):128. https://doi.org/10.1186/s13244-023-01462-1.
6. Boriani S, Weinstein JN, Biagini R. Primary bone tumors of the spine. Terminology and surgical staging. Spine (Phila Pa 1976). 1997;22(9):1036–44. https://doi.org/10.1097/00007632-199705010-00020.

7. Chang SY, Ha JH, Seo SG, Chang BS, Lee CK, Kim H. Prognosis of single spinal metastatic tumors: predictive value of the spinal instability neoplastic score system for spinal adverse events. Asian Spine J. 2018;12(5):919–26. https://doi.org/10.31616/asj.2018.12.5.919.

8. Fisher CG, DiPaola CP, Ryken TC, Bilsky MH, Shaffrey CI, Berven SH, Harrop JS, Fehlings MG, Boriani S, Chou D, Schmidt MH, Polly DW, Biagini R, Burch S, Dekutoski MB, Ganju A, Gerszten PC, Gokaslan ZL, Groff MW, Liebsch NJ, Mendel E, Okuno SH, Patel S, Rhines LD, Rose PS, Sciubba DM, Sundaresan N, Tomita K, Varga PP, Vialle LR, Vrionis FD, Yamada Y, Fourney DR. A novel classification system for spinal instability in neoplastic disease: an evidence-based approach and expert consensus from the spine oncology study group. Spine (Phila Pa 1976). 2010;35(22):E1221–9. https://doi.org/10.1097/BRS.0b013e3181e16ae2.

9. Rodallec MH, Feydy A, Larousserie F, Anract P, Campagna R, Babinet A, Zins M, Drapé JL. Diagnostic imaging of solitary tumors of the spine: what to do and say. Radiographics. 2008;28(4):1019–41. https://doi.org/10.1148/rg.284075156.

10. Tsukamoto S, Mavrogenis AF, Langevelde KV, Vucht NV, Kido A, Errani C. Imaging of spinal bone tumors: principles and practice. Curr Med Imaging. 2022;18(2):142–61. https://doi.org/10.2174/15734056176662103011110446.

11. Van Goethem JW, van den Hauwe L, Ozsarlak O, De Schepper AM, Parizel PM. Spinal tumors. Eur J Radiol. 2004;50(2):159–76. https://doi.org/10.1016/j.ejrad.2003.10.021.

12. Benndorf M, Bamberg F, Jungmann PM. The Lodwick classification for grading growth rate of lytic bone tumors: a decision tree approach. Skelet Radiol. 2022;51(4):737–45. https://doi.org/10.1007/s00256-021-03868-8. Epub 2021 Jul 24

13. Mechri M, Riahi H, Sboui I, Bouaziz M, Vanhoenacker F, Ladeb M. Imaging of malignant primitive tumors of the spine. J Belg Soc Radiol. 2018;102(1):56. https://doi.org/10.5334/jbsr.1410.

14. Ariyaratne S, Jenko N, Iyengar KP, James S, Mehta J, Botchu R. Primary osseous malignancies of the spine. Diagnostics (Basel). 2023;13(10):1801. https://doi.org/10.3390/diagnostics13101801. PMID: 37238285; PMCID: PMC10217758

15. Patnaik S, Jyotsnarani Y, Uppin SG, Susarla R. Imaging features of primary tumors of the spine: a pictorial essay. Indian J Radiol Imaging. 2016;26(2):279–89. https://doi.org/10.4103/0971-3026.184413.

16. Riahi H, Mechri M, Barsaoui M, Bouaziz M, Vanhoenacker F, Ladeb M. Imaging of benign tumors of the osseous spine. J Belg Soc Radiol. 2018;102(1):13. https://doi.org/10.5334/jbsr.1380.

17. Ariyaratne S, Jenko N, Iyengar KP, James S, Mehta J, Botchu R. Primary benign neoplasms of the spine. Diagnostics. 2023;13(12):2006. https://doi.org/10.3390/diagnostics13122006.

Index

© The Editor(s) (if applicable) and The Author(s) 2024
J. Hodler et al. (eds.), *Diseases of the Brain, Head and Neck, Spine 2024-2027*, IDKD Springer Series,
https://doi.org/10.1007/978-3-031-50675-8

Printed in the United States
by Baker & Taylor Publisher Services